Living Donor Advocacy

Jennifer Steel
Editor

Living Donor Advocacy

An Evolving Role Within Transplantation

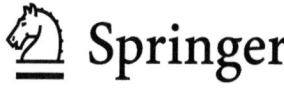

Editor
Jennifer Steel
University of Pittsburgh
Starzl Translpant Institute
Pittsburgh
Pennsylvania
USA

ISBN 978-1-4614-9142-2   ISBN 978-1-4614-9143-9 (eBook)
DOI 10.1007/978-1-4614-9143-9
Springer New York Heidelberg Dordrecht London

Library of Congress Control Number: 2013952768

© Springer Science+Business Media New York 2014
This work is subject to copyright. All rights are reserved by the Publisher, whether the whole or part of the material is concerned, specifically the rights of translation, reprinting, reuse of illustrations, recitation, broadcasting, reproduction on microfilms or in any other physical way, and transmission or information storage and retrieval, electronic adaptation, computer software, or by similar or dissimilar methodology now known or hereafter developed. Exempted from this legal reservation are brief excerpts in connection with reviews or scholarly analysis or material supplied specifically for the purpose of being entered and executed on a computer system, for exclusive use by the purchaser of the work. Duplication of this publication or parts thereof is permitted only under the provisions of the Copyright Law of the Publisher's location, in its current version, and permission for use must always be obtained from Springer. Permissions for use may be obtained through RightsLink at the Copyright Clearance Center. Violations are liable to prosecution under the respective Copyright Law.
The use of general descriptive names, registered names, trademarks, service marks, etc. in this publication does not imply, even in the absence of a specific statement, that such names are exempt from the relevant protective laws and regulations and therefore free for general use.
While the advice and information in this book are believed to be true and accurate at the date of publication, neither the authors nor the editors nor the publisher can accept any legal responsibility for any errors or omissions that may be made. The publisher makes no warranty, express or implied, with respect to the material contained herein.

Printed on acid-free paper

Springer is part of Springer Science+Business Media (www.springer.com)

Preface

This book has evolved as part of the 2000 Living Donor Consensus Conference, which recommended that all transplant centers have a living donor advocate "whose only focus is on the best interest of the donor." In 2007, the Department of Health and Human Services (DHHS) and the United Network for Organ Sharing (UNOS) included in their requirements that all transplant centers provide living donors with an advocate. I was appointed to be the independent living donor advocate (ILDA) at our transplant center and since that time have been interested in the development of guidelines to facilitate the best practices of ILDAs to decrease potential harm and bias to living donors and transplant candidates. This book was intended to provide ILDAs with information that would facilitate their understanding of the complexity of the living donor surgeries and medical contraindications, evaluation of the donor by the ILDA, and bioethics involved in living donation. However, the book may also be beneficial to other health care professionals, within as well as outside of transplant, and to potential transplant candidates and living donors.

The first section of the book includes chapters describing the five different types of living donor surgeries that are performed at this time—kidney, liver, intestine, lung, and pancreas—and the medical evaluation and contraindications for such surgeries. A chapter in this section is also devoted to the living donor kidney exchange program, which describes the complexities and nuances of those who participate in these exchanges. The authors who contributed each of these chapters are internationally recognized leaders in their field and graciously shared their time and expertise to provide an overview of these complex surgeries.

The next section of the book is devoted to issues regarding living donor advocacy, and these chapters are written by those who practice as ILDAs or who have donated an organ to a loved one. Many of the ILDAs who have written chapters for this section of the book also serve as leaders in their respective fields and are active in transplant organizations that are advancing the field of transplantation but also involved in the protection of living donors. The first chapter provides a history of living donation and specifically how the role of the ILDA has evolved. This is followed by a presentation of the findings of a national survey regarding the qualifications, practices, and ethical challenges faced by ILDAs. The next chapter describes the advantages and disadvantages of the independent living donor team versus an

ILDA. A subsequent chapter is dedicated to describing the different types of donors. This is followed by a chapter devoted specifically to unrelated donors, who are increasing in numbers at many centers. We have also included chapters describing the timing and components of the ILDA evaluation and contraindications for surgery from the ILDA perspective. This section concludes with a chapter devoted to how disagreements may be resolved between the ILDA and the transplant team, as well as a chapter written by a living donor who shares her experience.

The final section of the book includes chapters about ethical issues related to living donation that are written by ILDAs and others who have expertise in bioethics and are internationally recognized. The first chapter in this section addresses the informed consent process for donors, which is viewed as challenging owing to the Hippocratic Oath, "primum non nocere" or "do no harm," and the frequently unspoken pressures associated with the potential loss of a loved one. The next chapter provides considerations with regard to the assessment by the ILDA of pressure or coercion by the candidate, the candidate's family, and/or by the medical teams. Valuable consideration and financial risks of living donation are also discussed. A chapter is also devoted to the issue of donor autonomy and the balance between advocacy and protection of donors. A timely chapter on the health disparities that are observed within transplantation and, specifically, living donation is also included. Finally, recommendations for practice guidelines for the ILDA are proposed; however, these recommendations will continue to evolve owing to the constantly changing field of transplant and living donor advocacy.

Acknowledgments

This book owes a great deal to many people. First, the living donors, their families and friends who I have had the privilege to learn from and who have shared their great acts of generosity and love. To the authors of this book, who I have such great respect for and who have dedicated their lives to medicine and transplantation. These authors, in addition to their many other responsibilities of caring for patients, advancing science, and teaching, shared their valuable time and expertise for this book. I would also like to thank Diane Lamsback, who has provided the most timely support throughout the progress of this book, and to Drs. Carr, Geller, and Billiar, who have provided me the unique experience of working as a psychologist within a department of surgery. Also to James Bender, who has provided his support and patience for this, as well as other academic endeavors.

Contents

Part I Living Donation

1. **The Medical Selection of Live Donors** 3
   Christine Wu and Henkie P. Tan

2. **Kidney Paired Donation Programs for Incompatible Living Kidney Donors and Recipients** 17
   Sommer E. Gentry, Ron Shapiro and Dorry L. Segev

3. **Living Donor Liver Transplantation** 29
   Vikraman Gunabushanam, Abhideep Chaudhary and Abhinav Humar

4. **Intestinal Transplantation from Living Donors** 41
   Massimiliano Tuveri, Salvatore Pisu and Luca Cicalese

5. **Living Donor Lung Transplantation** 75
   Robbin G. Cohen, Mark L. Barr and Vaughn A. Starnes

6. **Live Donor Pancreas Transplantation** 91
   Miguel Tan

Part II Living Donor Advocacy

7. **The History of Living Donor Advocacy in Living Donor Transplantation** 103
   Talia B. Baker and Helen G. Spicer

8. **Findings from a National Survey of Living Donor Advocates** 119
   Jennifer L. Steel, Andrea Dunlavy, Maranda Friday, Mark Unruh, Chanelle Labash, Kendal Kingsley, Henkie P. Tan, Ron Shapiro and Abhinav Humar

9 The Independent Donor Advocate and the Independent
   Donor Advocate Team 131
   Dianne LaPointe Rudow

10 Classification of Living Organ Donors 139
   Andrew W. Webb, RN, BSN, CCTC

11 Unrelated Donors 149
   Mary Amanda Dew, Ginger Boneysteele and Andrea F. DiMartini

12 Education of the Donor by the ILDA (Psychosocial Aspects) 169
   Marjorie A. Clay

13 Components and Timing of the ILDA Evaluation 197
   Kathleen Swartz

14 Contraindications to Living Donation from an ILDA Perspective 205
   Rebecca Hays

15 Management of Conflict Between the Independent
   Living Donor Advocate and the Transplant Team 221
   Roxanne M. Taylor

16 Story Behind the Story 231
   Barbara L. Rutt

17 Living Donor Experience 253
   Donna M. Kinzler

Part III Living Donor Ethics

18 Informed Consent for Living Organ Donation 261
   Frank Chessa

19 Pressure and Coercion 275
   Cindy Koslowski Brown

20 Financial Considerations 293
   Jami Hanneman

21 Autonomy, Agency, and Responsibility: Ethical
   Concerns for Living Donor Advocates 301
   Rosamond Rhodes

22 A Practical Guide: Role of the Independent Living Donor Advocate: Protect or Advocate or Is it Both? 311
Betsy B. Johnson

23 Racial Disparities in Kidney Transplant and Living Donation 327
Tanjala S. Purnell and L. Ebony Boulware

24 The Evolution of the Role of the Independent Living Donor Advocates: Recommendations for Practice Guideline 347
Jennifer L. Steel, Andrea C. Dunlavy, Maranda Friday, Kendal Kingsley, Deborah Brower, Mark Unruh, Henkie P. Tan, Ron Shapiro, Mel Peltz, Melissa Hardoby, Christina McCloskey, Mark L. Sturdevant and Abhinav Humar

Index 357

Contributors

Talia B. Baker Department of Transplant Surgery, Northwestern Memorial Hospital, Chicago, IL, USA

Mark L. Barr Department of Cardiothoracic Surgery, USC Transplantation Institute, University of Southern California, Los Angeles, CA, USA

Ginger Boneysteele Department of Psychiatry, University of Pittsburgh Medical Center, Pittsburgh, PA, US

L. Ebony Boulware Department of Medicine/General Internal Medicine, Johns Hopkins School of Medicine, Baltimore, MD, USA

Deborah Brower Department of Surgery, University of Pittsburgh, Kaufman Building, Pittsburgh, PA, USA

Cindy Koslowski Brown Department of Social Work, University of Michigan Hospital and Health Systems, Ann Arbor, MI, USA

Abhideep Chaudhary Department of Surgical Gastroenterology and Liver Transplantation, Sir Ganga Ram Hospital, New Delhi, India

Frank Chessa Department of Clinical Ethics, Maine Medical Center and Tufts University School of Medicine, Portland, ME, USA

Luca Cicalese Department of General Surgery-Transplant, University of Texas Medical Branch, Galveston, TX, USA

Robbin G. Cohen Department of Cardiothoracic Surgery, Keck/USC University Hospital, USC Healthcare Consultation Center II, Los Angeles, CA, USA

Marjorie A. Clay University of Massachusettes Memorial Medical Center, Worcester, MA, USA

Mary Amanda Dew Department of Psychiatry, School of Medicine and Medical Center, University of Pittsburgh, Pittsburgh, PA, USA

Andrea F. DiMartini Department of Psychiatry, School of Medicine and Medical Center, University of Pittsburgh, Pittsburgh, PA, USA

Andrea Dunlavy Department of Surgery, University of Pittsburgh School of Medicine, Pittsburgh, PA, USA

Maranda Friday Department of Surgery, Starzl Translpant Institute and Liver Cancer Center, Montefiore Hospital, University of Pittsburgh, Pittsburgh, PA, USA

Department of Surgery, University of Pittsburgh Medical Center, Montefiore Hospital, Pittsburgh, PA, USA

Sommer E. Gentry Department of Mathematics, United States Naval Academy, Annapolis, MD, USA

Department of Surgery, Johns Hopkins University School of Medicine, Baltimore, MD, USA

Vikraman Gunabushanam Department of Transplant Surgery, University of Pittsburgh Medical Center, Pittsburgh, PA, USA

Jami Hanneman Kovler Organ Transplant center, Northwestern Memorial Hospital, Chicago, IL, USA

Melissa Hardoby UPMC, Pittsburgh, PA, USA

Department of Surgery, University of Pittsburgh, Pittsburgh, PA, USA

Rebecca Hays Transplant Clinic, University of Wisconsin Hospital and Clinics, Madison, WI, USA

Abhinav Humar Department of Surgery, University of Pittsburgh, Pittsburgh, PA, USA

Betsy B. Johnson Division of Transplantation, Baystate Medical Center, Springfield, MA, USA

Kendal Kingsley Department of Surgery, UPMC Montefiore Hospital, Pittsburgh, PA, USA

Donna M. Kinzler DMK Legal Nurse Consultants, LLC, Pittsburgh, PA, USA

Chanelle Labash Department of Surgery, University of Pittsburgh, Kaufman Building, Pittsburgh, PA, USA

Christina McCloskey Department of Surgery, University of Pittsburgh, Pittsburgh, PA, USA

Mel Peltz Department of Surgery, University of Pittsburgh, Pittsburgh, PA, USA

Salvatore Pisu Department of Bioethics, University of Cagliari, Cagliari, Italy

Tanjala S. Purnell Department of Medicine/General Internal Medicine, Johns Hopkins School of Medicine, Baltimore, MD, USA

Rosamond Rhodes Department of Medical Education, Icahn School of Medicine at Mount Sinai, New York, NY, USA

Dianne LaPointe Rudow Recanati Miller Transplantation Institute, Mount Sinai Medical Center, New York, NY, USA

Barbara L. Rutt Lehigh Valley Network, Allentown, PA, USA

Dorry L. Segev Department of Surgery, Johns Hopkins University School of Medicine, Baltimore, MD, USA

Department of Epidemiology, Johns Hopkins University School of Public Health, Baltimore, MD, USA

Ron Shapiro Department of Surgery, Division of Transplantation, Starzl Translpant Institute, University of Pittsburgh Medical Center, Pittsburgh, PA, USA

Helen G. Spicer Kidney Transplant Services, Henrico Doctors' Hospital, Richmond, VA, USA

Vaughn A. Starnes Department of Surgery, H. Russell Smith Foundation, Keck School of Medicine of the University of Southern California, Keck Medical Center of USC, Los Angeles, CA, USA

Department of Surgery, CardioVascular Thoracic Institute, Keck School of Medicine of the University of Southern California, Keck Medical Center of USC, Los Angeles, CA, USA

Jennifer L. Steel Department of Surgery, Psychiatry, and Psychology, University of Pittsburgh School of Medicine, Pittsburgh, PA, USA

Mark L. Sturdevant Department of Surgery, Starzl Transplant Institute, University of Pittsburgh, Pittsburgh, PA, USA

Kathleen Swartz Trauma Services, Beaumont Health System, Royal Oak, MI, USA

Henkie P. Tan Department of Surgery, Division of Transplant Surgery, University of Pittsburgh Medical Center, Veterans Hospital of Pittsburgh, Pittsburgh, PA, USA

Department of Transplant Surgery, Veterans Hospital of Pittsburgh, University of Pittsburgh Medical Center/Starzl Transplant Institute, Pittsburgh, PA, USA

Miguel Tan Kidney and Pancreas Transplantation, Piedmont Transplant Institute, Piedmont Hospital, Atlanta, GA, USA

Roxanne M. Taylor Maine Medical Center, Portland, ME, USA

Massimiliano Tuveri Department of General Surgery-Transplant, University of Texas Medical Branch, Galveston, TX, USA

Mark Unruh Department of Internal Medicine, Department of Nephrology, University of New Mexico, Albuquerque, NM, USA

Department of Nephrology, Internal Medicine, University of New Mexico, Albuquerque, NM, USA

Andrew W. Webb RN, BSN, CCTC Renal Transplant Office, University of Missouri Hospital and Clinics, Columbia, MO, USA

Christine Wu Department of Medicine, University of Pittsburgh Medical Center, Pittsburgh, PA, USA

Part I
Living Donation

Chapter 1
The Medical Selection of Live Donors

Christine Wu and Henkie P. Tan

Introduction

Living donation has been an integral part of transplantation since the field's inception, with the first successful kidney transplant taking place between identical twins in Boston, Massachusetts, in 1954. While there are many potential advantages to living donation, donation poses both short- and long-term risks to the donor.

Ethics

The first principal of medical ethics, *primum non nocere* ("first do no harm"), charges the medical profession with considering the potential harm of any medical intervention. However, living donation, as a procedure not undertaken to benefit the individual undergoing surgery, is associated with inherent harm to the donor, when interpreted in a broad sense of the word. Risks include blood loss, pain, temporary loss of wages, reduction in organ function, visible physical changes such has scarring, and loss of the whole self. The medical evaluation of live donors necessarily takes a more narrow interpretation of harm to mean *undue* risk, those that are modifiable or preventable that may be associated with substantial new morbidity, both perioperative and long term—occurrences such as inadequate remaining organ function, major cardiovascular events, infection, or even death. Some have advocated the complete separation of the donor evaluation from all recipient considerations as necessary to preserve an unbiased assessment of the donor; however, the medical

---

C. Wu (✉)
Department of Medicine, University of Pittsburgh Medical Center, Pittsburgh, PA, USA
e-mail: wucm@upmc.edu

H. P. Tan
Department of Transplant Surgery, Veterans Hospital of Pittsburgh, University of Pittsburgh Medical Center/Starzl Transplant Institute, Pittsburgh, PA, USA
e-mail: tanxhp@upmc.edu

selection of live donors must consider organ recipient issues such as transmission of infection or malignancy, the provision of adequate organ function, and the risk of recurrent disease. When an independent living donor team is not possible, the living donor advocate can serve only the living donor and is not involved in the evaluation of the transplant candidate.

While a primary goal of the medical evaluation of the live donor is to inform the potential donor of the short- and long-term medical risks involved with organ donation, the degree of risk acceptable to donors can vary widely, with emotionally committed donors such as parents potentially willing to accept even extreme risk [1]. Risk tolerance also differs between individual transplant medical centers; however, the implications of poor outcomes in today's media-rich society have the potential to widely affect society's view and trust of the transplant community as a whole. Thus, the medical selection of live donors involves the identification of donors with risk profiles that are acceptable from the multiple standpoints of the donor, the recipient, the transplant medical team, and the transplant community. In addition to patient autonomy, other nonmedical threats to donor safety, whether motivated by monetary incentive or altruistically motivated by the desire to expand access to transplantation, have led to an increasingly broader acceptance of individuals for organ donation. Those involved in the medical selection of living donors should recognize the limitations of currently available data in determining risks for individuals with medical comorbidity.

Available Data on Risk to Donors

There has been a general decrease in morbidity to living donors with improved operative technique and the advent of, and increasing experience with, laparoscopic techniques. Operative mortality from living kidney donation is reported to be on the order of 0.03 %, and for liver donors 0.1–0.5 % [1, 2]. Quantitative long-term risk assessment for donors is more difficult to interpret. Individual center data generally provide limited follow-up given the inadequate resources dedicated to accurate data collection and a disincentive to find poor outcomes. The issue of underreporting is of concern as the reporting of donor deaths is not universally mandated. Large data sources such as North European national registry data [3–6] and military data [7] are composed of populations that are not necessarily representative of an individual donor and cannot account for genetic differences due to race or familial predisposition. In general, however, published accounts to date have found that long-term survival of living kidney donors has exceeded expected survival. The same cannot be said definitively for nonrenal solid organ donors where donor risk is often much higher [8]. In addition, it remains to be seen, even for kidney donors, whether the long-term outlook for their health will change as stringent donor acceptance criteria are increasingly relaxed.

Medical Suitability

The ideal donor for any organ is someone who is young and in perfect health—taking no medications, with no significant personal or family history of significant or chronic illness, with normal body mass index, normal physical exam, and normal laboratory and other testing. However, the increasing gap between donor supply and demand has led to the cautious acceptance by transplant centers of individuals who are increasingly farther from the ideal. Acceptance criteria for living kidney donors with modified risk varies widely by organ and by transplant center, with guidelines based mostly on expert opinion or weak evidence [9]. For organs very rarely involving living donors (pancreas, intestine, and lung), and in the case of lung transplantation, possibly involving multiple donors, available data to inform decision-making are scarce.

The published discussion of risk, to date, has been mostly limited to those attendant to specific isolated comorbidities and medical conditions. However, current data lack reliable quantitative risk estimates for even the most common medical conditions such as hypertension or obesity [10]. A participant in the Amsterdam forum [11] outlined a method for semiquantitatively estimating risk by using the prevalence of specific medical conditions in the general population and the incidence of the outcome of interest associated with that condition with the following equation: (yearly risk of end-organ disease due to "A") divided by (prevalence of "A" in the population) multiplied by (number of years of expected life remaining). As an example, in the year 2000, 20,000 cases of end-stage renal disease (ESRD) were attributed to hypertension, which had a prevalence of 70 million. Thus, the raw yearly risk of 1/3,500 patient years can be multiplied by 20 years to obtain 1/175 as an estimate of the risk of developing ESRD due to hypertension in an individual over the next 20 years. Unfortunately, such an estimate does not factor in the effect of donation or the presence or future development of other comorbid conditions that may have an additive or synergistic effect on risk. In addition, there are no current data available on the effect of diminished renal function in previous organ donors on the risks associated with future diagnostic testing (e.g., radiologic procedures requiring the administration of intravenous contrast) or on the tolerability and dosing of drug therapies.

Age

As a general rule, most transplant centers agree that minors less than 18 years of age should not be used as living donors, and a number of centers consider age 18–21 to be a relative exclusion [9].

The population in the U.S. and in most of the developed world is aging [12]. Donor age has paralleled this trend [13]. A 2007 survey revealed that 59% (twice the percentage in the 1995 survey) of US transplant centers do not set an upper age limit for living kidney donation [9]. In general, the function of the organ to be donated as well as regenerative capacity decline with age while the number of comorbid conditions increases. In addition, while baseline function changes gradually as individuals age, a much steeper decline in functional reserve occurs with aging [14]. What is not known is whether organ donation affects the rate of expected age-related functional decline. Whether decline is inevitable with normal aging or due to environmental pressures is also unknown. The marked decline in graft survival with increased age seen in deceased kidney transplantation is not seen with living donation, where even older living donor outcomes exceed that of standard criteria deceased donor transplant outcomes [15]. The Scandinavian national health registry demonstrates preserved glomerular filtration rate (GFR) in older donors, no accelerated loss of kidney function in live donors with normal renal function at the time of nephrectomy, but age-expected decline [16]. Age has been associated with decreased hepatic volume, resistance to oxidative stress, drug metabolism, hepatobiliary function, and regenerative capacity, yet successful transplantation from donors in their seventh and eighth decades of life has been reported [17]. Thus, for kidney and liver donor evaluation, organ reserve may be less of a concern than donor comorbidity as the individual ages.

The optimal upper age limit for organs other than kidney or liver is even less clear. An individual reaches his maximal number of pulmonary alveoli by age 10–12 years, with maximum function by age 20–25. Dilatation of alveoli, airspace enlargement, decreased surface area for exchange, loss of tissue support for peripheral airways, and "senile emphysema" are all concerns with older lung donors and reportedly associated with inferior graft survival. Living lung donation is generally restricted to those less than 55 years of age [18]. Even less is known about the role of age in other living donor candidates.

Transmission of Infection

Donors are routinely screened for infections that can be transmitted through organ transplantation. These include infections that would constitute a contraindication to donation such as the viral hepatitides and human immunodeficiency virus (HIV). Hepatitis C positive (HCV+) donors can be considered for HCV+ recipients if the donor has an undetectable viral load (i.e., donor is polymerase chain reaction (PCR) negative), especially for donors infected by more easily treated genotypes and no evidence of chronic hepatitis or cirrhosis on biopsy. The recipient should be counseled regarding the possibility of reinfection or relapse and the implications that organ donation may have on the risk of disease progression and ability to tolerate available antiviral treatment. For potential donors who are found to be hepatitis B core antibody (HBcAb) and hepatitis B surface antibody (HBsAb) positive, total HBcAb (both IgG and IgM) is required to exclude low-level hepatitis B surface antigen (HBsAg) and escape mutants of hepatitis B virus (HBV) not detectable by current screening assays for HBsAg. If IgM+, donation should be delayed. A potentially infected donor who is HBV PCR negative may be considered for an immune (natural or immunized) recipient.

Prospective donors should also be screened for infections that would not be considered absolute contraindications to donation but may have a significant impact on the recipient's risk of disease and may require specific pre-, peri-, or postoperative treatment and/or prevention strategies. Such infections include the herpes viruses, cytomegalovirus (CMV), Epstein–Barr virus (EBV), and syphilis. Some viruses that fit this category may be incorporated into routine screening only in areas where endemic. For example, donors from endemic areas may be screened for additional infections such as Chagas disease (*Trypanosoma cruzi*), schistosomiasis, strongyloidiasis, brucellosis, malaria (*Plasmodium falciparum*), endemic fungal infections (coccidiomycosis, histoplasmosis, and cryptococcosis), human T-lymphotropic virus (HTLV), and tuberculosis. Routine screening of more unusual or rare infections that have been associated with disease transmission from deceased donors such as West Nile virus and rabies is not usually recommended for living donors [19]. Potential donors who resided in the UK during the bovine spongiform encephalopathy (BSE) risk period (1980s to 1990s) who ate meat or who have a family history of unexplained neurodegenerative disease are not permitted to donate blood in North America, Australia, and New Zealand. The remote risk of disease transmission should be discussed with any potential donor–recipient pair for which BSE is of concern.

Transmission of Malignancy

The lifetime risk of developing cancer, exclusive of nonmelanomatous skin cancer, has been estimated to be 40–45 % [20]. The risk of unidentified cancer increases with the aging of the donor population. Based on the deceased donor experience, the risk of donor transmission, even with a history of curative resection, for most cancers is high, particularly for certain cancers such as melanoma, choriocarcinoma, lung cancer, and advanced breast and renal cell carcinomas [21]. Thus, in general, any prior history of malignancy usually excludes live donation. Exceptions may be made for cancers considered to be cured, where both risk of disease recurrence and the potential risk of transmission can be reasonably excluded, and where the cancer does not decrease the reserve of the organ to be donated or increase operative risk (e.g., Dukes A colon cancer with disease-free survival of greater than 5 years, nonmelanomatous skin cancer, and in situ cervical cancer). Both donor and recipient should be informed that transmission cannot be excluded with absolute certainty.

All living donors should be screened by history for preexisting cancer and they should undergo age-appropriate cancer screening. Many centers adopt screening recommendations put forth by major cancer societies. The American Cancer Society recommends breast cancer screening with mammography beginning at age 40, colon cancer screening with one of various modalities including colonoscopy at age 50, cervical cancer screening with pap smear testing beginning at age 21, lung cancer screening only for high-risk individuals, and consideration of prostate cancer screening beginning at age 50. A careful skin exam should be performed on all potential donors.

Other Comorbid Illnesses

Uniform methods for defining and quantifying risk from isolated comorbid illness, even common conditions such as hypertension in kidney donors, have not been conclusively established. While the following is a discussion of select isolated co-morbidities, potential donors with a combination of minor conditions, such as a constellation that suggests the metabolic syndrome, are often discouraged from donating.

Obesity

Data suggest an association between obesity and kidney disease. Unilateral nephrectomy for nondonation is associated with an increased risk of proteinuria and chronic kidney disease (CKD) on long-term follow-up in patients with BMI ≥ 30 kg/m^2 [22]. These findings have led to a trend over the last decade toward stricter application of weight requirements for donors [9]. Potential donors with BMI ≥ 35 kg/m^2 should be discouraged from donating, and those with irreversible associated comorbidities should not proceed with donation. Obese individuals should be encouraged to lose weight prior to donation with, at minimum, provision of healthy lifestyle education, and they should be informed of both acute and long-term risks of being overweight.

Cardiovascular Disease

The majority of individuals being considered for living donation, according to the American College of Cardiology/American Heart Association (ACC/AHA) consensus guidelines for preoperative cardiac testing prior to noncardiac surgery [23], would not meet the criteria for testing, which recommend limiting preoperative cardiac testing to patients with "active cardiac conditions" (unstable coronary syndromes, decompensated heart failure, significant arrhythmia, or severe valvular disease) or patients with "clinical risk factors" (history of ischemic heart disease or congestive heart failure, cerebrovascular disease, diabetes, or kidney disease). Even minor predictors of ischemic heart disease, for which testing is not recommended because these factors have not been proven to be independently associated with higher perioperative risk, including age greater than 70, abnormal electrocardiogram (EKG), rhythm other than sinus, and uncontrolled hypertension, would also generally exclude an individual from consideration as a potential living donor.

However, because the donor surgery is not undertaken for the benefit of the individual undergoing surgery, and needs to consider not only immediate perioperative risk but also long-term donor health, transplant centers, in general, have adopted a much lower threshold for cardiac testing. While the guidelines published by the cardiovascular societies have increasingly narrowed the indications for preoperative stress testing, routine cardiac testing for donors has become more widespread in transplant centers [9]. At our center, all prospective organ donors are asked to obtain an EKG. Stress testing is requested for all potential donors aged greater than 50 years.

Pulmonary Disease

Routine preoperative pulmonary function testing (PFT) is not recommended in stable, asymptomatic donors, with the exception of lobar lung donors. Careful history and physical examination are generally sufficient to assess risk. In select individuals with concern for underlying lung disease, PFTs may be considered. There are no validated threshold values for the exclusion of living donors based on PFT testing. However, the risk of postoperative pulmonary complications increases with FEV1 or forced vital capacity (FVC) values of <70% predicted [24]. Patients at risk of developing progressive chronic lung disease should be excluded from donation.

Smoking

Pneumonia is the most serious complication after noncardiac surgery and the third most common postoperative infection [25]. Smoking increases the risk of perioperative death, pneumonia and respiratory failure, cardiovascular events, and infection [26, 27]. Even tobacco cessation interventions instituted within 4 weeks of surgery appear to significantly decrease perioperative risk [28]. A recent meta-analysis debunks the oft-cited concern that quitting too close to the date of surgery may have detrimental effects on surgical outcomes due to factors such as physiological response to nicotine withdrawal and increased stress and anxiety [29]. All potential donors who smoke should be offered tobacco cessation interventions and encouraged to quit smoking as soon as possible and to commit to lifelong abstinence. The Amsterdam Forum on the Care of the Live Donor advises abstinence from both smoking and alcohol for at least 4 weeks prior to donation [11].

Venous Thromboembolism

There are no consensus recommendations regarding the screening for hypercoagulopathy. It would be prudent to carefully examine family and personal history of hypercoagulable events (venous or arterial thrombosis, second or third trimester miscarriage). At our center, a comprehensive coagulation profile (testing for activated protein C (APC) resistance to detect Factor V Leiden mutation, antithrombin III, proteins C and S, prothrombin (Factor II) mutation, anticardiolipin antibodies, and lupus anticoagulants, prothrombin time (PT), and activated partial thromboplastin time (aPTT)) is requested only for individuals with a concerning personal or family history. Because the Factor V Leiden mutation is highly prevalent, present in 3–8% of the healthy White population [30], and its association with venous thrombosis increases markedly with the use of oral contraceptives, many transplant centers recommend that all women discontinue the use of oral contraceptives, substituting effective alternative birth control, for at least 4 weeks prior to surgery, with treatment resumption only when fully ambulatory following surgery.

Organ Reserve

No living organ donation should proceed without ensuring that the donor has sufficient organ reserve to allow for normal function for the remainder of the donor's expected life. The assessment of organ reserve necessarily varies by organ and may be complicated by competing methodologies as well as methodological flaws and limitations. The ability of a specific organ to either regenerate or accommodate, and how organ donation affects the rate of expected functional decline of aging, is important to consider. In addition, any potential extra-organ consequences associated with even moderate loss of function of the donated organ (e.g., association of cardiovascular disease with even moderate degrees of renal insufficiency) need to be considered and discussed with the potential donor. The detailed discussion of individual organ-specific testing is beyond the scope of this chapter.

Graft function and survival are related not only to donor organ size and function but also to recipient factors such as gender, size, and, for some organs such as the liver, disease severity. Recipient characteristics need to be considered to ensure adequate provision of creatinine clearance in the case of kidney transplantation, or to avoid "small-for-size" syndrome in liver recipients, or to determine the need for multiple donors in lung recipients. Size may also need to be considered for technical reasons, particularly in the case of adult donors to pediatric recipients where large organs may lead to difficulties with vascular compression and difficult wound closure.

Pregnancy

Very little is written about the reproductive concerns of potential donors beyond recommending against donation during pregnancy and need for pregnancy testing. The use of birth control and its associated risk of thromboembolism have previously been discussed. Several retrospective studies have found an increased risk of preeclampsia in previous kidney donors [31, 32]. However, overall pregnancy outcomes in prior kidney donors appear to be the same or better than outcomes found in the general non-donor population. Several published series report outcomes of pregnancies in previous kidney donors and provide guidelines for living kidney donors that generally advise delaying pregnancy following donation for at least 2 months to allow recovery, compensation, and establishment of stable renal function [11, 31–35].

Staging the Evaluation/Final Checklist

The medical evaluation of the potential living donor should be efficient and timely to minimize the burden on the prospective donor, while balancing the cost-effectiveness for the transplant center. In general, testing begins with simple screening tools and progresses through more costly and complex testing. A proposed testing algorithm is detailed in Table 1.1. Careful testing is for naught if the studies are not thoroughly reviewed prior to proceeding with living donation. While time consuming, duplicate independent review by more than one individual is recommended to minimize human error.

Counseling Regarding Follow-Up Care

Many potential donors are not up to date with recommended health maintenance and screening. The donor evaluation offers an opportunity to improve the health of the donor by addressing long-term health concerns such as routine cancer screening, obesity, tobacco smoking, and safe use of potentially organ-toxic medications, particularly those available over the counter. In general, the need and intensity of medical follow-up after living donation is dependent on the type of organ donated, donor age, and medical risk. Consensus guidelines for living donation recommend that donors should be actively followed for at least 24 months following donation by the transplant center, then lifelong by a primary-care physician [36].

Unmet Needs

In 2007, the Organ Procurement and Transplantation Network/United Network for Organ Sharing (OPTN/UNOS) notified transplant programs that federal regulations now require OPTN to develop policies regarding living donors and living donor recipients. Guidelines for the evaluation of kidney and liver donors are now posted on the OPTN website.

Table 1.1 Medical selection of live donors

1. Phone screening
   Age, weight
   History of medical or psychiatric illness/substance abuse
   Medications
2. Compatibility testing
   ABO
   HLA, crossmatching[a]
3. Assessment of functional reserve of donor organ, organ specific
4. Clinic evaluation
   a. Professional evaluations (surgery, medicine, behavioral health, social work, financial, dietician[b]) for history and physical to assess general medical conditions as well as organ-specific concerns
   b. Address risk modification—smoking cessation, weight loss, hypertension
   c. Determine appropriate testing
   d. Assess ability to comply (medical insurance, established PCP for follow-up)
   e. Independent donor advocate
   f. Discuss future risks, address reproductive health concerns, and obtain informed consent
5. Testing
   a. Preliminary laboratory work—chemistries, blood sugar, liver function, albumin, calcium, phosphorus, PT/PTT, HCG quantitative for premenopausal women without surgical sterilization
   b. Infection screening
      (i) Routine serologic testing (HIV, viral hepatitis, CMV, EBV, herpes virus, syphilis, tuberculosis)
      (ii) Additional testing for endemic exposure (Chagas disease (*Trypanosoma cruzi*), schistosomiasis, strongyloidiasis, brucellosis, malaria (*Plasmodium falciparum*), endemic fungal infections (coccidio, crypto), HTLV, West Nile, toxoplasmosis)
   c. Cancer screening
   d. Major comorbidity screening[c]
      (i) Cardiac—EKG, stress test, echocardiogram, carotids
      (ii) Pulmonary—PFTs, CXR
      (iii) Thrombophilia
      (iv) Metabolic—diabetes screening (FBS, OGTT, HbA1C), lipids
   e. Organ-specific imaging/testing
6. Final checklist—at least two independent reviewers

Cost/complexity increases from 1 to 5
HLA human leukocyte antigen, *CMV* cytomegalovirus, *EBV* Epstein–Barr virus, *PT* prothrombin time, *PTT* partial thromboplastin time, *HCG* human chorionic gonadotropin, *PCP* primary-care physician, *HTLV* human T-lymphotropic virus, *PFT* pulmonary function testing, *CXR* chest X-ray, *FBS* fasting blood sugar, *OGTT* oral glucose tolerance test
[a] Compatibility testing is not necessary for successful transplantation of most organs [37]
[b] As indicated for BMI < 18 or > 30
[c] The studies below may not all be required. Specific testing is determined at stage 4c during clinic evaluation

A consistent theme in this chapter is the need for more comprehensive and accurate data on donor outcomes. Several guidelines have been proposed over the years, but much of the work has been duplicative based on a paucity of good available data. The establishment of long-term comprehensive prospective studies and national registries would provide an important step toward this goal. Given the potential negative impact of reporting adverse outcomes on the reputation of individual hospital centers, the successful recruitment of future donors, and the ability to maintain and attract new insurance providers, universal reporting must be mandated. In addition, information on specific risks in minority populations, particularly ethnic subgroups with known health risk factors (i.e., African Americans, Native Americans, and Hispanics), is needed.

The ability to quantify risks associated with common conditions such as advanced age, obesity, hyperlipidemia, and tobacco use would help not only the donor but also the medical team, and the transplant community as a whole, to establish thresholds of acceptability and to develop appropriate recommendations for follow-up care. A better understanding of the interaction between these factors and recipient characteristics may be helpful not only in determining the acceptability of a donor, but also in choosing among donors for recipients who may have several potential options.

Medical outcomes like operative complications, readmission rates, development of disease, or death tell only part of the story. The impact of organ donation on quality of life may be just as important to an individual considering living donation. In the end, the medical selection of the living donor must recognize that the ultimate decision to proceed with living donation will be an individualized one made in a spirit of cooperation between the individual most affected, the donor, and the transplant medical team whose role is to safeguard the donor's health and well-being.

References

1. Tan HP, Marcos A, Shapiro R. Living donor transplantation. New York: Informa Healthcare; 2007.
2. Ringe B, Strong RW. The dilemma of living liver donor death: to report or not to report? Transplantation. 2008;85(6):790–3 [Epub 2008/03/25].
3. Fehrman-Ekholm I, Duner F, Brink B, Tyden G, Elinder CG. No evidence of accelerated loss of kidney function in living kidney donors: results from a cross-sectional follow-up. Transplantation. 2001;72(3):444–9 [Epub 2001/08/15].
4. Fehrman-Ekholm I. Life-span of living-related kidney donors. Transplant Proc. 1997;29(7):2801–2 [Epub 1997/11/20].
5. Fehrman-Ekholm I, Elinder CG, Stenbeck M, Tyden G, Groth CG. Kidney donors live longer. Transplantation. 1997;64(7):976–8 [Epub 1997/11/05]
6. Fehrman-Ekholm I, Johansson A, Konberg A, Tyden G. Long-term survival of living related kidney donors. Transplant Proc. 1997;29(1–2):1481 [Epub 1997/02/01].
7. Narkun-Burgess DM, Nolan CR, Norman JE, Page WF, Miller PL, Meyer TW. Forty-five year follow-up after uninephrectomy. Kidney Int. 1993;43(5):1110–5 [Epub 1993/05/01].
8. Khalaf H, Al-Sofayan M, El-Sheikh Y, Al-Bahili H, Al-Sagheir M, Al-Sebayel M. Donor outcome after living liver donation: a single-center experience. Transplant Proc. 2007;39(4):829–34 [Epub 2007/05/26].
9. Mandelbrot DA, Pavlakis M, Danovitch GM, Johnson SR, Karp SJ, Khwaja K, et al. The medical evaluation of living kidney donors: a survey of US transplant centers. Am J Transplant. 2007;7(10):2333–43 [Epub 2007/09/12].

10. Ommen ES, Winston JA, Murphy B. Medical risks in living kidney donors: absence of proof is not proof of absence. Clin J Am Soc Nephrol. 2006;1(4):885–95 [Epub 2007/08/21].
11. Delmonico F. A Report of the Amsterdam forum on the care of the live kidney donor: data and medical guidelines. Transplantation. 2005;79 Suppl 6:S53–66 [Epub 2005/03/24].
12. Siegel J. Aging into the 21st century. Washington, D.C.: U.S. Department of Health and Human Services; 1996.
13. Matas AJ, Smith JM, Skeans MA, Lamb KE, Gustafson SK, Samana CJ, et al. OPTN/SRTR 2011 Annual Data Report: kidney. Am J Transplant. 2013;13 Suppl 1:11–46 [Epub 2013/01/31].
14. Cook DJ, Rooke GA. Priorities in perioperative geriatrics. Anesth Analg. 2003;96(6):1823–36 [Epub 2003/05/23].
15. Gill J, Bunnapradist S, Danovitch GM, Gjertson D, Gill JS, Cecka M. Outcomes of kidney transplantation from older living donors 2 older recipients. Am J Kidney Dis 2008;52(3):541–52 [Epub 2008/07/26].
16. Fehrman-Ekholm I, Kvarnstrom N, Softeland JM, Lennerling A, Rizell M, Oden A, et al. Postnephrectomy development of renal function in living kidney donors: a cross-sectional retrospective study. Nephrol, Dialysis, Transplant. 2011;26(7):2377–81 [Epub 2011/04/05].
17. Darius T, Monbaliu D, Jochmans I, Meurisse N, Desschans B, Coosemans W, et al. Septuagenarian and octogenarian donors provide excellent liver grafts for transplantation. Transplant Proc. 2012;44(9):2861–7 [Epub 2012/11/14].
18. Starnes VA, Bowdish ME, Woo MS, Barbers RG, Schenkel FA, Horn MV, et al. A decade of living lobar lung transplantation: recipient outcomes. J Thoracic Cardiovasc Surg. 2004;127(1):114–22 [Epub 2004/01/31].
19. Razonable RR. Rare, unusual, and less common virus infections after organ transplantation. Curr Opin Organ Transplant. 2011;16(6):580–7 [Epub 2011/10/18].
20. Girard SL, Gauthier J, Noreau A, Xiong L, Zhou S, Jouan L, et al. Increased exonic de novo mutation rate in individuals with schizophrenia. Nat Genet. 2011;43(9):860–3 [Epub 2011/07/12].
21. Buell JF, Beebe TM, Trofe J, Gross TG, Alloway RR, Hanaway MJ, et al. Donor transmitted malignancies. Ann Transplant. 2004;9(1):53–6 [Epub 2004/10/14].
22. Praga M, Hernandez E, Herrero JC, Morales E, Revilla Y, Diaz-Gonzalez R, et al. Influence of obesity on the appearance of proteinuria and renal insufficiency after unilateral nephrectomy. Kidney Int. 2000;58(5):2111–8 [Epub 2000/10/24].
23. Fleisher LA, Beckman JA, Brown KA, Calkins H, Chaikof E, Fleischmann KE, et al. ACC/AHA 2007 Guidelines on Perioperative Cardiovascular Evaluation and Care for Noncardiac Surgery: Executive Summary: A Report of the American College of Cardiology/American Heart Association Task Force on Practice Guidelines (Writing Committee to Revise the 2002 Guidelines on Perioperative Cardiovascular Evaluation for Noncardiac Surgery): Developed in Collaboration With the American Society of Echocardiography, American Society of Nuclear Cardiology, Heart Rhythm Society, Society of Cardiovascular Anesthesiologists, Society for Cardiovascular Angiography and Interventions, Society for Vascular Medicine and Biology, and Society for Vascular Surgery. Circulation. 2007;116(17):1971–96 [Epub 2007/09/29].
24. Smetana GW. Preoperative pulmonary evaluation. N Engl J Med. 1999;340(12):937–44 [Epub 1999/03/25].
25. Arozullah AM, Khuri SF, Henderson WG, Daley J. Development and validation of a multifactorial risk index for predicting postoperative pneumonia after major noncardiac surgery. Ann Intern Med. 2001;135(10):847–57 [Epub 2001/11/20].
26. Moller AM, Villebro N, Pedersen T, Tonnesen H. Effect of preoperative smoking intervention on postoperative complications: a randomised clinical trial. Lancet. 2002;359(9301):114–7 [Epub 2002/01/26].
27. Turan A, Mascha EJ, Roberman D, Turner PL, You J, Kurz A, et al. Smoking and perioperative outcomes. Anesthesiology. 2011;114(4):837–46 [Epub 2011/03/05].

28. Lindstrom D, Sadr Azodi O, Wladis A, Tonnesen H, Linder S, Nasell H, et al. Effects of a perioperative smoking cessation intervention on postoperative complications: a randomized trial. Ann Surg. 2008;248(5):739–45 [Epub 2008/10/25].
29. Myers K, Hajek P, Hinds C, McRobbie H. Stopping smoking shortly before surgery and postoperative complications: a systematic review and meta-analysis. Arch Intern Med. 2011;171(11):983–9 [Epub 2011/03/16].
30. De Stefano VM, Casorelli I, et al. The risk of recurrent deep venous thrombosis among heterozygous carriers of both factor V Leiden and the G20210A prothrombin mutation. N Engl J Med. 1999;341(11):801–6 [Epub 1999/09/09].
31. Ibrahim HN, Akkina SK, Leister E, Gillingham K, Cordner G, Guo H, et al. Pregnancy outcomes after kidney donation. Am J Transplant. 2009;9(4):825–34 [Epub 2009/04/09].
32. Reisaeter AV, Roislien J, Henriksen T, Irgens LM, Hartmann A. Pregnancy and birth after kidney donation: the Norwegian experience. Am J Transplant. 2009;9(4):820–4 [Epub 2008/10/16].
33. Mackie F. The CARI guidelines. Potential child-bearing donors. Nephrology (Carlton). 2010;15 Suppl 1:S99–100 [Epub 2010/04/01].
34. Buszta C, Steinmuller DR, Novick AC, Schreiber MJ, Cunningham R, Popowniak KL, et al. Pregnancy after donor nephrectomy. Transplantation. 1985;40(6):651–4 [Epub 1985/12/01].
35. Wrenshall LE, McHugh L, Felton P, Dunn DL, Matas AJ. Pregnancy after donor nephrectomy. Transplantation. 1996;62(12):1934–6 [Epub 1996/12/27].
36. Tong A, Chapman JR, Wong G, Bruijn J de, Craig JC. Screening and follow-up of living kidney donors: a systematic review of clinical practice guidelines. Transplantation. 2011;92(9):962–72 [Epub 2011/10/01].
37. Terasaki PI, Cecka JM, Gjertson DW, Takemoto S. High survival rates of kidney transplants from spousal and living unrelated donors. N Engl J Med. 1995;333:333–336.

Chapter 2
Kidney Paired Donation Programs for Incompatible Living Kidney Donors and Recipients

Sommer E. Gentry, Ron Shapiro and Dorry L. Segev

Rationale

About one-third of people who offer to donate a kidney will be either blood type incompatible or human leukocyte antigen (HLA) incompatible with their intended recipient. Kidney paired donation (KPD), or kidney exchange, circumvents the incompatibility between donor and intended recipient by redistributing organs among two or more donors before the transplants [1]. In the simplest type of KPD, two donors exchange kidneys so that their two candidates can each receive a compatible transplant (Fig. 2.1). The donor operations are usually started simultaneously, to prevent the situation in which one donor decides not to donate after that donor's intended recipient has already received a kidney.

Many extensions to this concept, such as three-way and larger exchanges, compatible paired donation, and use of nondirected (altruistic) donors, have allowed greater numbers of people to find matches. KPD is the fastest-growing modality of living donation in the U.S., growing from just a handful of transplants in 2000 to

---

S. E. Gentry (✉)
Department of Mathematics, United States Naval Academy, Annapolis, MD, USA
e-mail: gentry@usna.edu

Department of Surgery, Johns Hopkins University School of Medicine, Baltimore, MD, USA

R. Shapiro
Starzl Translpant Institute, University of Pittsburgh, Pittsburgh, PA, USA
e-mail: shapiror@upmc.edu

Department of Surgery, Division of Transplantation, University of Pittsburgh Medical Center, Pittsburgh, PA, USA

D. L. Segev
Department of Surgery, Johns Hopkins University School of Medicine, Baltimore, MD, USA
e-mail: dorry@jhmi.edu

Department of Epidemiology, Johns Hopkins University School of Public Health, Baltimore, MD, USA

Fig. 2.1 A two-way kidney paired donation. The donor in *blue* is not compatible with his or her intended recipient, and the donor in *gray* is not compatible with his or her intended recipient, but, through KPD, both recipients can be transplanted

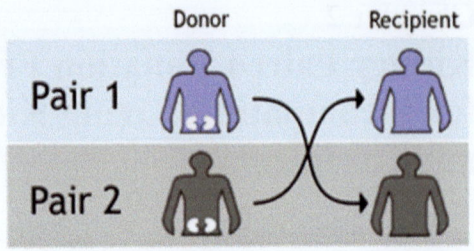

surpass 500 transplants per year in 2010 [2]. Kidney exchange accounted for nearly 10 % of living kidney transplants in 2011.

History

KPD was first suggested in the literature by Rapaport in 1986 [3], but some observers argued that this modality would help only a small number of people [4]. The earliest functioning exchange programs may have been those in Korea that accomplished more than 100 transplants by 1997 [5]. In the U.S., single-center programs were performing KPD at a low rate until 2005, when a national consensus conference was held to discuss the possibility of larger registries that would combine incompatible pairs from many transplant centers to find more matches. Because the National Organ Transplantation Act of 1984 forbade acquiring or transferring a kidney for valuable consideration, members of the transplant community pressed the US Congress to pass the Charlie W. Norwood Living Organ Donation Act of 2007 clarifying that kidney exchange was legal. The current landscape for KPD in the U.S. includes several single-center programs [6], multicenter consortia [7–9], and a registry operated by the organization that administers deceased donation in the U.S., the United Network for Organ Sharing. Recently, a second consensus conference produced detailed recommendations for developing KPD in the U.S. [10].

Mathematical and Computational Considerations

Once a paired donation program exceeds about 10 or 20 pairs, it requires a nontrivial mathematical optimization to find the combination of matches that achieves the greatest number and the most optimal transplants. Two possible combinations of matches for the same ten pairs are shown in Figs. 2.2a and b. Each small numbered circle represents two people: a kidney transplant candidate and his incompatible donor. The lines that connect some of the circles show cases in which a paired exchange is possible; that is, if a line connects two circles, then the donor of each pair

2 Kidney Paired Donation Programs for Incompatible Living Kidney Donors ... 19

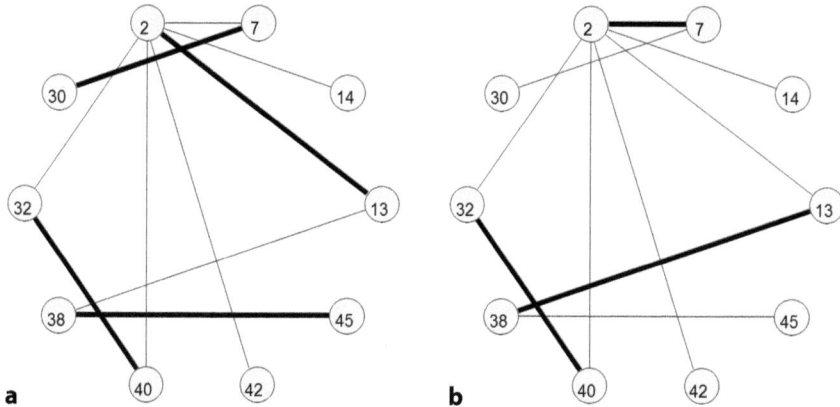

Fig. 2.2 **a** One possible combination of two-way KPD matches is shown with *dark lines*, representing eight transplants among ten incompatible pairs. Each small arbitrarily numbered *circle* represents two people: a kidney transplant candidate and his incompatible donor. The *lines* that connect some of the *circles* show which two-way KPD matches are possible. If a *line* connects two *circles*, then the donor of each pair is compatible with the recipient of the other pair. **b** A different combination of two-way KPD matches is shown in the *dark lines*, representing six transplants among the same ten incompatible pairs as in (**a**). There are no feasible KPD matches for the remaining four incompatible pairs

is compatible with the recipient of the other pair. Sophisticated mathematical algorithms are required, in general, to find the optimal matching in Fig. 2.2a, in which the dark lines show how four exchanges could result in transplantation for eight of these ten participants. All of the decisions in any paired exchange registry affect the opportunities for other pairs in the group. For instance, after performing the three exchanges shown in Fig. 2.2b, only six people out of these same ten have been transplanted, and there is no way to find compatible transplants for the remaining four.

Many considerations besides the absolute number of transplants are important in choosing which incompatible pairs should be matched with more optimal donors and candidates. Matches that involve pediatric candidates, highly sensitized candidates, or matches in the same transplant center are preferred, as are matches for the pairs that have been waiting the longest. KPD registries generally use optimization methods like integer programming to maximize the benefit afforded to all pairs in the registry.

These static optimization methods require all donors and recipients to wait for some period of time before any matches are made, or else the entire advantage will be lost. KPD registries that do not wait for 25–100 registrants to accumulate between matches are predicted to achieve about 10–20 % fewer transplants than would otherwise be possible [11]. Competition among multiple registries might predictably lead to just this outcome, in which the drive to make matches earlier means fewer matches overall. A more advanced mathematical technology called dynamic optimization could alleviate this trade-off, but these methods for KPD matching are still being developed [12, 13].

An expanded definition of KPD would include exchanges among three or more pairs. The donor of one pair gives the recipient of the next pair, whose donor gives to the recipient of the next pair, and so on, until the last pair's donor gives to the recipient of the first pair in the cycle. Moving to three-way or larger exchanges significantly increases the likelihood that any pair will find a match.

Desensitization protocols using high-dose intravenous immunoglobulin (IVIg) or plasmapheresis and low-dose IVIg have enabled successful transplants against either human leukocyte antigen (HLA) or blood type incompatibilities. Thus, desensitization might be viewed as an alternative to KPD. However, some incompatible pairs can only be transplanted through a combination of desensitization and KPD. This situation arises when a transplant candidate has very high donor-specific antibody levels against the intended donor, but the candidate has a lower level of donor-specific antibody for some other donor in the exchange pool. To offer one example, more than half of all KPD recipients in the Johns Hopkins Hospital Incompatible Kidney Transplant program have required desensitization.

One complicating factor in all paired donation registries is imperfect prior information about exactly which donors are compatible with which candidates. Even with proper histocompatibility testing, which includes donor and recipient HLA typing and recipient antibody testing to identify unacceptable antigens, unexpected positive crossmatches will occur. An unexpected positive crossmatch will cancel all of the transplants in a planned kidney exchange. These unexpected positive crossmatches are very disruptive to the operations of a KPD registry, causing delays and disappointment for enrolled incompatible pairs. Strict standards for histocompatibility laboratories might mitigate this difficulty. Histocompatibility experts play a vital role in managing KPD, especially for centers that combine KPD with desensitization.

Blood Type Distribution and the Role of Compatible Pairs

Because a selection bias skews blood types among incompatible pairs, the pairs who have overrepresented blood types will find it difficult to match to a complementary pair. For example, the population of incompatible pairs will be enriched for O blood type recipients because O recipients are blood type incompatible with all A, B, and AB donors. On the other hand, pairs with O blood type donors would only seek KPD in the comparatively rare circumstance that the donors were HLA incompatible with their intended recipients. The 28% of incompatible pair donors who have O blood type will not be sufficient to match the 59% of incompatible pair recipients who have O blood type [14]. Simulation studies suggest that O blood type recipients with non-O donors and all recipients with AB donors will wait longer and match at lower rates [15].

If donors who are compatible with their intended recipients also participated in KPD, the blood type imbalance could be corrected and twice as many incompatible pairs would find a match [16]. Compatible pairs might join a kidney exchange pool to find a donor who is a better size match, HLA match, or age match for the intended

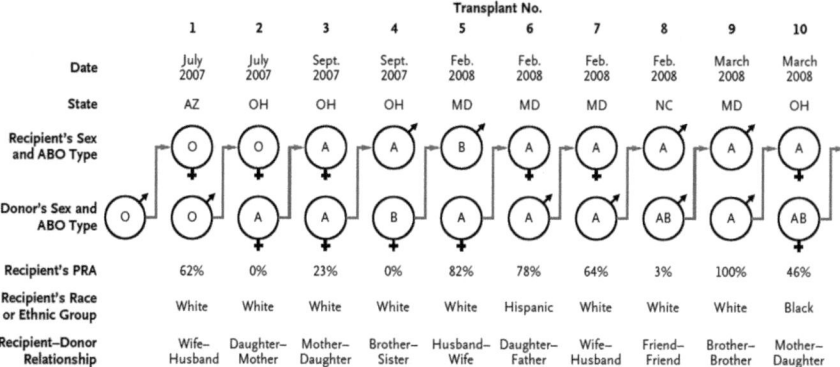

Fig. 2.3 A nonsimultaneous extended altruistic donor chain, initiated by a nondirected donor from Michigan. The recipients of transplants 6 and 9 required desensitization in conjunction with donor exchange. (From Rees et al. [19], Copyright © 2009, Massachusetts Medical Society. Reprinted with permission)

recipient; recent evidence supports this practice, particularly in the case of older living donors [17]. Compatible pairs also might offer to participate in kidney exchange out of an altruistic desire to help candidates with incompatible donors. The largest single-center KPD program in the U.S., at Methodist Specialty and Transplant Hospital in San Antonio, makes extensive use of compatible pairs and 35% of its transplant volume is paired donation [6].

Role of Nondirected Donors

Nondirected donors, or altruistic donors, are people who volunteer to donate a kidney without naming any intended recipient. After appropriate screening and counseling, a nondirected donor might give to a candidate on the deceased donor waiting list. Alternatively, a nondirected donor might give to the recipient of an incompatible pair, and the incompatible donor's kidney can go to another pair, and so on, thereby multiplying the gift of the nondirected donation. Figure 2.3 illustrates one such chain. A consensus conference recently urged that all nondirected donors be informed about KPD and their potential to trigger multiple transplants through these programs [10].

Nondirected donors are especially empowered to enable transplants for incompatible pairs. In many operating KPD programs, a majority of the transplants are accomplished in exchanges started by nondirected donors [18]. This is true both because of a favorable blood type distribution among nondirected donors, with 48% of nondirected donors having O blood type, and because nondirected donors relax the reciprocality requirement that otherwise constrains the last donor to match the intended recipient of an initiating pair. Further, kidney exchanges that start with a nondirected donor can relax the restriction of simultaneity.

At the end of a chain of transplants initiated by a nondirected donor, the donor of the last pair might donate a kidney to a candidate on the deceased donor waiting list, or might be asked to wait a few months as a bridge donor. The bridge donor delays his donation so that he or she can serve as the starting donor for another chain of transplants after new incompatible pairs join the program. A chain that is always continued with a bridge donor after a delay is called a nonsimultaneous extended altruistic donor (NEAD) chain [19]. A chain of donations started by a nondirected donor that ends with a donation to a deceased donor waiting list candidate is called a domino paired donation [20]. A simultaneous domino paired donation ends immediately with a donation to the waiting list; a nonsimultaneous domino paired donation incorporates one or more bridge donors who extend the domino through time until it ultimately ends with a donation to the waiting list.

When the donations are performed in succession starting with a nondirected donor, there is less risk associated with nonsimultaneous operations. Because none of the donor operations in the chain occurs before the intended recipient of that donor has received a transplant, there is no way for a candidate to remain untransplanted after his bargaining chip, his intended donor, has already given a kidney. If a bridge donor decides not to donate, then the incompatible pairs farther down the chain can be matched into a different KPD arrangement, because every candidate still has his incompatible donor. This observation holds only for operations performed in the natural sequence. At least one group has reported performing a successful out-of-sequence nonsimultaneous chain [21].

In theory, each nondirected donor could begin a very long NEAD chain of donations extending over time. In practice, the bridge donors become increasingly difficult to match to the next recipient. In fact, the reason someone is designated as a bridge donor is usually that he or she does not match any of the recipients presently in the incompatible pairs registry. Transplant 9 in Fig. 2.3, for example, required desensitization across a blood type barrier to use an AB blood type donor, and the sequence of transplants halted again at an AB blood type donor after transplant 10. It might be the case that bridge donors who are difficult to match and who have to wait longer are more likely never to donate in the long run. Every KPD registry using bridge donors that we are aware of has had at least one bridge donor who ultimately did not donate.

It is not entirely clear whether extending all NEAD chains indefinitely, or ending domino paired donations with the deceased donor waiting list, will yield a larger number of transplants [22, 23]. The preferred strategy depends on the precise characteristics of the incompatible pairs, the relative prevalence of nondirected donors, and the probability of bridge donor withdrawal. The usual practice in registries that use bridge donors is to ask the bridge donor to donate to someone on the deceased donor waiting list if no opportunity has been found for that donor to match an incompatible pair candidate within some reasonable span of time.

Ethical concerns about nondirected donors in KPD include fears of coercion for bridge donors who promise to donate later, and the permanent diversion of transplants from nondirected donors away from the deceased donor waiting list in NEAD chains [24].

Donor Travel Versus Living Donor Kidney Transport

Long-distance kidney exchanges between pairs who live hundreds or thousands of miles apart are becoming more frequent in the era of large multicenter paired donation registries. A recent study found that 44 % of matches involved transplant centers in different states [2]. In the earliest days, physicians worried about degrading the performance of living donor kidneys by delaying the transplants to allow transportation time. Thus, physicians would ask donors in a paired transplant to travel to the hospital where the other pair's candidate would receive his transplant.

However, a retrospective review of transplant registry data showed that moderately prolonged cold ischemia times had no impact on long-term outcomes for live donor kidney transplant [25]. In the first long-distance transport of a live donor kidney that we are aware of, surgeons transported a kidney by charter jet from San Francisco, California, to Baltimore, Maryland [26]. Later, a series of 56 transported live donor kidneys was reported with cold ischemia times up to 14.5 h, and with no incidence of delayed graft function [27]. Today, the majority of kidney exchanges among multiple transplant centers in the U.S. are accomplished by shipping the kidneys rather than by requiring donors to travel.

Donor Education and Other Considerations

All potential living donors should be advised of the possibility of KPD early in the counseling process, even before tests of compatibility are completed. Potential donors should have time to consider their preferences regarding donor exchange, to prevent feelings of coercion if KPD is only mentioned after a finding of incompatibility [10].

Donors considering KPD should receive the standard counseling offered to all living donors, but should additionally be informed of the unique aspects of multicenter KPD registries [10]. When joining a paired donation registry, donors and their intended recipients should know that delays in finding a paired exchange opportunity are common. If a provisional match for paired donation arises, there are many reasons that it might not culminate in an exchange transplant, including logistical, medical, or compatibility contraindications that could not have been anticipated. Each donor should know that details of his or her medical history and health status, but not his or her identity, likely need to be disclosed to potential matching candidates and those candidates' care providers.

The donor consent process for KPD should cover the risks of kidney transport, the possibility of last-minute cancellations, and the potential for redirecting the kidney to another recipient under rare circumstances.

In kidney exchanges, donor and recipient pairs are kept anonymous to the other people involved in the exchange, at least until the transplants are completed. After that, donors and recipients often arrange to meet each other, or keep each other informed of their health status, by mutual consent. In some cases, donors involved in paired exchanges might never learn of the outcome for the person who received their organ. Alternatively, if exchange partners decide to share information and if any recipient in a kidney exchange has an unfavorable outcome, it could have an adverse psychological impact on donors.

Financing KPD

KPD, particularly between different transplant centers, presents novel challenges for administrators and payers [28]. Every exchange transplant necessitates individual financial negotiations and contracts, which might or might not align with the guidelines for recipient payers. Many prospective donors who require workups before they can be entered into KPD registries will not actually donate. There may be additional costs for organ transport or donor travel, as well as out-of-network pricing for the donor operations. There are also costs, which are not directly related to the number of transplants performed, for the administrative and logistical coordination of a multicenter paired donation registry. There is an effort under way to establish a national KPD standard acquisition charge (SAC), which would accumulate all costs associated with evaluating KPD donors and possibly donor-related professional fees [29].

International Programs

Many other countries have established KPD programs, which can vary substantially from the US-centric description of kidney exchange presented in this chapter. For instance, in Germany anonymous donation is strictly forbidden; therefore, the exchange donors always meet their paired recipients prior to the transplants [30]. In geographically compact Netherlands, rather than transporting the organs after recovery, as in the U.S., donors in a paired exchange always travel to the transplant center of their actual recipient [31]. In Canada, some regulatory difficulties have stalled the widespread use of live donor kidney transports.

Some of the earliest kidney exchanges occurred in Korean transplant programs, as well as the first known report of a donor hesitating to donate after his intended recipient had received a kidney transplant [5]. In those early days, researchers also had to address concerns that allografts from unrelated donors might not perform as well as those from related donors [32]. With local variations that derive from differing laws or differing transplant practices, KPD programs are flourishing in many countries: Canada, Korea, the UK, Romania, India, the Netherlands, and Australia. A kidney exchange between two countries has even been reported [33].

Conclusion

Paired donation offers many donors a path to helping a loved one receive a kidney transplant, and is the fastest-growing arena of living donation. As exciting as the numbers are, studies suggest that KPD has room to grow. There are still some transplant centers where kidney transplant candidates who present with an incompatible living donor do not have access to a KPD registry. At other centers, there may be transplant candidates who have been on the deceased donor waiting list for some time who know about a potential living incompatible donor, but have not been enrolled for KPD. If all US transplant centers were as active in promoting and pursuing kidney exchanges as the highest-performing centers, researchers estimate that an additional 1,000 kidney transplants could be achieved every year [34].

This modality is incredibly promising, and many groups working in KPD are at the forefront of clinical innovation to eliminate histocompatibility, transport, logistical, and mathematical barriers to performing more transplants. To reduce the number of provisional matches refused for compatibility or donor criteria, many registries have employed a preselection step for transplant centers to specify which of the potential donors are acceptable for each candidate. Coordination of HLA laboratories is also important, and was responsible for decreasing the unexpected positive crossmatch rate from 57 to 9% in one registry [8]. Cryobanking of preserved donor lymphocytes might enable prescreening of crossmatch compatibility for highly sensitized candidates.

There are a dozen or more different KPD registries operating in the U.S., and many incompatible pairs are enrolled in more than one of these registries. This can lead to disappointment if a pair starts to move forward with an exchange opportunity available through one program while another program tries to match that same pair to a conflicting arrangement. Further, the highest proportion of incompatible pairs find a transplant when exchanges are considered among the largest possible group of exchange partners [11]. That is, if the same 1,000 incompatible pairs are all enrolled in the same registry, then more transplants will be possible than if 500 pairs join one registry and the other 500 join a separate registry. As this emerging field matures, candidates with incompatible donors would gain the most benefit from a unified KPD registry in the U.S. [10].

References

1. Montgomery RA, Zachary AA, Ratner LE, Segev DL, Hiller JM, Houp J, et al. Clinical results from transplanting incompatible live kidney donor/recipient pairs using kidney paired donation. JAMA. 2005;294(13):1655–63.
2. Segev DL, Kucirka LM, Gentry SE, Montgomery RA. Utilization and outcomes of kidney paired donation in the United States. Transplantation. 2008;86(4):502–10.
3. Rapaport FT. The case for a living emotionally related international kidney donor exchange registry. Transplant Proc. 1986;18(3) Suppl 2:5–9.

4. Terasaki PI, Gjertson DW, Cecka JM. Paired kidney exchange is not a solution to ABO incompatibility. Transplantation. 1998;65(2):291.
5. Park K, Moon JI, Kim SI, Kim YS. Exchange donor program in kidney transplantation. Transplantation. 1999;67(2):336–8.
6. Bingaman AW, Wright FH Jr, Kapturczak M, Shen L, Vick S, Murphey CL. Single-center kidney paired donation: the Methodist San Antonio experience. Am J Transplant. 2012;12(8):2125–32.
7. Delmonico FL. Exchanging kidneys—advances in living-donor transplantation. N Engl J Med. 2004;350(18):1812–4.
8. Veale J, Hil G. National Kidney Registry: 213 transplants in three years. Clin Transpl. 2010:333–44.
9. Akkina SK, Muster H, Steffens E, Kim SJ, Kasiske BL, Israni AK. Donor exchange programs in kidney transplantation: rationale and operational details from the north central donor exchange cooperative. Am J Kidney Dis. 2011;57(1):152–8.
10. Feng S, Melcher ML, Blosser CD, Baxter-Lowe LA, Delmonico F, Gentry SE, et al. Dynamic challenges inhibiting optimal adoption of kidney paired donation: findings of a consensus conference. Am J Transplant. 2013;13(4):851–60.
11. Segev DL, Gentry SE, Warren DS, Reeb B, Montgomery RA. Kidney paired donation and optimizing the use of live donor organs. JAMA. 2005;293(15):1883–90.
12. Ünver MU. Dynamic kidney exchange. Rev Econ Stud. 2010;77(1):372–414.
13. Awasthi P, Sandholm T. Online stochastic optimization in the large: application to kidney exchange. In International Joint Conference on Artificial Intelligence, 2009.
14. Gentry SE, Segev DL, Montgomery RA. A comparison of populations served by kidney paired donation and list paired donation. Am J Transplant. 2005;5(8):1914–21.
15. Segev DL, Gentry SE, Melancon JK, Montgomery RA. Characterization of waiting times in a simulation of kidney paired donation. Am J Transplant. 2005;5(10):2448–55.
16. Gentry SE, Segev DL, Simmerling M, Montgomery RA. Expanding kidney paired donation through participation by compatible pairs. Am J Transplant. 2007;7(10):2361–70.
17. Berger JC, Muzaale AD, James N, Hoque M, Wang JM, Montgomery RA, et al. Living kidney donors ages 70 and older: recipient and donor outcomes. Clin J Am Soc Nephrol. 2011;6(12):2887–93.
18. Melcher ML, Leeser DB, Gritsch HA, Milner J, Kapur S, Busque S, et al. Chain transplantation: initial experience of a large multicenter program. Am J Transplant. 2012;12(9):2429–36.
19. Rees MA, Kopke JE, Pelletier RP, Segev DL, Rutter ME, Fabrega AJ, et al. A nonsimultaneous, extended, altruistic-donor chain. N Engl J Med. 2009;360(11):1096–101.
20. Montgomery RA, Gentry SE, Marks WH, Warren DS, Hiller J, Houp J, et al. Domino paired kidney donation: a strategy to make best use of live non-directed donation. Lancet. 2006;368(9533):419–21.
21. Butt FK, Gritsch HA, Schulam P, Danovitch GM, Wilkinson A, Del Pizzo J, et al. Asynchronous, out-of-sequence, transcontinental chain kidney transplantation: a novel concept. Am J Transplant. 2009;9(9):2180–5.
22. Gentry SE, Montgomery RA, Swihart BJ, Segev DL. The roles of dominos and nonsimultaneous chains in kidney paired donation. Am J Transplant. 2009;9(6):1330–6.
23. Ashlagi I, Gilchrist DS, Roth AE, Rees MA. Nonsimultaneous chains and dominos in kidney-paired donation-revisited. Am J Transplant. 2011;11(5):984–94.
24. Woodle ES, Daller JA, Aeder M, Shapiro R, Sandholm T, Casingal V, et al. Ethical considerations for participation of nondirected living donors in kidney exchange programs. Am J Transplant. 2010;10(6):1460–7.
25. Simpkins CE, Montgomery RA, Hawxby AM, Locke JE, Gentry SE, Warren DS, et al. Cold ischemia time and allograft outcomes in live donor renal transplantation: is live donor organ transport feasible? Am J Transplant. 2007;7(1):99–107.
26. Montgomery RA, Katznelson S, Bry WI, Zachary AA, Houp J, Hiller JM, et al. Successful three-way kidney paired donation with cross-country live donor allograft transport. Am J Transplant. 2008;8(10):2163–8.

27. Segev DL, Veale JL, Berger JC, Hiller JM, Hanto RL, Leeser DB, et al. Transporting live donor kidneys for kidney paired donation: initial national results. Am J Transplant. 2011;11(2):356–60.
28. Irwin FD, Bonagura AF, Crawford SW, Foote M. Kidney paired donation: a payer perspective. Am J Transplant. 2012;12(6):1388–91.
29. Rees MA, Schnitzler MA, Zavala EY, Cutler JA, Roth AE, Irwin FD, et al. Call to develop a standard acquisition charge model for kidney paired donation. Am J Transplant. 2012;12(6):1392–7.
30. Giessing M, Deger S, Roigas J, Schnorr D, Fuller F, Liefeldt L, et al. Cross-over kidney transplantation with simultaneous laparoscopic living donor nephrectomy: initial experience. Eur Urol. 2008;53(5):1074–8.
31. Ferrari P, de klerk M. Paired kidney donations to expand the living donor pool. J Nephrol. 2009;22(6):699–707.
32. Kim BS, Kim YS, Kim SI, Kim MS, Lee HY, Kim YL, et al. Outcome of multipair donor kidney exchange by a web-based algorithm. J Am Soc Nephrol. 2007;18(3):1000–6.
33. Segev DL, et al. Case report: a trans-national kidney paired donation. 2013 [in press]
34. Massie AB, Gentry SE, Montgomery RA, Bingaman AA, Segev DL. Center-level utilization of kidney paired donation. Am J Transplant. 2013;13(5):1317–22.

Chapter 3
Living Donor Liver Transplantation

Vikraman Gunabushanam, Abhideep Chaudhary and Abhinav Humar

Introduction

The shortage of organs for transplant is the major limiting factor in liver transplantation. Nearly 17,000 people are actively listed for a liver transplant in the U.S. The number of deceased donor liver transplants (DDLTs) performed each year is around 6,000. This has not significantly changed since 2004. The mortality on the waiting list is around 10–15 % [1]. Living donor liver transplant (LDLT) provides potential recipients the benefit of reduced wait-list times and survival. The advantages of LDLTs are even more evident in parts of the world where deceased donation is nonexistent.

The concept of LDLT emerged from experience gained from the use of reduced-size and split grafts in DDLT. The first reported LDLT from adult to child was performed in Brazil (by Raia in 1988), while the first successful adult-to-child LDLT was performed in Australia (by Strong in 1989) [2, 3]. The positive outcomes of LDLT led to its application in adults, mostly by utilization of the right lobe from the donor. The first right lobe liver donation was performed in a child in Japan, due to anatomical reasons, while the first successful adult-to-adult right lobe transplant was performed in Hong Kong in 1996 [4, 5]. Wachs et al. performed the first successful adult right lobe LDLT in the U.S. in 1998 [6]. LDLT has been widely accepted and adopted in Asia and the rest of the world. Around 4 % of all liver transplants

---

A. Humar (✉)
Department of Surgery, University of Pittsburgh, Room 725, 3459 Fifth Ave.,
Pittsburgh, PA 15213, USA
e-mail: humara2@upmc.edu

V. Gunabushanam
Department of Transplant Surgery, University of Pittsburgh Medical Center,
3459 Fifth Ave, UPMC Montefiore 7S, Pittsburgh, PA 15206, USA
e-mail: gunabushanamv@upmc.edu

A. Chaudhary
Department of Surgical Gastroenterology and Liver Transplantation,
Sir Ganga Ram Hospital, Rajinder Nagar, New Delhi 110060, India
e-mail: drabhideep@yahoo.com

Table 3.1 Stages in living donor evaluation

Phase I
Phone interview with transplant coordinator

Phase II
Evaluation by hepatologist, social worker, medical psychologist, and coordinator
Complete medical history and physical examination
Laboratory tests

Phase III
Surgical evaluation of donor
Preoperative anesthesia evaluation
CT/MRI to assess vascular/biliary anatomy
Other tests: based on results of initial testing
Presentation at liver transplant-selection conference

Phase IV
Final meeting with surgeon
Informed consent

performed in the U.S. are LDLTs [1]. The proportion is significantly higher in the rest of the world. With improved donor safety and recipient results, this modality has continued to emerge as a possible alternative or additional option to DDLT.

Donor Evaluation

The evaluation of a potential donor is a very critical part of the LDLT process. The evaluation process can vary depending on the intended recipient (adult or pediatric), planned liver resection (right, left, or left lateral), and transplant center preference; one possible evaluation process is shown in Table 3.1 [7]. Key to evaluation is the involvement of a multidisciplinary team including a hepatologist, surgeon, psychologist, social worker, and transplant coordinator. The entire evaluation process should be thorough yet efficient. Invasive and expensive tests are reserved for the latter part of the evaluation process.

The basic components of the evaluation process include

- medical,
- surgical, including radiologic, and
- psychological and social.

Medical Evaluation

The purpose of performing a medical evaluation is twofold. The first is identifying an underlying medical disorder that would jeopardize the potential donor's health; the second is to determine the suitability of the liver for transplantation, including screening for chronic liver disease and viral pathogens [8]. The initial part of this evaluation is similar to that of any patient undergoing a major abdominal surgery.

The initial screening of this evaluation can be performed by an experienced transplant coordinator, and often a phone interview is adequate. A general questionnaire includes obtaining information on age, height, weight, blood type, and a medical, surgical, and psychosocial history (including a history of alcohol and substance abuse). Potential donors with obesity and significant comorbidities can often be excluded at this stage. Age is an important screening variable at the initial encounter and potential donors falling outside the center's accepted age criteria are excluded. The lower limit of age for donation is determined by the ability to give legal consent. The upper age limit for donation can vary from center to center but generally is between 55 and 60 years. Screening blood work can be performed at a center that is closest to the potential donor. Based on the results of the screening history and blood work, a potential donor is then brought to the transplant center for a complete evaluation.

The next phase of the evaluation begins with a complete history and physical examination by a physician. Individuals with significant underlying cardiac, respiratory, or renal problems are excluded from donation. Individuals with underlying risk factors for these specific organ systems (e.g., age >40 and family history of cardiac disease) may require specialist consultation and tests. A more thorough and complete set of blood tests are now obtained assessing organ functions, potential risk factors (including risk of clotting), and potential for viral transmissions (Table 3.2). Special considerations include the following:

- Donor obesity: Obese individuals are at an increased risk of surgical complications including bleeding, wound infection, and cardiopulmonary problems. The incidence of hepatic steatosis is greater in obese individuals. One study suggested that 78% of potential donors with a body mass index (BMI) greater than 28 kg/m^2 had over 10% steatosis on liver biopsy [9]. However, not all studies have shown this degree of correlation. A BMI greater than 35 would exclude living liver donation for most centers. While many centers exclude donors with BMI >30, a few selectively evaluate these donors and perform a liver biopsy to exclude hepatic steatosis [10].
- Hepatitis B Core Antibody (HBcAb) positive donors: The concerns of using HBcAb positive donors are twofold—risk to the donor and risk of transmission to the seronegative recipient [11]. The proportion of donors who are HbcAb positive is variable. In Asia, over half of evaluated donors test positive, and results from these areas have shown that the risk to seropositive donors is not different from HbcAb-negative donors. A liver biopsy is performed in HbcAb-positive donors to exclude hepatic inflammation and fibrosis. The concerns for the recipient are similar to that of a deceased donor who is HbcAb positive. The risk to a seronegative recipient can be nearly eliminated by the use of appropriate hepatitis B virus (HBV) prophylaxis.
- Evaluation for thrombophilia: Deep venous thrombosis with subsequent pulmonary embolism is a serious postoperative complication that can be potentially life threatening. Several cases of pulmonary embolism have been reported with at least one or two cases of mortality due to this complication. Known risk factors

Table 3.2 Blood tests obtained from the potential donor

Initial screen
Complete blood count
Serum electrolytes
Renal function tests
Liver function tests
Lipid profile
Blood type
Viral serologic evaluation
Hepatitis C
Hepatitis B
CMV
EBV
HIV
Screening for thrombophilia disorders
Protein C/S
Antithrombin III
Factor V Leiden mutation
Prothrombin gene mutation
Tests to exclude underlying chronic liver disease
Serum transferrin saturation
Ferritin
α-1 Antitrypsin
Other tests
EKG
Chest X-ray

CMV cytomegalovirus, *EBV* Epstein-Barr virus, *HIV* human immunodeficieny virus, *EKG* electocardiogram

for thromboembolic complications include obesity, use of oral hormone therapy, older age, smoking, positive family history, and an identified underlying procoagulation disorder. These risk factors should be addressed during the evaluation process, including screening tests to identify a procoagulation disorder. Tests should include testing Factor V Leiden and prothrombin gene mutations.

Surgical and Radiological Evaluation

This component of the evaluation determines the surgical suitability of the potential donor and specifically whether the anatomy and size of the donor liver is suitable for donation.

Anatomy

Evaluation of the vascular anatomy includes imaging of the hepatic artery, portal vein, and hepatic veins (Fig. 3.1). Most transplant centers routinely use computed tomography (CT) or magnetic resonance imaging (MRI) with 3-D reconstructions as a single test [12, 13]. While some vascular variations may preclude donation,

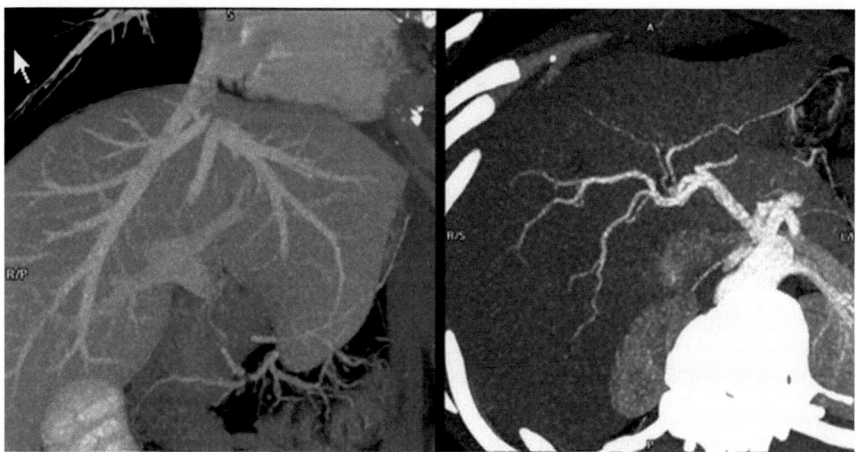

Fig. 3.1 Vascular anatomy, including the hepatic veins, portal vein, and hepatic artery, can be determined with a single noninvasive test such as a CT scan with contrast

most can be handled with vascular reconstruction techniques. However, knowledge of these variations is important for operative planning and dissection. Possible vascular variations include a replaced or accessory left hepatic artery (LHA) or right hepatic artery (RHA), trifurcation of the main portal vein, and accessory hepatic veins. Depending on the planned liver resection, these anatomical variations may either have no impact or significantly complicate surgery.

Some centers routinely obtain magnetic resonance cholangiopancreatogram (MRCP) or endoscopic retrograde cholangiopancreatogram (ERCP) as part of the evaluation to look at biliary anatomy. A CT cholangiogram may also be performed. These tests do not always provide the detail required, as a result of which many centers routinely perform an intraoperative cholangiogram.

Liver Volume

An accurate assessment of liver volumes is necessary to determine if the size of the transplanted liver graft is of adequate size for the recipient and if the size of the remnant liver is sufficient in the donor to prevent acute liver failure. A CT or MRI provides a reasonable estimate of the liver volume (Fig. 3.2). Most living donor transplants in adults are performed using the right lobe. Most centers prefer a graft weight to recipient weight (GW/RW) ratio greater than 0.8, or an estimate of graft weight as a percentage of standard liver mass exceeding 40%. Smaller grafts may be associated with small-for-size syndrome and have worse outcomes.

The important concern in a pediatric recipient is not usually if the liver volume is too small, but rather too large. A large graft (GW/RW ratio >5%) can cause difficulty in abdominal closure in the recipient. With regard to residual volume in the donor, an important part of the evaluation process is to ensure that the donor is not

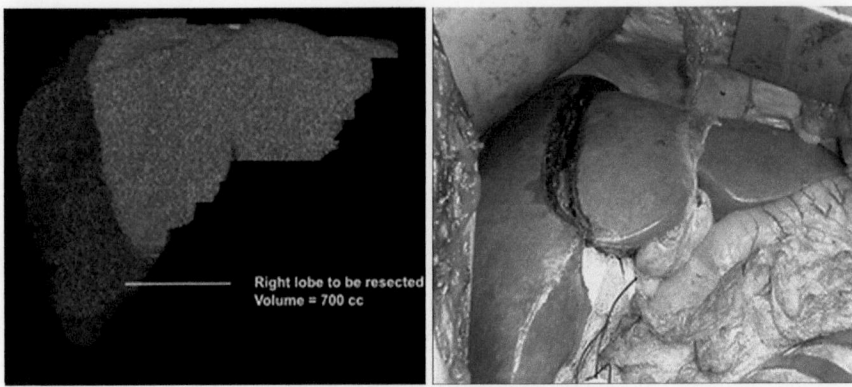

Fig. 3.2 Determination of the volume of liver to be resected is an important component of the preoperative surgical evaluation and usually correlates well with intraoperative findings

left with too small a liver volume. The donor should be left with at least 30% of the measured total liver volume. The left lateral segment is most commonly used in pediatric recipients, and the adequacy of remnant liver size in the donor is not a concern. However, when a larger portion of the liver is removed (such as the right lobe), liver failure has been reported postdonation. There have been at least three reported cases of living donors in the U.S. requiring an urgent liver transplant for liver failure after donation [14].

Liver Parenchyma

Some centers routinely biopsy all potential donors, while others biopsy only on a selective basis [15, 16]. The benefits of obtaining a liver biopsy are to assess for steatosis, and exclude chronic liver disease. Steatosis is more common in donors with a history of alcohol use, elevated triglyceride levels, higher BMI, or abnormal appearance on CT imaging. Some centers use these criteria to selectively biopsy the donors. Liver biopsy, with its risk for bleeding, remains an invasive test. Additional studies are needed to better define the role for liver biopsy. The presence of fibrosis, inflammatory changes, nonalcoholic steatohepatitis (NASH), and steatosis > 10–20 % (for right lobe liver donors) precludes donation. Steatosis identified on a predonation biopsy can be reversed with a program of dieting and exercise.

Psychological and Social Evaluation

This component of the evaluations assesses the potential donor's willingness and competence to donate. It also ensures that the decision to donate is voluntary and free from coercion or inducement. It assesses the donor's coping strategies and support structures. The formal part of this evaluation is multidisciplinary and is performed by a psychiatrist, psychologist or other mental health care professional, and a social worker [17, 18]. There are several components to this part of the evaluation, which can be broadly divided into:

- Mental health assessment: This includes obtaining a history of psychiatric disorders, substance abuse (if any), and assessment of competence to make the decision to donate.
- Psychosocial history and assessment: This includes evaluation of life stressors, coping strategies, support structures, stability of living arrangements, finances, and work/school issues.
- Motivation: The potential donor's reasons for donation are determined, including an assessment to ensure that there is no coercion or inducement.
- Knowledge of the process: An assessment of the understanding and knowledge of the donation process, surgery, complications, and recovery is carried out.

Operative Procedure

A left lateral segment of the donor's liver is removed for a pediatric recipient, and a left lobe for a larger or older child. Just about every portion of the liver has been used for an adult recipient including the left lobe (with or without the caudate lobe), right lobe, and extended right lobe; even dual left lobe grafts from separate donors have been used [19]. Donor safety is the most important consideration in deciding which portion is the best. In the U.S., most centers use the right lobe for adult-to-adult LDLT. The use of the left lobe had initially fallen into disfavor due to a higher incidence of small-for-size syndrome. More recently, there has been an increasing interest in using the left lobe, as studies suggest that the donor complication rate associated with left lobe donation is generally lower compared to right lobe donation.

Two factors are important in deciding whether a graft is of sufficient size: (1) severity of recipient disease and (2) size of donor graft relative to recipient size [20–22]. Graft size is expressed as the ratio of graft weight to recipient weight (GW/RW: $\geq 0.8\%$) or as the percentage of the calculated ideal liver weight of the recipient (CILW $\geq 40\%$). Recipients with compensated cirrhosis and recipients without cirrhosis can possibly tolerate a smaller graft size.

Left Lateral Segmentectomy

The abdomen is opened through a subcostal or midline incision. The falciform and left triangular ligaments are divided till the anterior aspect of the left hepatic vein (LHV) is visualised. The gastrohepatic ligament is divided from the hilum posteriorly to the LHV superiorly.

The LHV is then encircled with an umbilical tape. The left hepatic artery (LHA) is identified at the ligamentum teres and traced distally to where it enters the liver, and proximally to the segment IV branch. The left portal vein (LPV) is mobilized along its extrahepatic course. The branches of the portal vein supplying segment IV are identified and divided. The umbilical tape previously passed around the LHV is brought in the ligamentum groove, and anteriorly to the LHA and LPV. The 'hanging maneuver' is used by pulling on the ends of the umbilical tape to guide the plane of transection. The parenchyma of the liver is then transected to the right of the falciform ligament. The biliary drainage from segments II and III are sharply divided at the base of the lateral segment.

Left Lobectomy

The left caudate lobe is dissected from the inferior vena cava (IVC) ligating minor hepatic veins. A large caudate hepatic vein, if encountered, may be preserved for implantation. Cholecystectomy and a transcystic cholangiogram are performed to identify biliary anatomy. The LHA is dissected proximally, preserving segment IV artery, and the LPV is identified medial and posterior to the LHA and dissected circumferentially. The umbilical tape is then passed behind the caudate lobe between the right hepatic vein (RHV) and middle hepatic vein (MHV), to facilitate parenchymal transection. An intraoperative ultrasound (IUS) is performed to delineate the course of the MHV. The parenchyma of the liver is then transected just to the right of MHV. The left hepatic duct (LHD) is sharply transected. Careful inspection is made for any caudate hepatic ducts.

When the recipient team is ready, the graft is removed by dividing the vascular structures. Clamps are placed proximally on the LPV and LHA. A stapling device is used to transect the hepatic veins. The graft is flushed and given to the recipient team. The cut surface of the donor is carefully inspected for any evidence of bleeding or bile leak, and the abdomen is closed in layers. We prefer to leave a drain, while many centers do not.

Right Lobectomy

The falciform ligament is divided posteriorly to the RHV. The right lobe of the liver is mobilized by dividing the right triangular ligament and exposing the bare area Small Short hepatic veins are divided while branches larger than 5 mm are preserved for implantation in the recipient. The RHV is encircled using an umbilical tape. Cholecystectomy and transcystic cholangiogram are performed. The junction of the right hepatic duct and LHD is defined. The RHA is identified where it enters the liver and is then traced proximally to the bile duct. The right portal vein (RPV) is then identified. The junction with the LPV is clearly defined so as not to compromise the latter when the RPV is eventually divided. The RHA and the RPV are retracted inferiorly and the right hepatic duct is identified. IUS is performed to identify the course of the MHV and its tributaries from segments V and VIII. We prefer to perform the parenchymal transection just to the right of the MHV, preserving the MHV in the donor. The technique of performing the parenchymal transection to the left of the MHV has also been described.

The central venous pressure in the donor is kept low, so as to minimize bleeding. Larger tributaries (>4 mm) of the MHV are preserved for reimplantation in the recipient. When the recipient team is ready, the vascular and biliary structures of the right graft are divided. The RHV is divided using a laparoscopic stapler. The right lobe is flushed and given to the recipient team. The cut surface of the left lobe is carefully inspected for any evidence of bile leak or bleeding. The falciform ligament is reattached to prevent torsion of the remnant left lobe.

Outcomes

In an uncomplicated postoperative course, most donors are in hospital for an average of 4–7 days. Liver enzymes peak between 48 and 72 hours after surgery. The synthetic function of the liver returns to normal by 1 week. The remnant liver reaches 80–90% of its volume by 3 months [23]. Most donors are able to return to employment by 6–12 weeks postdonation. Complications after surgery can alter the recovery course and time.

Donor Mortality

The greatest concern with LDLT—in fact, with any living donor procedure—is the risk of death to the donor. Unfortunately, there is some risk of mortality associated with any surgical procedure, but the magnitude of risk associated with this procedure has been difficult to determine. In the U.S., there have been five deaths that were early in the postoperative period and directly related to the surgery. Of these, four were in right lobe donors and one was after left lateral hepatectomy [14]. There have been additional deaths, but these have been late and likely not related to the donation surgery. The number of deaths worldwide, however, is more difficult to know, as there is no mandatory reporting. Most centers will quote a 0.5% risk of mortality associated with this procedure, though the quoted rate may vary from 0.1 to 1.0% at different centers [24]. Based on the deaths described in the world literature, the overall mortality rate is of the order of 0.2–0.5%. The estimated mortality for donation for pediatric recipient is lower compared to donation for adult recipient, likely a result of the magnitude of liver resection involved for the donor. Similarly, the risk associated with left lobe donation may be lower than that of right lobe donation.

Donor Morbidity

The reported incidence of complications in the donor varies in the literature from 9 to 67%, but likely is in the 30% range [25–30]. A number of different complications have been reported in donors. The vast majority of these complications tend to occur in the early postoperative period (usually within 1 month postdonation). The modified Clavien classification is commonly used to describe, report, and compare donor morbidity:

- Grade I—a complication that is not life threatening, does not result in residual disability, and does not require a therapeutic invasive intervention.
- Grade II—a complication that is potentially life threatening, that requires the use of drug therapy or foreign blood units.
- Grade III—a complication that is potentially life threatening that requires a therapeutic invasive intervention.
- Grade IV—a complication with residual or lasting disability or that leads to death [31].

The Adult Living Donor Liver Transplantation Cohort Study (A2ALL), funded by the National Institutes of Health with nine liver transplant centers, reported a donor complication rate of 38%, of which 21% donors had one complication and 17% had two or more [30]. Complications were graded using the modified Clavien system described earlier: 27% had grade I (minor), 26% had grade II (potentially life threatening), 2% had grade III (life threatening), and 0.8% had grade IV (leading to death) complications. Common complications included biliary leaks beyond postoperative day 7 (9%), bacterial infections (12%), incisional hernia (6%), pleural effusion requiring intervention (5%), neuropraxia (4%), re-exploration (3%), wound infections (3%), and intra-abdominal abscess (2%). Two donors developed portal vein thrombosis, and one had inferior vena caval thrombosis. As much as 13% of donors required hospital readmission, and 4% required two to five readmissions.

Biliary problems are the most common major complication after donor surgery [32]. Bile leaks and strictures have been reported in roughly 15% and 5% of the donors, respectively. Bile may leak from the cut surface of the liver or from the site where the bile duct is divided. This site may later become strictured. Generally, bile leaks resolve spontaneously with simple drainage. Strictures and sometimes bile leaks may require an endoscopic procedure and stenting. If the above measures fail, a reoperation may be required. Intra-abdominal infections developing in donors are usually related to a biliary problem. Hemorrhage is another major complication which can be intraoperative or postoperative. Intraoperative blood loss is usually in the range of 250–750 cc for uncomplicated cases and depends on transection surface, anatomy of vessels, and, most importantly, experience and skill of the surgeon. Blood loss can be reduced by keeping the central venous pressure low. The risk of postoperative blood loss requiring nonautologous blood and need for reoperation is usually less than 5% [25, 26].

Pulmonary complications like aseptic basal atelectasis, right pleural effusion, or pneumonia are also a significant source of morbidity, though the incidence is the same as any other major upper abdominal surgery. Other complications after donor surgery may include incisional problems such as pain, wound infections and hernias, urinary infections, and ileus. The risk of deep venous thrombosis and pulmonary embolism is the same as for other major abdominal procedures. Overall, the risk of complications for right lobe donors is felt to be significantly higher compared to that for left lateral segment or left lobe donors.

Conclusion

In summary, LDLT is an acceptable option for select recipients. While there is no obvious benefit for donors, there are advantages for recipients of living donor transplants. In countries without DDLT, the survival benefits associated with LDLT are obvious. Even in areas with DDLT, the potential risk of mortality associated with waiting for a deceased donor is avoided. Additionally, patients can be transplanted before they develop far advanced liver disease associated with marked overall decompensation. While the advantages of live donor transplants for potential recipients are obvious, this must be carefully balanced against the risk of mortality and morbidity for the donor. Short- and long-term results in the donor must be carefully tracked and the technique refined to try to minimize this risk as much as possible.

References

1. Health Resources and Service Administration. Organ Procurement and Transplantation Network. http://www.optn.org.
2. Raia S, Nery JR, Mies S, et al. Liver transplantation from live donors. Lancet. 1989;2:497.
3. Strong RW, Lynch SV, Ong TH, Matsunami H, Koido Y, Balderson GA, et al. Successful liver transplantation from a living donor to her son. N Engl J Med. 1990;322:1505–7.
4. Hashikura Y, Makuuchi M, Kawasaki S, Matsunami H, Ikegami T, Nakazawa Y, et al. Successful living-related partial liver transplantation to an adult patient. Lancet. 1994;343:1233–4.
5. Lo CM, Fan ST, Liu CL, Lo RJ, Lau GK, Wei WI, et al. Extending the limit on the size of adult recipient in living donor liver transplantation using extended right lobe graft. Transplantation. 1997;63:1524–8.
6. Wachs ME, Bak TE, Karrer FM, Everson GT, Shrestha R, Trouillot TE, et al. Adult living donor liver transplantation using a right hepatic lobe. Transplantation. 1998;66:1313–6.
7. Tuttle-Newhall JE, Collins BH, Desai DM, Kuo PC, Heneghan ME, et al. The current status of living donor liver transplantation. Curr Prob Surg. 2005;42:144–83.
8. Rudow DL, Brown RS. Jr. Evaluation of living liver donors. Prog Transplant. 2003;13:110–6.
9. Rinella ME, Alonso E, Rao S, Whitington P, Fryer J, Abecassis M, et al. Body mass index as a predictor of hepatic steatosis in living liver donors. Liver Transpl. 2001;7:409–14.
10. Trotter JF. Selection of donors and recipients for living donor liver transplantation. Liver Transpl. 2000;6:S52–8.

11. Chen YS, Cheng YF, De Villa VH, Wang CC, Lin CC, Huang TL, et al. Evaluation of living liver donors. Transplantation. 2003;75:S16–9.
12. Alonso-Torres A, Fernandez-Cuadrado J, Pinilla I, Parron M, Vicente E de, Lopez-Santamaria M, et al. Multidetector CT in the evaluation of potential living donors for liver transplantation. Radiographics. 2005;25:1017–30.
13. Valentin-Gamazo C, Malago M, Karliova M, Lutz JT, Frilling A, Nadalin S, et al. Experience after the evaluation of 700 potential donors for living donor liver transplantation in a single center. Liver Transpl. 2004;10:1087–96.
14. Muzaale AD, Dagher NN, Montgomery RA, Taranto SE, Mcbride MA, Segev DL, et al. Estimates of early death, acute liver failure, and long-term mortality among live liver donors. Gastroenterology. 2012;142:273–80.
15. Nadalin S, Malago M, Valentin-Gamazo C, Testa G, Baba HA, Liu C, et al. Preoperative donor liver biopsy for adult living donor liver transplantation: risks and benefits. Liver Transpl. 2005;11:980–6.
16. Nakamuta M, Morizono S, Soejima Y, Yoshizumi T, Aishima S, Takasugi S, et al. Short-term intensive treatment for donors with hepatic steatosis in living-donor liver transplantation. Transplantation. 2005;80:608–12.
17. Jacobs C, Johnson E, Anderson K, Gillingham K, Matas A, et al. Kidney transplants from living donors: how donation affects family dynamics. Adv Ren Replace Ther. 1998;5:89–97.
18. Schover LR, Streem SB, Boparai N, Duriak K, Novick AC. The psychosocial impact of donating a kidney: long-term follow-up from a urology based center. J Urol. 1997;157:1596–601.
19. Lee SG, Park KM, Hwang S, Lee YJ, Kim KH, Ahn CS, et al. Adult-to-adult living donor liver transplantation at the Asan Medical Center, Korea. Asian J Surg. 2002;25:277–84.
20. Ben-Haim M, Emre S, Fishbein T, Sheiner P, Bodian C, Kim-Schluger L, et al. Critical graft size in adult-to-adult living donor liver transplantation: impact of the recipient's disease. Liver Transpl. 2001;7:948–53.
21. Taketomi A, Kayashima H, Soejima Y, Yoshizumi T, Uchiyama H, Ikegami T et al. Donor risk in adult-to-adult living donor liver transplantation: impact of left lobe graft. Transplantation. 2009;87:445–50.
22. Kanoh K, Nomoto K, Shimura T, Shimada M, Sugimachi K, Kuwano H, et al. A comparison of right-lobe and left-lobe graft for living-donor liver transplantation. Hepatogastroenterology. 2002;49:222–4.
23. Humar A, Kosari K, Sielaff TD, Glessing B, Gomes M, Dietz C, et al. Liver regeneration after adult living donor and deceased donor split-liver transplants. Liver Transpl. 2004;10:374–8.
24. Middleton PF, Duffield M, Lynch SV, Padbury RT, House T, Stanton P, et al. Living donor liver transplantation—adult donor outcomes: a systematic review. Liver Transpl. 2006;12:24–30.
25. Trotter JF, Adam R, Lo CM, Kenison J, et al. Documented deaths of hepatic lobe donors for living donor liver transplantation. Liver Transpl. 2006;12:1485–8.
26. Salvalaggio PR, Baker TB, Koffron AJ, Fryer JP, Clark L, Superina RA, et al. Comparative analysis of live liver donation risk using a comprehensive grading system for severity. Transplantation. 2004;77:1765–7.
27. Brown RS Jr, Russo MW, Lai M, Shiffman ML, Richardson MC, Everhart JE, et al. A survey of liver transplantation from living adult donors in the United States. N Engl J Med. 2003;348:818–25.
28. Lo CM. Complications and long-term outcome of living liver donors: a survey of 1508 cases in five Asian Centers. Transplantation. 2003;75:S12–5.
29. Broering DC, Wilms C, Bok P, Fischer L, Mueller L, Hillert C, et al. Evolution of donor morbidity in living related liver transplantation: a single-center analysis of 165 cases. Ann Surg. 2004;240:1013–26.
30. Ghobrial RM, Freise CE, Trotter JF, Tong L, Ojo AO, Fair JH, et al. A2ALL Study Group. Donor morbidity after living donation for liver transplantation. Gastroenterology. 2008;135:468–76.
31. Dindo D, Demartines N, Clavien PA, et al. Classification of surgical complications: a new proposal with evaluation in a cohort of 6336 patients and results of a survey. Ann Surg. 2004;240:205–13.
32. Yuan Y, Gotoh M. Biliary complications in living liver donors. Surg Today. 2010;40:411–7.

Chapter 4
Intestinal Transplantation from Living Donors

Massimiliano Tuveri, Salvatore Pisu and Luca Cicalese

Introduction

Intestinal transplantation (ITx) represents the physiologic alternative to total parenteral nutrition (TPN) for patients suffering from life-threatening complications of irreversible intestinal failure. The number of transplants performed worldwide has been increasing for several years until recently (Fig. 4.1) [1]. ITx has recently become a valid therapeutic option with a graft survival rate between 80% and 90% at 1 year, in experienced centers [1]. These results have been achieved due to a combination of several factors: better understanding of the pathophysiology of intestinal graft, improved immunosuppression techniques, more efficient strategies for the monitoring of the bowel graft, as well as control of infectious complications and posttransplant lymphoproliferative disease (PTLD). In fact, this procedure is associated with a relatively high rate of complications, such as infections, acute rejection, graft versus host disease (GVHD), and PTLD, if compared to the transplantation of other organs [2–5]. These complications may be, at least in part, the consequence of the peculiarity of this graft, which contains gut-associated lymphoid tissue and potentially pathogenic enteric flora. Furthermore, in these patients, the existing disease and the relative malnutrition could predispose them to infectious complications. Additionally, other factors associated with the procedure, such as laparotomy, preservation injury, abnormal motility, and lymphatic disruption, could all be implicated in the development of complications.

M. Tuveri (✉) · L. Cicalese
Department of General Surgery-Transplant, University of Texas Medical Branch, Galveston, TX 77555–0533, USA
e-mail: matuveri@UTMB.EDU

L. Cicalese
e-mail: lucicale@utmb.edu

S. Pisu
Department of Bioethics, University of Cagliari, SS554 Sestu, Cagliari 09028, Italy
e-mail: Salvatore.pisu@libero.it

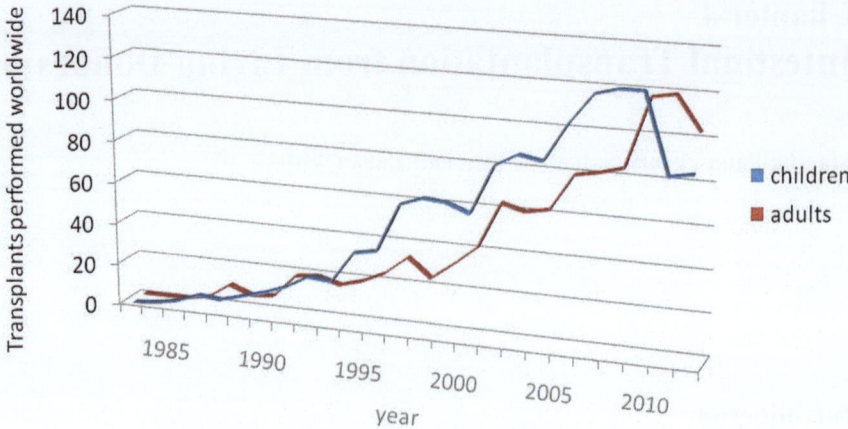

Fig. 4.1 Intestine transplant performed worldwide since 1985

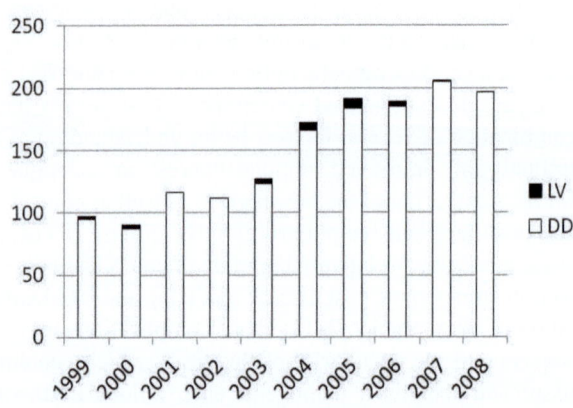

Fig. 4.2 Growth of living donor and deceased donor intestinal transplantation worldwide by era. *LV* living donors, *DD* deceased donors

Data from the Scientific Registry of Transplant Recipients (SRTR) show that most of the intestinal transplants have been performed in the U.S. using intestinal graft obtained from cadaver donors (Fig. 4.2) [6]. Differently to what occurred in liver and kidney transplantation, the use of living donors for ITx has been limited mostly because deceased intestinal donors are available. However, optimal deceased intestinal donors are not common either. In fact, despite the fact that the number of patients waiting for ITx is limited, the time spent on the waiting list increased compared to previous years for all candidates on the waiting list. In 2011, 41.7 % of patients listed waited less than 1 year for ITx, while 25.1 % waited between 1 and 2 years, and 33.2 % waited for more than 2 years [6]. Despite the fact that mortality on the waiting list has decreased in the U.S. in recent years compared to the past, it is still reported to be up to 20 % per year on the waiting list [6, 7]. All this suggests that despite the fact that many cadaver donors are available, they are often not utilized because they are not adequate to satisfy the need of patients waiting for ITx.

Table 4.1 Potential advantages and disadvantages using intestinal grafts from living compared to deceased donors

Advantages
Eliminates waiting time in cadaver donor list
Can be used in countries where TPN and deceased donors are not available
Use of hemodynamically stable donors
Elective case, allows better donor bowel preparation and optimization of recipient clinical condition
Short cold ischemia time
Optimal donor–recipient HLA matching
Small graft can be accommodated in retracted abdominal cavity
Disadvantages
Risk for the donor
Short graft and smaller vascular pedicle

HLA human leukocyte antigen, *TPN* total parenteral nutrition

Intestinal Transplant Registry data show that patient and graft survival rates after living donor ITx (LD-ITx) are similar to those obtained with cadaver organs [1, 7–10]. However, it is important considering that most of the LD-ITx surgeries were performed in low-volume centers (often as isolated cases in low-experience centers), while the best results obtained with ITx from cadaver donors are obtained in high-volume centers, suggesting that increasing the use of LD-ITx could further improve outcome. In fact, the use of intestinal grafts from living donors, when compared to cadaver donors, offers important advantages with low risks, and these are summarized in Table 4.1.

As mentioned above, LD-ITx virtually eliminates waiting time and could further decrease morbidity and mortality on the waiting list compared to the activity seen on the deceased donor list. LD-ITx also would allow transplantation in developing countries where TPN and deceased donor are not easily available. Furthermore, because LD-ITx is an elective procedure, it can be performed when the donor and the recipient conditions are optimal, and the donor bowel preparation can be easily performed, leading to a decreased risk of infectious complications. In an analysis of 50 pediatric ITx recipients, it has been shown that the length of graft preservation was the most significant factor in inducing bacterial translocation [11, 12]. This phenomenon can contribute to the high rate of infections seen during the early posttransplant period also considering that this coincides with the timing of maximum amount of immunosuppression given to the patient.

The Achilles' heel of bowel transplantation remains its extreme sensitivity to preservation injury. Deceased donors are often subject to either cardiac arrest or resuscitation, to prolonged periods of hypotension, or use of vasopressors. All these could result in splanchnic hypoperfusion, which can trigger ischemia/reperfusion injury even before the intestine is procured from the donor. Cold preservation of the graft can be also extended due to the distance between procurement and transplant centers. This can further increase such injury considering that specific preservation solutions designed for intestinal grafts are not yet available. The use of living donors can obviate these problems, since the donor is a healthy individual, hemodynamically stable, and with consequent normal intestinal perfusion. Furthermore, the short cold ischemic time prior to revascularization also improves graft quality, virtually eliminating ischemia/reperfusion injury, and may reduce the rate of posttransplant infections [12].

Another not negligible benefit of LD-ITx is immunologic [8, 9]. A living donor is often a relative of the recipient due to the strong emotional involvement that justifies the donation. Living related donors have a closer distribution of human leukocyte antigens (HLAs) with the recipient that could contribute to an immunologic advantage. This is supported by the experience of HLA-matched transplants performed between homozygote twins [13]. This point might be challenged since in recent times, a significant decreased rate of rejection has been also observed using HLA-unmatched deceased donors [1, 14]. However, this improvement has been accomplished using more potent immunosuppression and induction therapy with polyclonal antibodies. However, a similarly low rate of rejection is seen using living related HLA-matched donors using a less potent immunosuppressive regimen [8, 9, 15]. An additional benefit can be offered performing LD-ITx at an earlier stage of the disease, since long-term TPN and indwelling venous catheters can be associated with priming of the immune system, as recently suggested [16–18].

Naturally, potential disadvantages are also associated with the use of living donors. The main disadvantage remains the risk for the donor, which includes early surgical complications of bowel resection as well as potential long-term impairment of intestinal absorption. The procedure-specific risks for the live intestinal donor are given in Table 4.2. Specific data on living intestinal donors are limited at this time, and no serious complications have been reported. The potential risk can be hypothetically calculated, using a parallelism with general surgery-related data of small bowel resection; about 3–5% of the donors could develop a small bowel obstruction [19–24]. In large series, the mortality rate for patients with small bowel obstruction is approximately 2% for the lifetime of the patient [25]. A brief and self-limited period of diarrhea has been reported after intestinal donation for LD-ITx [15]. Although weight loss and dysvitaminosis are not reported, they represent potential risks of this procedure.

Another disadvantage is associated with the increased risk of vascular thrombosis, related to the smaller vascular pedicle used compared to grafts obtained from cadaver donors. Nevertheless, these risks can be reduced with a careful and appropriate surgical technique [26, 27].

Donor Selection and Evaluation

General Considerations

The potential donor should be an individual in good health with no history of previous intestinal or abdominal surgery, and with no underlying chronic medical illnesses that would increase the surgical operative risk.

Table 4.2 Potential procedure-specific risk for the live intestinal donor	Short bowel syndrome
	Small bowel obstruction
	3–8%
	3% mortality
	Dysvitaminosis
	Weight loss
	Diarrhea

Once a potential donor is identified, the initial step should consist of a meeting with the surgeon to describe the procedure, as well as risks and benefits and the steps involved in the workup. During this initial visit, the potential donor can be screened with an ABO blood type determination. If this is compatible and the candidate is willing to continue the workup, an HLA test and histocompatibility testing by T-cell crossmatch should be performed. Crossmatch should be negative, and among multiple donor candidates, the one with the best HLA match should be preferred and should be directed to continue the workup. The cornerstone of success is the identical or compatible HLA. For this reason, it is preferred that living donors be relatives of the recipients. The donor can also be unrelated to the recipient but should have a compatible HLA and close emotional relationship. This condition and the absence of any financial interest or coercion for donation are of paramount importance in LD-ITx, just like any other type of live organ donation. The screening process should exclude active or uncontrolled psychiatric disorders, and ensure the altruistic nature of the donation. The institution's ethical committee should separately evaluate the donor to ensure that there is full understanding of the limited information regarding the short- and long-term risks associated with intestinal donation.

Full Evaluation

Once the potential donor has completed these initial steps, a series of tests are mandatory for the live donor evaluation (Table 4.3). Based on the available clinical experience with LD-ITx, a limit of 60 years of age is advisable. The minimal age is only determined by legal ability to consent to the procedure. High body mass index (>30) may not affect graft quality and does not constitute, per se, an absolute contraindication to live donation, though general surgical experience indicates that a high body mass index (>30 kg/m^2) may increase the risk of surgical complications after intestinal resection.

A comprehensive metabolic panel should be obtained. Blood test results that confirm donor infection with HIV, HCV, or HBV are contraindications for living intestine donation.

Specific considerations must be used for genetically related donors of potential recipients who have a genetic or familial intestinal disease. Despite the fact that no data are available at this time, it is possible that the related donor might develop the same condition later in life. At the present time, it is advisable not to consider these donors and eventually to screen them to rule out the same genetic disorder.

Table 4.3 Donor and recipient preoperative workup

Workup	Donor	Recipient
Laboratory tests	Blood group system (ABO) and HLA CBC with differential Coagulation panel (PT/INR, PTT) Liver chemistries, amylase, lipase Renal chemistries and electrolytes Basic metabolic panel Urinalysis and culture Stool culture Vitamin A, D, E, K, and B_{12} Ammonia, alpha fetoprotein, lipid profile	Blood group system (ABO) and HLA CBC with differential Coagulation panel (PT/INR, PTT) Liver chemistries, amylase, lipase Renal chemistries and electrolytes Basic metabolic panel Urinalysis and culture Stool culture Vitamin A, D, l, K, and B_{12} Ammonia, alpha fetoprotein, lipid profile Baseline serum citrullin level Hypercoagulable workup (i.e., protein C, protein S, antithrombin III, factor V Leiden mutation) when indicated
Serology	Hepatitis screen, HIV, CMV IgM and IgG, EBV IgM and IgG, ZVZ IgA EIA,	Hepatitis screen, HIV, CMV IgM and IgG, EBV IgM and IgG, ZVZ IgA EIA, syphilis For pediatric patients also: lgG and IgM titers for herpes, varicella, mumps, measles, and rubella
Cardiac assessment	Chest X-ray EKG (12 lead) and electrocardiography	Chest X-ray EKG (12 lead) and electrocardiography
GI assessment	D-xylose and fecal fat absorption studies Screen for celiac sprue	D-xylose and fecal fat absorption studies
Imaging studies	CT abdomen with intravenous contrast 3D angio CT scan or SMA angiogram	CT abdomen with intravenous contrast Barium enema Upper GI with small bowel follow through Gastric emptying study Venogram
Other	Formal psychosocial assessment Ethics committee evaluation	Liver biopsy Colonoscopy

HLA human leukocyte antigen, *PT* prothrombin time, *PTT* partial thromboplastin time, *INR* international normalized ratio, *HIV* human immunodeficiency virus, *CMV* cytomegalovirus, *EBV* Epstein-Barr virus, *ZVZ* varicella zoster, *EKG* electocardiogram, *SMA* superior mesentric artery

Imaging studies are performed to rule out underlying or occult pathology and to specifically delineate the intestinal vascular anatomy. A computed tomography (CT) or magnetic resonance (MR) angiography is performed, possibly with computerized three-dimensional (3D) reconstruction, if available. In case, these techniques are not available or are inadequate, a traditional angiogram can be also performed.

Fig. 4.3 Mesenteric angiography

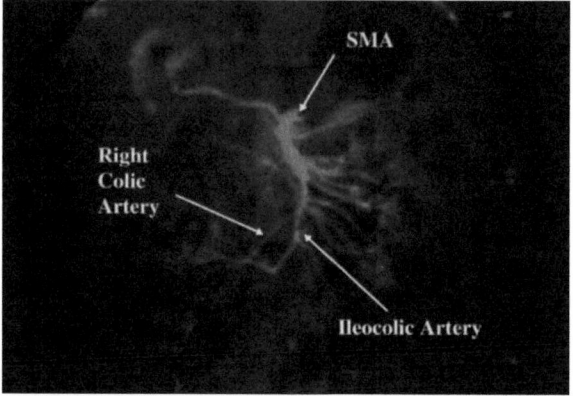

Angiography is performed to evaluate the superior mesenteric artery (SMA) anatomy, to ensure a normal vascular distribution to the small bowel with particular attention to the right colic and ileocolic arteries and the terminal branches of the SMA, and to exclude the presence of atherosclerotic disease and abnormal anatomy. If more than one donor is available, patients with a single distal arterial pedicle should be preferred to patients with multiple vessels. These vessels usually originate caudal to the takeoff of the right colic artery and must be spared during procurement to provide adequate blood supply to the cecum, terminal ileum, and ileocecal valve (Fig. 4.3).

Indications and Recipient Selection

The indications for ITx are identical using either a living or a deceased donor. This transplant should be considered for patients with irreversible intestinal failure requiring TPN. This can be caused by short gut syndrome (Figs. 4.4 and 4.5) related to the loss of over 70% of the native small bowel length (<100 cm of residual intestine), defective gastrointestinal (GI) motility, impaired enterocyte absorptive capacity, genetic malformations of the GI tract or abdominal wall, or neoplastic disease [1]. The irreversibility of intestinal failure is based on the length and function of the remaining native bowel and its inability to provide sufficient fluid and nutritional support. Intestinal rehabilitation can correct this condition in up to 50% of patients requiring chronic TPN, and should be always attempted before considering transplantation [28, 29].

Inclusion Criteria

A patient diagnosed with intestinal failure is not automatically considered an ITx candidate. Usually, these patients are considered transplant candidates only when TPN-related complications arise. These criteria are summarized in Table 4.4.

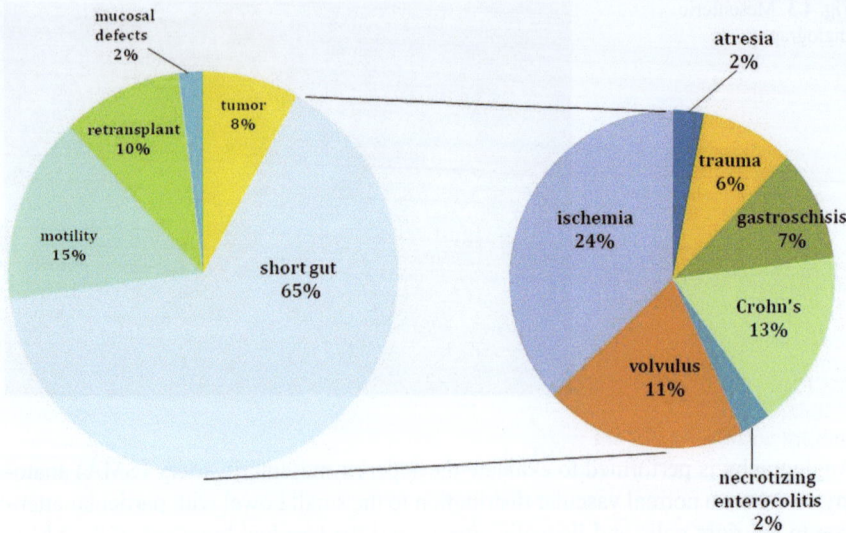

Fig. 4.4 Indications for intestinal transplantation in adults

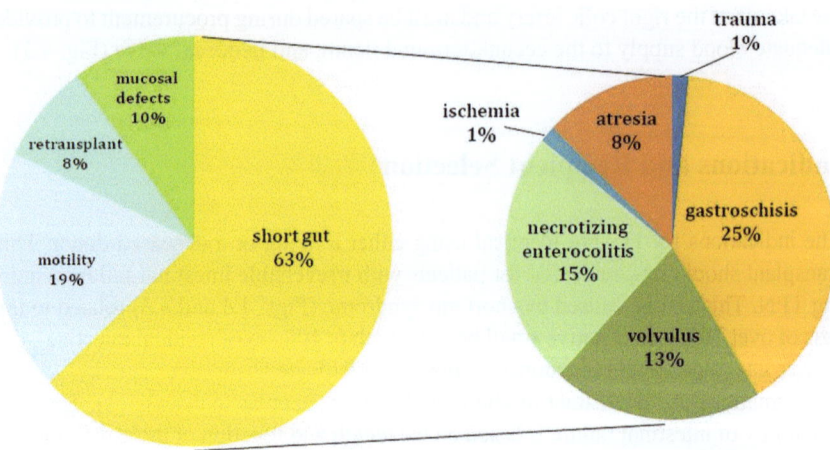

Fig. 4.5 Indications for intestinal transplantation in children

Impending Liver Failure Due to TPN-Induced Cholestasis

TPN-induced cholestasis is a condition of impaired canalicular secretion of bile, characterized by bile duct regeneration, portal inflammation, and fibrosis. It is diagnosed in patients receiving TPN who develop cholestasis not due to other liver diseases or biliary obstruction. The clinical manifestations include elevated serum

Table 4.4 Potential procedure-specific risk for the live intestinal donor

Failure of parenteral nutrition, as defined by the Centers for Medicare and Medicaid Services
Impending or overt liver failure due to TPN-induced liver injury
Thrombosis of two or more central veins
Two or more episodes per year of catheter-related systemic sepsis that requires hospitalization
A single episode of line-related fungemia, septic shock, or acute respiratory distress syndrome
Frequent episodes of severe dehydration despite intravenous fluid supplementation in addition to TPN

TPN total parenteral nutrition

bilirubin and/or liver enzymes, splenomegaly, thrombocytopenia, gastroesophageal varices, coagulopathy, stomal bleeding, or hepatic fibrosis/cirrhosis. Its progression could be very rapid, and in some patients, liver cirrhosis may develop in a few months [30].

Vascular Access

This can be consequent to the thrombosis of the major central venous system, such as jugular, subclavian, and femoral veins. Thrombosis of two or more of these vessels is considered a life-threatening complication and a failure of TPN therapy. The sequelae of central venous thrombosis are the lack of access for TPN infusion, fatal sepsis secondary to infected thrombi, pulmonary embolism, superior vena cava syndrome, or chronic venous insufficiency.

Frequent Line Infections and Sepsis

The development of two or more episodes per year of systemic sepsis, secondary to line infection that requires hospitalization, also indicates failure of TPN therapy. A single episode of line-related fungemia, septic shock, and/or acute respiratory disease syndrome (ARDS) is considered TPN failure.

Frequent Episodes of Severe Dehydration Despite Intravenous Fluid Supplement in Addition to TPN

Under certain medical conditions, such as secretory diarrhea, in GI tract that cannot be reconstructed, the loss of the GI and pancreatobiliary secretions exceed the maximum intravenous infusion rates that can be tolerated by the cardiopulmonary system.

Table 4.5 Contraindications for live donor intestinal transplant

Relative contraindications
Age less than 6 months or greater than 70 years
Human immunodeficiency virus (HIV) seropositive
Active substance abuse
Absolute contraindications
Significant uncorrectable cardiopulmonary insufficiency
Incurable malignancy
Active systemic infections
Severe systemic autoimmune disease
Acquired immune deficiency syndrome

Exclusion Criteria

Several conditions also preclude intestinal transplant. The exclusion criteria are summarized in Table 4.5.

Preoperative Workup

Once a patient with intestinal failure is considered for a transplant, a specific evaluation is performed. The purpose of the evaluation is to determine if the patient would benefit from ITx; to rule out contraindications; and to improve, if possible, the current medical management of these patients. The workup performed in the recipient is similar for either a deceased donor or a live donor (see Table 4.3). The workup is performed by a multidisciplinary team consisting of a transplant surgeon, gastroenterologist, nutrition specialist, cardiologist, anesthesiologist, infectious disease specialist, psychiatrist, and social worker. A multidisciplinary committee discussion and presentation of each case are advisable.

Radiographic Imaging Studies

It is imperative to know the anatomy of the recipient pretransplant. If numerous intestinal resections have been performed over a long period of time, often previous medical records are not available or are inaccurate in recording the remaining portion of the intestine and its length after each surgery. In addition, intraoperative evaluation of the anatomy is often difficult due to the scarring and adhesions found. Upper and lower GI series with contrast will allow one to visualize the portion of residual gut, its position in the abdominal cavity, and its length. It is not uncommon that during a workup, a longer-than-expected segment of small or large intestine is identified, and this might allow different strategies than transplantation, such as surgical recanalization of the residual intestine, intestinal rehabilitation, or other surgical elongation procedures. Abdominal CT scan (or MR imaging) with contrast is also used to rule out malignancies or other undiagnosed diseases.

Patency of the upper and lower body veins must be established by venogram, since duplex scan might not be sufficiently sensitive for this purpose. Thrombosis of these vessels is not uncommon in patients receiving TPN. Thrombosis can cause inability to cannulate the vessels, and can cause superior vena cava syndrome when the inferior vena cava (IVC) is clamped. The patient may have patency only of the femoral veins. Complete lack of venous access could be a contraindication for ITx.

Electrocardiography and echocardiogram are used to determine the cardiac function and any valvular lesions, and should be accompanied by a cardiologic evaluation and clearance for surgery. Stress test or cardiac catheterization may also be performed, if indicated.

Additional Diagnostic Procedures

Liver biopsy may be indicated in patients with intestinal failure and hepatic dysfunction. TPN-induced cholestatic liver injury can be reversed by isolated intestinal transplant or by restoring intestinal integrity [31]. However, in the presence of liver cirrhosis or portal hypertension, a patient with intestinal failure requires a combined liver–ITx. This can be performed using a deceased donor. However, as an option, liver transplant from a deceased donor can be followed by intestinal transplant from a living donor, if an intestinal graft is not attainable from the same donor at the same time. In addition, in pediatric patients, combined liver–ITx from a living donor has been recently reported [10].

Further assessment of associated liver disease (portal hypertension, coagulopathy, ascites, hyperdynamic circulation, hepatopulmonary syndrome, and hepatic encephalopathy) should be done, if indicated.

Patients with familial polyposis should be evaluated for the presence of polyps in the remaining portion of the Gl tract. Patients with dysmotility disorders may require an assessment of the stomach to evaluate functional abnormalities. Children with pseudo-obstruction may require urologic assessment because as many as a third may have a dysfunctional urinary tract. Children with necrotizing enterocolitis may require a full neurologic and pulmonary workup to exclude the possibility of associated intraventricular hemorrhage and bronchopulmonary dysplasia.

Surgical Technique

Background

The transplantation of an intestinal graft from a live donor, by definition, involves the transplantation of a segment of the small intestine. Central caveat of the donor operation is to provide adequate length of intestine to the recipient to ensure enteral autonomy, while preserving enough small bowel length in the donor. The appropriate length and the anatomic origin of the segmental graft to harvest is the cornerstone of a successful transplant.

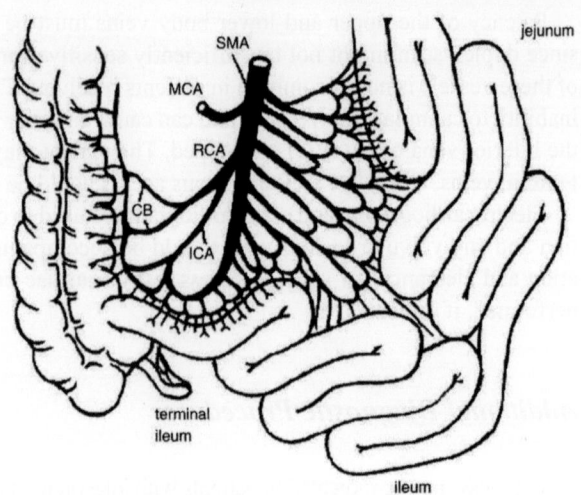

Fig. 4.6 Vascular supply to the small intestine from SMA. The terminal ileum, ileocecal valve, and right colon receive blood supply also from the right colic and ileocolic arteries, and are connected by the marginal artery of Drummond. *CB* colic branches, *ICA* ileocolic artery, *MCA* middle colic artery, *RCA* right colic artery, *SMA* superior mesenteric artery. (From Tan HP, Marcos A, Shapiro R, Living donor organ transplantation, 1st edition, copyright © 2007, Informa Healthcare. Reproduced with permission of Informa)

Anatomical Considerations

The arterial blood supply to the small intestine is from the superior mesenteric artery (SMA). The basic pattern of distribution of the intestinal arteries generally includes 5 arteries arising on the left of the SMA above the origin of the ileocolic artery and 11 below that level. Eight additional arteries usually originate from the ileal branch of the ileocolic artery [32]. These intestinal vessels branch a few centimeters from the border of the intestine to form arterial arcades connecting the intestinal arteries with one another. Proximally, a single set of arcades is present; distally, there are usually several sets of arcades. These arches form the primary interconnections of the arterial supply. From arches and arcades, the vasa recta arise and pass without cross-communication to enter the intestinal wall. A complete channel may also exist from the posteroinferior pancreaticoduodenal artery that is parallel to the intestine and joins the marginal artery of Drummond of the colon. The terminal ileum, ileocecal valve, and right colon receive blood supply also from the right colic artery and ileocolic artery, often sharing a common origin, connected by the marginal artery of Drummond to the terminal branches of the SMA (Fig. 4.6). In 5 % of the population, blood supply to these structures is guaranteed only by the ileocolic artery, as the marginal artery is incomplete (Fig. 4.7). The venous drainage of the small intestine is less complex than the arterial vessels, merging in the jejunal and ileal veins, and into the superior mesenteric vein and portal vein.

From a technical standpoint, the ileum offers the advantage of a larger vascular pedicle if the distal portion of the SMA is used. This vessel can be transected below the takeoff of the right colic artery to avoid hypoperfusion of the terminal ileum, and the preservation of the ileocecal valve in the donor (Fig. 4.8). At this level, this artery is commonly single, but could also consist of two or more branches.

Fig. 4.7 Vascular supply to the small intestine from SMA. The marginal artery is incomplete in 5% of the population. IMA incomplete marginal artery, ICA ileocolic artery, MCA middle colic artery, RCA right colic artery, SMA superior mesenteric artery. (From Tan HP, Marcos A, Shapiro R, Living donor organ transplantation, 1st edition, copyright © 2007, Informa Healthcare. Reproduced with permission of Informa)

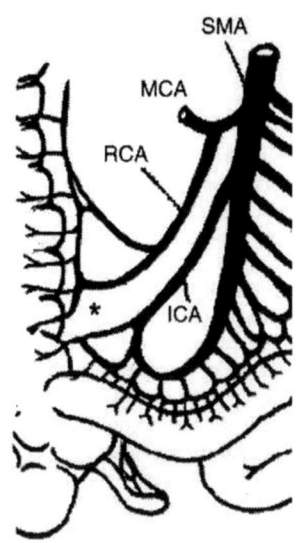

Additionally, despite the fact that both jejunum and ileum have the ability to adapt following intestinal resection, the ileum has the advantage of allowing structural and functional adaptation [33, 34].

Despite these advantages, the jejunum has been also used in early experience for the possible immunologic advantages, since it has been reported, from small-animal studies, that acute rejection is less severe in the jejunum [35, 36]. However, the vascular distribution to the jejunum makes the operation more complex, as the segmental graft obtained has numerous arterial branches needing multiple anastomoses in the recipient to obtain adequate revascularization for the graft (Fig. 4.9). Jaffe et al. reported attempts at proximal small bowel transplantation involving complex vascular reconstruction that resulted in vascular complications [35]. In addition, the early clinical experience from the same group did not show a clear immunologic advantage with the use of jejunal segmental grafts.

Optimal Length of the Segmental Graft

The appropriate length of the human alimentary tract to be resected has proven to be surprisingly difficult to measure. The length of the small intestine in deceased donors was reported to be from 10 to 40 feet, with an average of 20.5 feet or 624.8 cm [37]. *In vivo* measurements using an intraluminal method provided an average of 8.5 feet or 258 cm [38]. This discrepancy is attributed to the postmortem loss of longitudinal muscle tune of the small intestine that can lead to an increase in length, up to 135% in a few hours, as shown in animal studies [39]. For the purpose of ITx, intestinal measurements are performed in a live subject, but being under general

Fig. 4.8 From a technical standpoint, the ileum offers the advantage of a larger pedicle if the distal portion of the superior mesenteric artery is used. This vessel can be transected below the takeoff of the right colic artery to avoid hypoperfusion of the terminal ileum and ileocecal valve, which are always preserved in the donor. *CB* colic branches, *ICA* ileocolic artery, *MCA* middle colic artery, *RCA* right colic artery, *SMA* superior mesenteric artery. (From Tan HP, Marcos A, Shapiro R, Living donor organ transplantation, 1st edition, copyright © 2007, Informa Healthcare. Reproduced with permission of Informa)

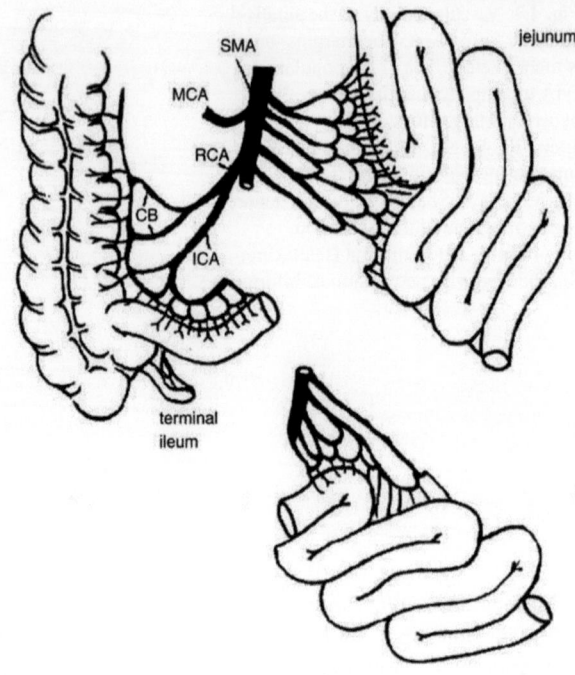

Fig. 4.9 The vascular distribution to the jejunum makes the operation more complex as the segmental graft obtained has numerous arterial branches needing multiple anastomoses in the recipient to obtain adequate revascularization of the graft. *CB* colic branches, *ICA* ileocolic artery, *MCA* middle colic artery, *RCA* right colic artery, *SMA*, superior mesenteric artery. (From Tan HP, Marcos A, Shapiro R, Living donor organ transplantation, 1st edition, copyright © 2007, Informa Healthcare. Reproduced with permission of Informa)

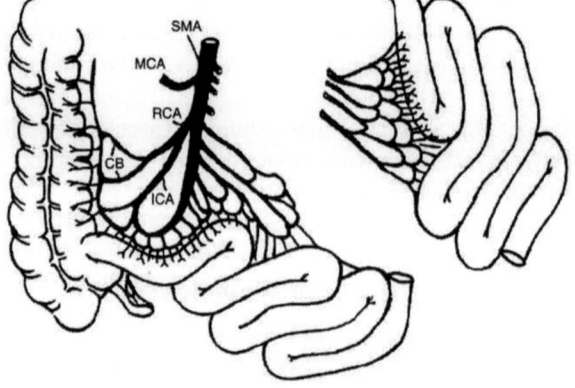

anesthesia, the effect of the pharmacologic agents used might affect the intestinal distension, motility, and length [40–43]. For these reasons, the calculation of a generic optimal length of small bowel graft to resect can be difficult. In each individual case, the entire small bowel should be measured from the ligament of Treitz to the ileocecal valve, using a sterile surgical tape. Once the length of the entire small bowel is determined in a particular patient under a specific anesthetic agent, a final determination of the segment to be removed is made. Although it is relatively easy to determine when an intestinal segment is too short, the long-term impact to the donor of the resection of a longer segment is unknown. Deltz reported a transplant of a 60-cm segment of distal jejunum and proximal ileum, whereas, Morris used a similarly long segment of distal ileum, ileocecal valve, and a portion of the cecum [44, 45]. Despite these early successes, a length of 60-cm small bowel has been generally inadequate to provide a TPN-free condition [44], and resection of the ileum, ileocecal valve, and cecum can have a negative impact on the function of the remaining donor bowel (e.g., increased transit time and vitamin B_{12} deficiency) [45].

From the short-bowel syndrome literature, a segment of approximately 1 m has been reported to be sufficient to ensure adequate absorption [29]. However, this depends on the presence of the ileocecal valve or part of the colon. Considerations in the recipient anatomy also play an important role in determining the length of the intestinal segment to remove in the donor. A recipient with no colon or ileocecal valve, for example, will require a longer segment compared with a patient where these structures are present.

Donor safety is, of course, paramount, and this will determine the upper limit of the length of resection. The resection of a long segment might induce malabsorption and weight loss, and the removal of terminal ileum might induce the malabsorption of bile salts, vitamin B_{12}, and chronic diarrhea. It is clear that the ileocecal valve and terminal ileum should be preserved in the donor, and that the segment of intestine to be removed should be the ileum. Only 20–30 % of the total length of the small intestine should be resected to minimize risk to the donor, as no data are available to determine the ideal length of the intestine to preserve. The successful use of ileal segments between 150 and up to 200 cm of length has been reported, with no sign of long-term complications in the donors [15]. Generally, the expectation is that the adaptation of the residual intestine will take place, compensating for the segment removed, and reestablishing a completely normal functional condition. However, although data exist about posttransplant adaptation in the recipient, such evidence is not yet available in the donor [26, 27].

Pollard was the first to report the use of a segment of ileum with the distal mesenteric artery and vein for an LD-ITx; however, no information was given regarding the distal terminal ileum and blood supply to the remaining cecum and ileocecal valve [46]. Subsequently, Gruessner reported a case describing the surgical technique utilized to preserve these structures [47].

Table 4.6 Preoperative orders for intestinal donor

Orders	
Labs on admission	
Chest X-ray (2 views)	
Stool culture	Ova and parasites, fecal leukocytes, *Clostridium difficile*, fungus, bacteria
Final crossmatch	
Type and cross, 2 units	
Golytely Prep	Mixed with 1 gallon of water at 16:00 before surgery
Selective digestive contamination	Nystatin 500,000 U PO BID + Tobramycin 80 mg PO BID + Polimixin B 125 mg PO BID
Antibiotics, or if allergic to penicillin	Ceftriaxone 1 g IV once Aztreonam 1 g IV once + Clindamycin 600 mg IV once

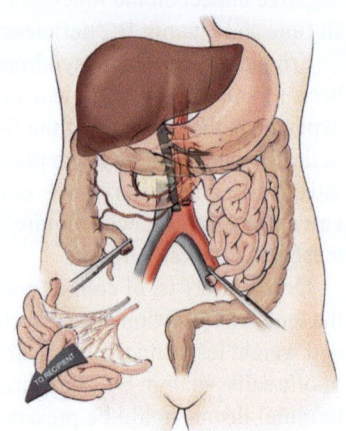

Fig. 4.10 A schematic illustration of the donor operation is shown. (From Tan HP, Marcos A, Shapiro R, Living donor organ transplantation, 1st edition, copyright © 2007, Informa Healthcare. Reproduced with permission of Informa)

Donor

Preoperative Orders

Preoperative orders are individualized by each transplant center. A mechanical bowel preparation and preoperative intestinal decontamination are preferred. A final crossmatch should be performed and stool cultures obtained. An example of these orders is shown in Table 4.6.

Surgical Procedure

A schematic illustration of the donor operation is shown in Fig. 4.10. The donor operation is performed with the patient in a supine position, using a midline incision

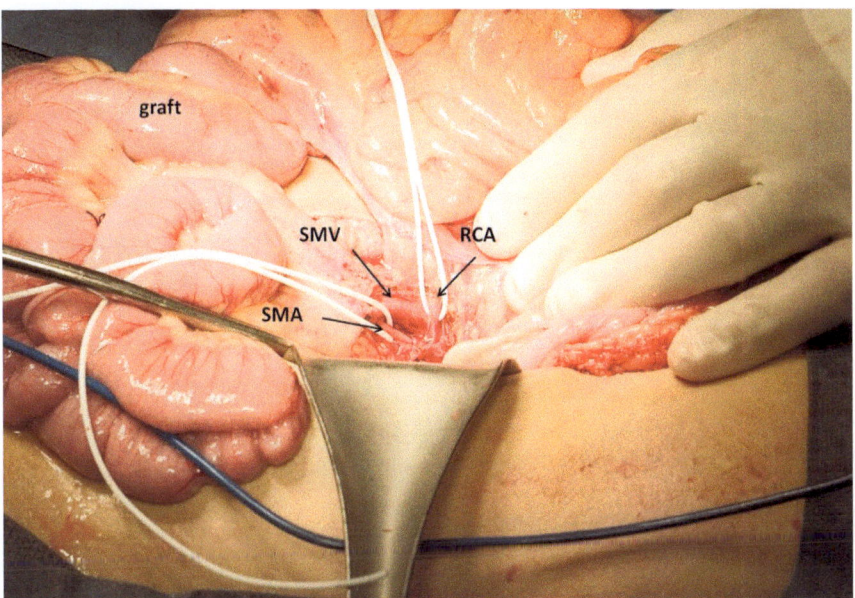

Fig. 4.11 The terminal branches of the superior mesenteric artery and vein are identified and dissected from the surrounding tissue and identified with vessel loops near the origin of the right colic artery. *SMV* superior mesenteric vein, *RCA* right colic artery, *SMA* superior mesenteric artery

from approximately 4 cm above the umbilicus to 2 cm above the pubis. The small intestine is inspected and measured from the ligament of Treitz to the ileocecal valve. The terminal ileum is identified, and a mark is placed at 15–20 cm from the ileocecal valve using a silk stitch in the serosal layer. This segment of terminal ileum is preserved and its blood supply maintained by the ileal branches of the ileocolic artery, usually originating from the right colic artery. The total length of the intestinal segment to be removed is based on the recipient anatomic characteristics and donor total intestinal length. This measurement starts at the previously placed mark proceeding cranially in the ileum, and is marked with another silk stitch in the serosal layer. At this point, the segment of ileum to be removed is identified, and is included between the two marks. Different marks should be used proximally and distally to identify later the orientation of the intestinal graft. The terminal branches of the SMA and vein are identified and dissected from the surrounding tissue, and identified with vessel loops near the origin of the right colic artery (Fig. 4.11). The origin of the right colic artery is also identified with a vessel loop. The line of transection of the SMA will be below this point to preserve the right colic artery in order to provide blood supply to the terminal ileum, ileocecal valve, and cecum with its ileocolic branches.

Careful inspection by transillumination of the vascular arcades is performed (Fig. 4.12). The peritoneum of the mesentery is initially scored with electrocautery, and the mesenteric tissue is dissected; the vascular arcades encountered are ligated

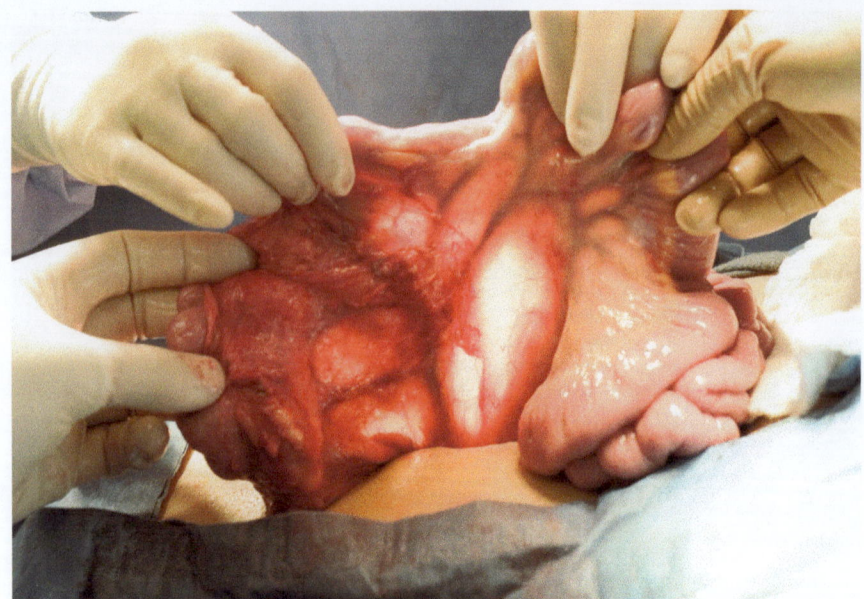

Fig. 4.12 Careful inspection by transillumination of the vascular arcades is performed. (From Tan HP, Marcos A, Shapiro R, Living donor organ transplantation, 1st edition, copyright © 2007, Informa Healthcare. Reproduced with permission of Informa)

and divided between silk ties. The line of dissection of the mesentery starts from the marks on the ileum and is directed toward the previously dissected and looped blood vessels. Once all the dissection is performed, the intestinal segment is still vascularized through a triangle of mesentery containing the distal superior mesenteric vessels (Fig. 4.13). Once the recipient is ready in the adjacent operating room, the intestine is transacted using a gastrointestinal anastomosis (GIA) stapler. Adequate blood supply to the proximal and the distal stumps of the ileum is confirmed when it is transected by GIA stapler (Fig. 4.14). The ileocolic vessels are clamped and transacted, and the vasculature of the intestinal segment is flushed using 4°C cold preservation solution on the back table. As the graft is transported to the recipient operating room for transplantation, the vascular stumps in the donor are ligated using nonabsorbable monofilament stick ties. The proximal and distal segments of the ileum are re-anastomosed primarily using either a GIA or a manual technique. To avoid intraperitoneal spillage of intestinal content, the intestine is clamped using linen-shod noncrushing Doyen clamps closed at one to two clicks. If the manual technique is used, our preference is to use an absorbable monofilament for the mucosal layer and a nonabsorbable monofilament for the sero-muscular layer using Lambert or Cushing stitches. A side-to-side technique is preferred to minimize the risk of stenosis. The mesenteric defect should be closed carefully. The abdomen is then closed using absorbable monofilament for the fascia and subcuticular for skin closure; the surgical drain is not necessary.

Fig. 4.13 Once the dissection is completed, the intestinal segment is still vascularized through a triangle of mesentery containing the distal superior mesenteric vessels. (From Tan HP, Marcos A, Shapiro R, Living donor organ transplantation, 1st edition, copyright © 2007, Informa Healthcare. Reproduced with permission of Informa)

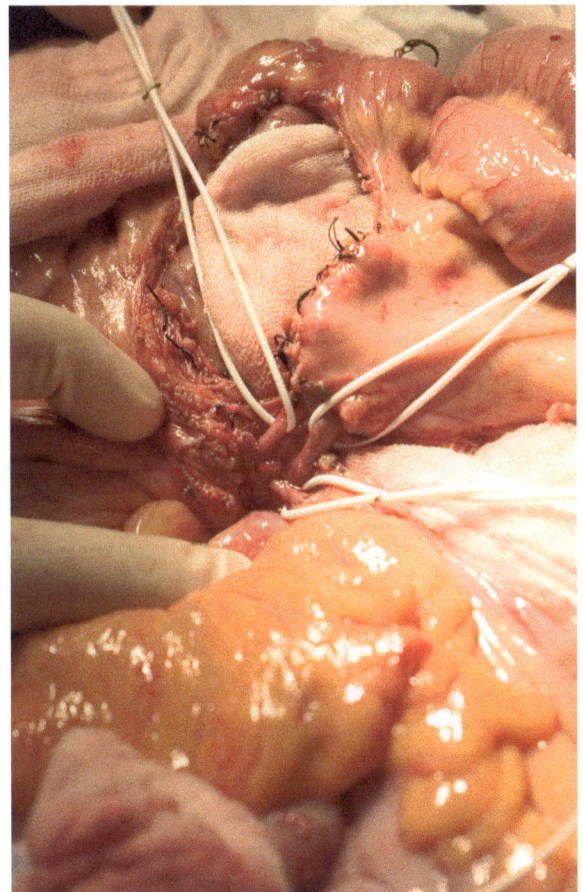

Postoperative Management and Follow-Up

Postoperative orders are substantially similar to the orders used for a general surgical patient undergoing small intestinal resection.

The recommended minimum follow-up includes postoperative visits for the first 4 weeks. There are several risks potentially associated with the donor operation that could occur early in the postoperative period, such as diarrhea, weight loss, dysvitaminosis, and small bowel obstruction, whereas the long-term risk of small bowel resection primarily involves small bowel obstruction. Donors should be followed until all procedure-related symptoms have been resolved. B_{12} deficiency can be monitored by performing serum levels at 6 months and annually for 3 years. Donor data should be collected and submitted to the intestinal transplant registry.

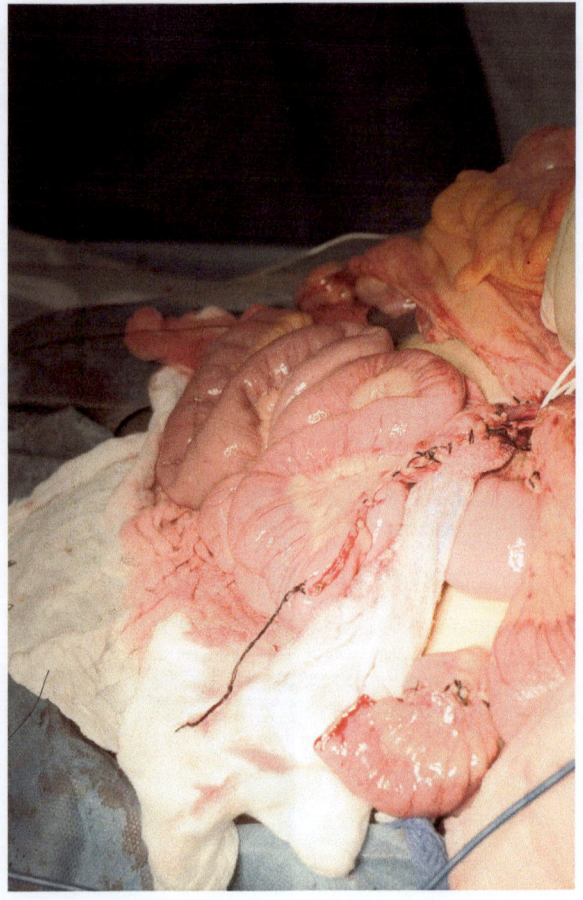

Fig. 4.14 The picture shows adequate blood supply to the proximal and distal stumps of the graft. (From Tan HP, Marcos A, Shapiro R, Living donor organ transplantation, 1st edition, copyright © 2007, Informa Healthcare. Reproduced with permission of Informa)

Recipient

Preoperative Orders

Preoperative orders are, again, individualized by each transplant center. An example of our preference is shown in the preoperative orders exhibited in Table 4.7.

Surgical Procedure

A schematic illustration of the recipient operation is shown in Fig. 4.15. The recipient operations for isolated ITx from living or deceased donors are not different, except for the length of the intestinal graft and the vascular pedicle. These patients can present with a variety of anatomic differences in their native intestine.

Table 4.7 Preoperative orders for intestinal recipient

Orders	
Labs on admission	
Chest X-ray (2 views)	
Stool culture	Ova and parasites, fecal leukocytes, *Clostridium difficile*, fungus, bacteria
Blood cultures × 2	
Nasal swab culture for r/o MRSA	
CMV IgG, EBV IgG	
Urine cultures	
ImmuKnow blood test	
Final crossmatch	
Type and cross, 4 units	
Golytely Prep	@16:00 before surgery
Selective digestive contamination	Nystatin 500,000 U PO BID + Tobramycin 80 mg PO BID + Polimixin B 125 mg PO BID
Antibiotics	Piperacillin/Tazobactam 3.375 g IV once + Vancomycin 1 g IV once + Liposomal Amphotericin B (10 mg/kg) IV once
Or if allergic to penicillin	Aztreonam 1 g IV once + Vancomycin 1 g IV once + Liposomal Amphotericin B (10 mg/kg) IV once
Immunosuppression induction	Dexamethasone 100 mg IV once, or Methylprednisolone 500 mg IV once Anti-thymocite globulin 1.5 mg/kg once

MRSA methycillin resistant *Staphylococcus aureus*, *CMV* cytomegalovirus, *EBV* Epstein-Barr virus

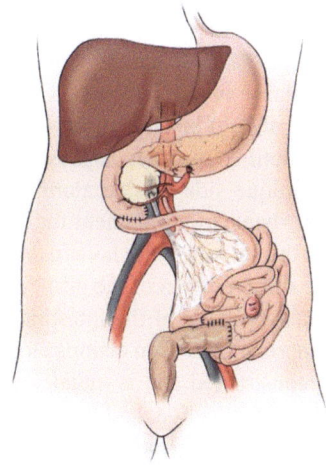

Fig. 4.15 The picture shows a schematic illustration of the recipient operation. (From Tan HP, Marcos A, Shapiro R, Living donor organ transplantation, 1st edition, copyright © 2007, Informa Healthcare. Reproduced with permission of Informa)

These can go from the presence of the entire dysfunctional intestine in patients with pseudo-obstruction, to the ultra-short gut syndrome with only a portion of the duodenum intact. In all cases, the anatomy should be well identified pretransplantation to plan the best surgical approach. The goal of the operation is to reestablish intestinal continuity by transplanting the segment of ileum recovered from the donor.

The proximal and distal (if present) segments of intestine in the recipient should be always preserved and used for the anastomosis. The presence of a segment of colon or ileocecal valve in these patients would decrease the transit time and increase absorption and would allow a shorter ileal graft to be transplanted.

Often, these patients develop short bowel syndrome as a consequence of multiple surgical resections. In this case, the presence of diffuse intra-abdominal adhesions requires a long and careful dissection to identify vascular and intestinal structures and anomalies. For this reason, we start the recipient operation first and initiate the procedure in the donor in the adjacent operating room only when the recipient anatomy is identified. A midline incision from the xiphoid process to the pubis is used. The operation is carried out to identify the aorta, vena cava, and the proximal and distal intestinal stumps. Once this is accomplished, the graft is removed from the donor and is transported in the recipient operating room. The previously dissected aorta and vena cava are used for the anastomoses. The vena cava is clamped in its infrarenal portion with a Satinsky vascular clamp. The ileocolic vein is anastomosed end to side with running nonabsorbable monofilament. The mesenteric artery is anastomosed end to side to the aorta after this vessel is also clamped using a vascular clamp. In this case, a running or interrupted anastomosis is performed, depending on the size of the vessel using nonabsorbable monofilament. If the vascular pedicle consists of multiple arteries, these are anastomosed individually. Once the vascular anastomoses have been completed, the intestinal graft is reperfused (Fig. 4.16). The proximity of the vena cava and aorta allows anastomosis without tension, as the vascular pedicle of the graft can be short. However, an alternative vascular approach, for example, using the portal vein, could also be utilized.

Intestinal continuity is immediately reestablished anastomosing the proximal end of the graft, previously marked in the donor, to the proximal intestinal stump available in the recipient. Often, this is the duodenum or the proximal jejunum. Care should be taken not to shorten the native intestine unless pseudo-obstruction or motility disorder is present. The intestine is anastomosed using a hand-sewn technique side to side along its anti-mesenteric border. Our preference is to use absorbable monofilament for the mucosal layer and a nonabsorbable monofilament for the seromuscular layer using Lambert or Cushing stitches. The same is done for the distal portion of the graft if a segment of colon is available. To avoid intraperitoneal spillage of the intestinal content, the intestine is clamped using linen-shod noncrushing Doyen clamps closed at one to two clicks. A temporary loop ileostomy is constructed and is maintained for 6 months. This is used for endoscopy, feces sample collection, and the evaluation of the graft mucosa visible in the stoma. Construction of the loop ileostomy is performed after the intestinal anastomoses have been completed, and intestinal continuity is reestablished. At this point, a site in the lower quadrant is identified to perform the ileostomy without tension, depending on the length of the mesenteric vessels, the anatomy of the recipient, and the intestinal reconstruction performed. This is performed excising a 2-cm diameter circle of skin followed by a 2-cm incision of the fascia. The muscle fibers are spread and the tips of two fingers should be easily introduced into the opening. The loop should be gently exteriorized using a Babcock clamp, and a rod is introduced in a small

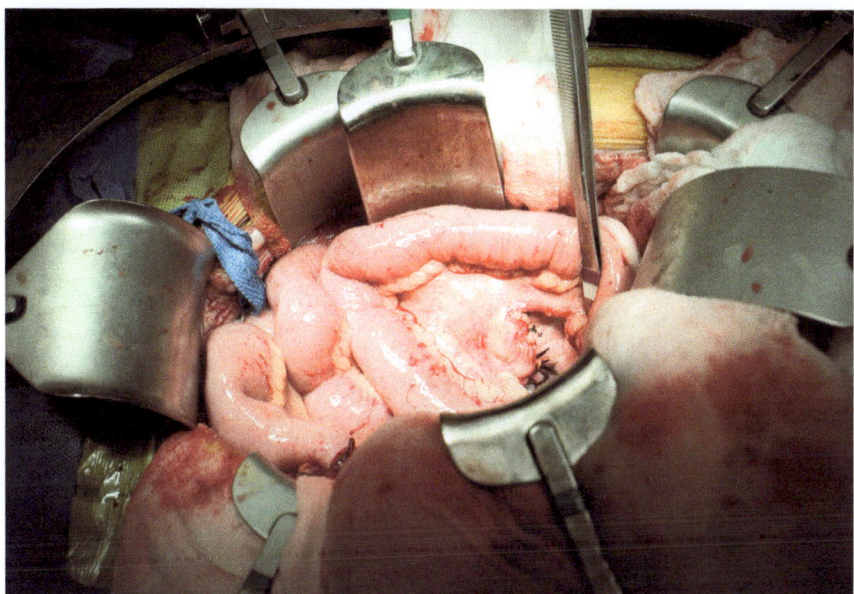

Fig. 4.16 Once the vascular anastomoses have been completed, the intestinal graft is reperfused. (From Tan HP, Marcos A, Shapiro R, Living donor organ transplantation, 1st edition, copyright © 2007, Informa Healthcare. Reproduced with permission of Informa)

opening of the mesentery to keep the loop in position. The anterior wall of the ileum is opened slightly more than 50% of its circumference. The proximal stoma is larger and is kept cephalad. The ileostomy is matured with mucocutaneous fixation using interrupted sutures. Sutures are also used to secure the graft to the peritoneum to prevent herniation, and to help in identifying the proximal and distal end of the ileostomy for future endoscopy.

If no colon is available, a permanent end ileostomy is constructed. If possible, this is performed approximately 5 cm to the right of the midline incision and about 4 cm below the umbilicus. The presence of scar from previous surgeries might mandate a different location. The end ileostomy is performed excising a 2-cm diameter circle of skin followed by a 2-cm incision of the fascia. After spreading the muscle, two fingers should be easily introduced into the opening. The distal end of the graft should be gently exteriorized using a Babcock clamp, preserving the marginal artery and with the mesentery cephalad. The end ileostomy is matured with mucocutaneous fixation using interrupted sutures. Intraperitoneal sutures are used to secure the graft to prevent herniation or prolapse of the stoma.

Abdominal closure is performed in two layers using nonabsorbable monofilament for the fascia and surgical staples for the skin. If tension exists on the fascia at the time of closure, this should not be attempted to reduce the risk of thrombosis. The skin can be approximated leaving the fascia open. This approach may require a complex plastic reconstruction later [48]. The abdominal wall fascia can be

Table 4.8 Postoperative orders for intestinal recipient

Orders	
Labs on admission and daily	
Chest X-ray (1 view)	
Vitals	
Oostomy drain monitoring	
Stool culture once a week	
GI consult	
Biopsy of proximal and distal bowel	
Duplex of ileocolic artery	
Selective Digestive Contamination	Nystatin 500,000 U PO BID + Tobramycin 80 mg PO BID + Polimixin B 125 mg PO BID x 7 days
Antibiotics	Piperacillin/tazobactam 3.375 g IV q4h x 3 days,
Or if allergic to penicillin	Aztreonam 1 g IV q8h + Clindamycin 600 mg IV q8h x 3 days
Steroid taper	Methylprednisolone 300 mg IV POD#1
	Methylprednisolone 200 mg IV POD#2
	Methylprednisolone 100 mg IV POD#3
	Methylprednisolone 75 mg IV POD#4
	Methylprednisolone 60 mg IV POD#5
	Methylprednisolone 40 mg IV POD#6
	Methylprednisolone 20 mg IV POD#7
	Anti-thymocite globulin 1.5 mg/kg IV q24h x 7 days
Immunosuppression	Tacrolimus PO q12h, start on POD#1
Prophylaxis	Ganciclovir 5 mg/kg IV daily x 7 days, then Valganciclovir 900 mg PO daily
	Bactrim SS half dose PO daily

GI gastrointestinal

alternatively closed without tension using a biological acellular dermal matrix that has been previously described to be safe in this setting [49].

Postoperative Orders

Postoperative orders are individualized by each transplant center. Several protocols of immunosuppression can be used. Our preference is shown in the postoperative and transfer orders shown (Table 4.8).

Current Outcome of ITx and LD-ITx

Intestinal transplant outcome drastically improved over time, and 1-year graft survival in the U.S. now exceeds 80% [1]. Unfortunately, longer-term outcomes have failed to improve over time and the 5-year patient survival rates for all types of ITx are approximately 50%. Graft rejection and/or infection are still the most common causes of early and late deaths. The inability to completely control rejection has resulted in heavier immunosuppression; consequently, infectious complication and malignancy were the cause of death in a substantial percentage of patients. LD-ITx offers theoretical advantages that could help to address these problems [8–10].

In fact, even among the early attempts made to transplant the intestine in the 1960s and early 1970s in the pre-cyclosporine era, the longest survivor (76 days after transplantation) received an HLA-identical ileal segment from her sister [50]. However, of 2,611 ITxs performed worldwide until 2009, only 66 (2.5%) were performed from living donors [1, 6]. Indeed, the potential benefits of live donation must be weighed against the potential disadvantages of LD-ITx, which include risk to the donor, shorter segment of the intestinal graft, and the limited experience available [51, 52].

Donors

At this time, no donor deaths or long-term morbid complications in intestinal donors have been reported. Only a 1–2-week period of postoperative diarrhea has been described [15]. However, this is usually self-limited and does not require aggressive therapy. In our experience, donors maintain their presurgical weight and, in some instances, tend not to gain weight even after increasing their caloric intake during the first few months. This is probably because of an adaptation of the remaining shorter segment of ileum left in the donor. No studies have been published at this time regarding bowel adaptation or absorption in donors following the donor enterectomy, probably a function of lack of symptoms and an understandable desire to minimize postoperative visits in these otherwise healthy individuals. Additionally, no data have been collected on vitamin absorption. However, even if the distal ileum has been utilized, most of the LD-ITx performed in recent years have been performed with careful preservation of the terminal ileum, which should prevent these problems.

Unfortunately, these patients are followed only for a limited period of time. It has been recently recommended that data on long-term follow-up of these donors should be collected. For example, vitamin B_{12} should be monitored with serum levels at 6 months, and annually for 3 years. In addition, recent recommendations have been developed to create a donor registry in conjunction with the existing International Intestinal Transplant Registry to evaluate the long-term risk of the procedure to the donor [53].

Recipient Outcomes

LD-ITx is not routinely performed; therefore, few reports of short- and long-term outcomes exist. The largest series, reported by the University of Illinois at Chicago, included 13 patients who underwent transplantation of 150–200 cm of terminal ileum proximal to the ileocecal valve [10]. Five of them had a combined liver–ITx.

The 1- and 3- year actuarial patient and graft survival rates in patients with LD-ITx only were 60 and 50%, respectively. In combined liver–LD-ITx recipients the patient survival rates at 1 and 2 years were 100%; the liver graft survival rate was 100%, and the bowel graft survival 80%. Three LD-ITx recipients developed acute rejection, and another recipient developed chronic rejection 3.5 years after the original transplant and died after re-transplantation [46, 47].

Intestinal graft survival has steadily improved over time. Close to half of the patients who have undergone LD-ITx are currently alive today [9, 10]. This is probably an underestimated survival, considering the high rate of failure of the early attempts (historical data). Causes of death included sepsis (29%), liver failure (5%), rejection (5%), and other causes (10%). Only one patient lost the intestinal graft to vascular thrombosis (2.5%). This suggests that the small vascular pedicle in LD-ITx is not a significant risk factor for graft loss when compared with deceased donor grafts, as the technical results are at least comparable with those seen with deceased donors (2.5% vs. 15–20% graft loss, respectively). In previous reports, center volume had no effect on graft survival, but this may reflect the small number of procedures performed worldwide. There was no difference in graft survival or patient survival when comparing LD-ITx and ITx. However, with increased center experience in LD-ITx, it is possible that an improved survival might be obtained, like it is observed in large centers performing ITx from cadaver donors.

Rejection and Immunosuppression

The rate of rejection in ITx from deceased donors has been higher than that observed with other organs, and possible benefits may exist with HLA-matched live donors.

Grafts obtained from deceased donors have not been HLA-matched, mostly because intestinal grafts have been at least initially transplanted in association with the liver. However, living-related donors often have a better HLA match. This benefit is supported by the experience of ITx performed between homozygous twins [54]. In addition, low or no rejection has been documented in living-donor HLA-matched intestinal grafts during the first year posttransplantation, and have had good long-term graft function [55].

Rejection was a cause of death in 3.8% of the patients transplanted with deceased donor organs, and 4.8% in patients transplanted with LD-ITx. However, graft loss was related to rejection in 56% of the transplants performed from deceased donors and 30% in patients transplanted from living donors.

To date, no additional data are available, as donor and recipient tissue typing information has not been collected and analyzed. A recent improvement in the rate of rejection has been reported in deceased donor transplants using antibody induction therapy with anti-interleukin-2 (IL-2) receptor blockers due to their powerful antirejection properties combined with the lack of side effects in terms of direct toxicity and development of infection or malignancy [56].

Posttransplant Lymphoproliferative disease

PTLD is a serious complication of intestinal transplantation, and is related to the heavy immunosuppression that is required to prevent rejection. Recent data show that the overall incidence of PTLD was 11.8% with a median onset 21 months after transplantation. A total of 50% of cases resulted in graft failure or death. In contrast, PTLD was never reported as the cause of death in LD-ITx recipients. In these patients, the ability to use a less aggressive immunosuppressive regimen could have a beneficial impact on the incidence of PTLD [57].

Graft Adaptation

Deltz et al. reported a successful transplant of a 60-cm segment of distal jejunum and proximal ileum, and Morris et al. successfully used a 60-cm segment of distal ileum, ileocecal valve, and a portion of the cecum [44, 45]. Despite these early successes, a length of 60 cm of the bowel is generally inadequate [45]. From the short bowel syndrome literature, a segment of approximately 1 m has been reported to be sufficient to ensure adequate absorption [58], depending on the presence of ileocecal valve or part of the colon. The successful use of ileal segments of length between 150 and 200 cm have been reported, with no sign of long-term complication for either the donors or the recipients [59]. Furthermore, adaptation of the remaining intestine occurs, compensating for the segment removed and reestablishing completely normal function.

Intestinal grafts show evidence of functional adaptation in recipients (see Table 4.3). This occurs because of a morphologic adaptation characterized by increased length and size of the villi (see Figs. 4.8 and 4.9) [26].

Given the experience reported thus far, it seems that ileal grafts measuring 150–200 cm of the distal ileum (without the ileocecal valve) will provide sufficient nutrient absorption to achieve independence from TPN, once adaptation is complete approximately 6 months after LD-ITx.

Ischemic Injury

Intestinal grafts are extremely sensitive to preservation injury. In an analysis of 50 pediatric ITx recipients, it has been shown that the ischemia time was the most significant factor in inducing bacterial translocation [11]. This phenomenon can contribute to the high rate of infections seen during the early posttransplant period, and, of course, also coincides with the timing of the maximum amount of recipient immunosuppression. With living donation, this problem is obviated, if the donor is a healthy individual who is hemodynamically stable, and this minimizes prerecovery gut hypoperfusion. Furthermore, the short cold ischemia time, limited to a few minutes' transport of the graft between donor and recipient operating rooms, virtually eliminates ischemia/reperfusion injury. This is documented by the fact that mucosal biopsies and zoom-endoscopy evaluation performed early after LD-ITx show no evidence of ischemic injury [60].

Ileal Compared with Jejunal Segmental Graft

In the early clinical experience, both jejunum and ileum were used. Jaffe et al. [59] reported attempts at proximal small bowel transplantation involving complex vascular reconstruction that resulted in vascular complications. Furthermore, the early clinical experience from the same group did not show an immunologic advantage for jejunal grafts. Currently, most transplant surgeons today prefer using distal ileal grafts.

Cost-Effectiveness

A cost analysis in the U.S. for TPN reveals that the cost per patient in 1992 was approximately US$ 150,000 per year only for supplies, not including the cost of frequent hospitalizations, medical equipment, and nursing care, and that the national cost of home TPN for Medicare was US$ 780 million in 1992 [61]. The cost of an intestinal transplantation performed from a deceased donor has been analyzed in the U.S. and varies according to the type of transplant performed. This was estimated in 1994–1998 to average US$ 132,285 for isolated intestinal transplant, US$ 214,716 for combined liver–ITx, and US$219,098 for multivisceral transplants [62]. The cost of LD-ITx was estimated to be US$ 16,000±2,000 for the donor workup and hospitalization, US$ 113,000±26,000 for the recipient hospitalization, US$3,900±750 for yearly routine follow-up, and US$ 20,000 for the first year, followed by US$ 3,000 per year thereafter for immunosuppression [22]. Compared with the cost of TPN, LD-ITx is cost-effective after the first year, and it is also less expensive than deceased donor-isolated ITx.

Quality of Life

The quality of life of recipients undergoing LD-ITx has been evaluated before the injury, while TPN-dependent, and following transplantation [63–68]. The premorbid period was defined as the patient's normal state of health prior to becoming TPN-dependent. The morbid phase was the period when patients were TPN-dependent.

Quality of life was measured with the Quality of Life Inventory (QOLI), designed for transplant recipients, and previously validated in liver transplant patients and in ITx patients at the T.E. Starzl Translpant Institute at the University of Pittsburgh Medical Center [69, 70]. These patients, when comparing "before illness" with "during illness" (while on TPN), reported disruption in most areas of their lives, except for marital relationships, medical compliance, and medical satisfaction, which were unchanged from before illness. After transition from TPN dependence to posttransplant TPN independence, when comparing posttransplant status with that during illness (while on TPN), patients reported a significant improvement in most areas of quality of life: psychological (less anxiety, less depression, better mental status, increased stress experience, improved optimism, less impulsiveness and improved control, increased sexuality, and improved coping); physical (better mobility, better appearance, decreased gastrointestinal and genitourinary symptoms, improved sleep, and improved energy); and social (more ability to perform and enjoy recreation activities, improved quality of social support, and improved quality of relationships). The patients did not report worsened quality of life in any area. These patients reported that their posttransplant status compared favorably with their pre-illness condition. Of the 26 domains, only 5 areas of functioning were statistically worse than (pretransplant or TPN patients: loss of control, poorer sleep, increased pain and discomfort, poor quality of social supports, and difficulty in parenting. Regarding employment, all were working full time before becoming TPN-dependent. When they became TPN-dependent, none maintained their working status. All these patients recovered their working status, and one also achieved paternity 36 months after the LD-ITx.

Specific Ethical Considerations

When we are faced with a healthy person, invading a healthy body to obtain an organ for another, the ethical problem is most obvious. Certainly, removal of a kidney from a living person donor was partially justified by the fact that kidneys are paired organs, but what about intestine? To remove an organ from a living donor, as is the case in LD-ITx, ethical problems can arise; the first is the hurdle of the ancient medical maxim, "do not harm," taking in account that "even identical twins do not require a living donor" [71]. Father Bert Cunningham anticipated its possibility with a thesis on the morality of organic transplantation. He considered the living donor a model of virtue for the reason that "there exist an ordination of men to one another and as a consequence, an order of their members to one another, thus we contend that men are ordinate to society as a part to the whole and, as such, are in some way ordinate to one another" [72]. Aquinas, too, had seen the sacrifice of one's life for the good of another as an act of charity. Much more was the undertaking of a risk for a proportionate benefit to another [73].

Kidney transplantation became a routine operation, and we know that we can live well with one kidney; therefore, it does not raise particular ethical problems anymore. However, LD-ITx is a novelty in the field of transplant surgery. We believe that Daube gave a correct formulation of the ethical problem presented by

LD-ITX. He suggested that more than consent is required. A medical judgment of relative risks to donor and recipient, a high degree of caution and concern for the donor, and the absence of alternatives "place on the transplanting surgeon a far greater responsibility" [74]. This is exactly what informed consent, or conscious consent, as we prefer to call it, means [75]. We must consider three actors involved in the setting: the doctor, the recipient, and the donor. The doctor has the technical knowledge, and then he can act in the way marked out by Daube. The recipient is at risk of dying if the donor does not give a segment of its gut. Therefore, the point of view of the recipient is completely in favor of transplant. Certainly, the long-term mortality among recipients is high, but the all or nothing perspectives compel us to do good for the patient. Therefore, the only perspective that can give rise to an ethical question is the particular condition of the donor. As the donor is a healthy person, the operation could represent a sort of mutilation. However, in the perspective given by Cunningham and considering the rule "do not harm" as a relativistic norm, where the imperative is beneficence, also for the others, we have the duty to consider living donor transplantation as an important tool in the field of surgery. All the existing data summarized in the chapter lean on the side of transplant. First of all, there are some problems, as the chapter pointed out, with deceased donors, taking into account that they are often subject to either cardiac arrest or resuscitation. Using living donors, we can obviate to these problems. Furthermore, LD-ITx can be performed and the recipient conditions are optimal and the donor bowel preparation can be easily performed, lessening the risk of infection complications. Not least, often a living donor is a relative of the recipient. This fact is not marginal, representing an unquestionable immunologic advantage. Furthermore, we have to consider that optimal deceased intestinal donors are not common, the waiting list is increasing, and the mortality for all candidates on the waiting list is reported to be up to 20%. Besides, LD-ITx would improve the possibility to obtain transplant in developing countries, where TNP and deceased donors are not easily available. Considering that the principle of beneficence compels us to do what is best for the patient, LD-ITx represents the best treatment for patients. Finally, but not in order of importance, we must consider the risks to the donor, which include early surgical complications, such as small bowel obstruction, diarrhea, weight loss, and vascular thrombosis. These seem to be acceptable risks compared with the benefit to the recipient, which are going to be resolved in a short period of time. We must consider that with a careful and appropriate surgical technique, these risks can be still further reduced. Unfortunately, we do not have long-term follow-up of these patients. This fact could be a dilemma from an ethical point of view, but we have a lot of data from patients who opted for intestinal obstruction or abdominal infarction. Despite the fact that they had even wider resections, the long-term effects are acceptable. In light of these reasons, we believe that the LD-ITx represents a valid and ethical alternative to ITx from a deceased donor.

References

1. Intestinal TR, Toronto, ONT, Canada. Available at www.intestinaltransplant.org/itr Accessed March 2013.
2. Adam R, McMaster F, O'Grady JG, Castaing D, Klempnauer JL, Jamieson N, et al. European Liver Transplant Association. Evolution of liver transplantation in Europe: report of the European Liver Transplant Registry. Liver Transpl. 2003;9(l2):1231–43.
3. Dharnidharka VR, Sullivan EK, Stablein DM, Tejani AH, Harmon WE, et al. North American Pediatric Renal Transplant Cooperative Study (NAFRTCS). Risk factors for posttransplant lymphoproliferative disorder (PTLD) in pediatric kidney transplantation: a report of the North American Pediatric Renal Transplant Cooperative Study (NAPRTCS). Transplantation. 2001;71(8):1065–68.
4. Caillard S, Lachat V, Moulin B, et al. Posttransplant lymphoproliferative disorders in renal allograft recipients: report of 53 cases of a French multicenter study. PTLD French Working Group. Transplant Int. 2000;13 (suppl 1):S338–93.
5. Loinaz C, Kato T, Nishida S, Weppler D, Levi D, Dowdy L, et al. Bacterial infections after intestine and multivisceral transplantation. The experience of the University of Miami (1994–2001). Hepatogastroenterology. 2006;53(68):234–42.
6. Smith JM, Skeans MA, Thompson B, Horslen SP, Edwards EB, Harper AM, et al. OPTN/SRTR 2011 annual data report: intestine. Am J Transplant. 2013;13 Suppl 1:103–18.
7. Mazariegos GV, Steffick DE, Horslen S, Farmer D, Fryer J, Grant D, et al. Intestine transplantation in the United States, 1999–2008. Am J Transpl. 2010;10:1020–34.
8. Tzvetanov IG, Oberholzer J, Benedetti E, et al. Current status of living donor small bowel transplantation. Curr Opin Organ Transplant. 2010;15:346–8.
9. Benedetti E, Holterman M, Asolati M, Di Domenico S, Oberholzer J, Sankary H, et al. Living related segmental bowel transplantation. From experimental to standardized procedure. Ann Surg. 2006;244:694–9.
10. Testa C, Holterman M, John E, Kecskes S, Abcarian H, Benedetti E, et al. Combined living-donor liver/small bowel transplantation. Transplantation. 2005;79(10):1401–4.
11. Cicalese L, Sileri I, Green M, Abu-Elmagd K, Kocoshis S, Reyes J, et al. Bacterial translocation in clinical intestinal transplantation. Transplantation. 2001;71(11):1414–7.
12. Cicalese L, Sileri P. Asolati M, Rastellini C, Abcarian H, Benedetti E, et al. Low infectious complications in segmental living related small bowel transplantation in adults. Clin Transplant. 2000;14(6):567–71.
13. Berney T, Genton L, Buhler LH, Raguso CA, Charbonnet P, Pichard C, et al. Five-year follow-up after pediatric living-related small bowel transplantation between two monozygotic twins. Transplant Proc. 2004;36(2):316–8.
14. Grant D, Abu-Elmagd K, Reyes J, Tzakis A, Langnas A, Fishbein T, et al. 2003 report of the intestine transplant registry: a new era has dawned. Ann Surg. 2003;2005;241:607–13.
15. Cicalese L, Rastellini C, Sileri P, Abcarian H, Benedetti E, et al. Segnientii living-related small bowel transplantation in adults. J Gastrointest Surg. 2001;5(2):168–72.
16. Okada Y, Klein NJ, Van-Saene HK, Webb G, Holzel H, Pierro A, et al. Bactericidal activity against coagulasenegative staphylococci is impaired in infants receiving long-term parenteral nutrition. Ann Surg. 2000;231:276–31.
17. Okada Y, Papp E, Klein NJ, Pierro A, et al. Total parenteral nutrition directly impairs cytokine production after bacterial challenge. J Pediatr Surg. 1999;34:277–80.
18. Okada Y, Klein NJ, Pierro A, et al. Neutrophil dysfunction: the cellular mechanism of impaired immunity Turing total parenteral nutrition in infancy. J Pediatr Surg. 1999;34:242–5.
19. Ellozy SH, Harris MT, Bauer JJ, Gorfine SR, Kreel I, et al. Early postoperative small-bowel obstruction: a prospective evaluation in 242 Consecutive abdominal operations. Dis Colon Rectum. 2002;45(9):1214–7.
20. Fraser SA, Shrier I, Miller G, Gordon PH, et al. Immediate postlaparotomy small-bowel obstruction: a 16-year retrospective analysis. Am Surg. 2002;68(9):780–2.

21. Matter I, Khalemsky L, Abrahamson J, Nash E, Sabo E, Eldar S, et al. Does the index operation influence the course and outcome of adhesive intestinal obstruction? Eur J Surg. 1997;163(10):767–2.
22. Menzies D, Ellis H. Intestinal Obstruction from adhesions—how big is the problem? Ann R Coll Surg Engl. 1990;72(1):60–3.
23. Ellis H, Moran BJ, Thompson JN, Parker MC, Wilson MS, Menzies D et al. Adhesion-related hospital admission after abdominal and pelvic surgery: a retrospective cohort study. Lancet. 1999;353(9163):1476–80.
24. Fevang BT, Fevang J, Lie SA, Søreide O, Svanes K, Viste A, et al. Long-term prognosis after operation for adhesive small bowel obstruction. Ann Surg. 2004;240(2):193–201.
25. Miller G, Boman J, Shrier 1, Cordon PH. Natural history of patients with adhesive small bowel obstruction. Br J Surg. 2000;87(9):1240–7.
26. Benedetti B, Baum C, Cicalese I, Brown M, Raofi V, Massad MG, et al. Progressive functional adaptation of segmental bowel graft from living related donor. Transplantation. 2001;71(4):569–71.
27. Jao W, Sileri P, Holaysan J, Morini S, Chejfec G, Rastellini C, et al. Morphologic adaptation following segmental living related intestinal transplantation. Transplant Proc. 2002;34(3):924.
28. Fishbein TM, Matsumoto CS. Intestinal replacement therapy: timing and indications for referral of patients to an intestinal rehabilitation and transplant program. Gastroenterology. 2006;130 (2 suppl 1):S147–51.
29. DiBaise JK, Young RJ, Vanderhoof JA, et al. Intestinal rehabilitation and the short bowel syndrome part 1. Am J Gastroenterol. 2004;99(7):1386–1395; part 2, Am J Gastroenterol. 2004;99(9):1823–32.
30. Guglielmi FW, Regano N, Mazzuoli S, Fregnan S, Leogrande G, Guglielmi A, et al. Cholestasis induced by total parenteral nutrition. Clin Liver Dis. 2008;12:97–110.
31. Scolapio JS, Fleming CR, Kelly G, Wick DM, Zinsmeister AR, et al. Survival of home parenteral nutrition-treated patients: 20 years of experience at the Mayo Clinic. Mayo Clin Proc. 1999;74:217–22.
32. Michels N, Siddhart P, Kornblith L, Horslen SP, Edwards EB, Harper AM, et al. The variant blood supply to the small and large intestines: its import in regional resections. J Int Coll Surg. 1963;39:127.
33. Dowling RI-I, Booth C. Structural and functional changes following small bowel resection in the rat. Clin Sci. 1967;32:139–49.
34. Thompson JS, Ferguson DC. Effect of the distal remnant on ileal adaptation. J Gastrointest Surg. 2000;4:430–4.
35. Tesi R, Beckj R, Lamblase I, Haque S, Flint L, Jaffe B, et al. Living-related small bowel transplantation: donor evaluation and outcome. Transplant Proc. 1997;29:686–7.
36. Kimura K, Money S, Jaffe IT, et al. The effect of size and site of origin of intestinal grafts on small-bowel transplantation in the rat. Surgery. 1987;101:618–22.
37. Bryant J. Observations upon the growth and length of the human intestine. Am J Med Sci. 1924;167:499.
38. Blankehorn DH, Hirsch J, Ahrens EH, et al. Transintestinal intubation: technique to measure the gut length and physiologic sampling of known loci. Proc Soc Exp Biol Med. 1995;88:356.
39. Reis VderV, Schembra IW. Lange and Lage des Verdauungsrohres beim Lebenden. Z Ges Exp Med. 1924;43:94.
40. Reinelt II, Schirmer U, Marx T, Topalidis P, Schmidt M, et al. Diffusion of xenon and nitrous oxide into the bowel. Anesthesiology. 2001;94:475–7; discussion 6A.
41. Akca O, Lenhardt R, Fleischmann E, Treschan T, Greif R, Fleischhackl R, et al. Nitrous oxide increases the incidence of bowel distension in patients undergoing elective colon resection. Acta Anaesthesiol Scand. 2004;48:894–8.
42. Ogilvy Al SG. The gastrointestinal tract after anaesthesia. Eur J Anaesthesiol Suppl. 1995;111:35–42. Review.
43. Torjman MC, Joseph JI, Munsick C, Morishita M, Grunwald Z, et al. Effects of isoflurane on gastrointestinal motility after brief exposure in rats. Int J Pharm. 2005;294(1–2):65–71.

44. Deltz B, Schroeder F, Gehbardt H, et al. Successful clinical bowel transplantation. Clin Transplant. 1989;3:89.
45. Morris JA, Johnson DL, Rimmer JA, Kuo PC, Alfrey EJ, Bastidas JA, et al. Identical-twin small-bowel transplant or desmoid tumor. Lancet. 1995;345:1577–8.
46. Pollard SG, Lodge P, Selvakumar S, Heatley RV, Wyatt J, Wood R, et al. Living-related small bowel transplantation: the first United Kingdom case. Transplant Proc. 1996;28:2733.
47. Gruessner R, Sharp H. Living-related intestinal transplantation: first report of a standardized surgical technique. Transplantation. 1997;64:1605–7.
48. Tzoracoleftherakis E, Cohen M, Sileri P, Cicalese L, Benedetti E, et al. Small bowel transplantation and staged abdominal wall reconstruction after shotgun injury. J Trauma. 2002;53:770.
49. Asham F, Uknis M, Rastellini C, Elias G, Cicalese L, et al. Acellular dermal matrix provides a good option for abdominal wall closure following small bowel transplantation: a case report. Transplant Proc. 2006;38(6):1770–1.
50. Fortner JG, Sichuk G, Litwin SD, Beattie EJ Jr, et al. Immunological responses to an intestinal allograft with HL-A-identical donor-recipient. Transplantation. 1972;14:531–5.
51. Fishbein TM. Intestinal transplantation. N Engl J Med. 2009;361:998–1008.
52. Cicalese L, Sileri P, Gonzales O, Asolati M, Rastellini C, Abcarian H, et al. Cost-effectiveness of early living related segmental bowel transplantation as therapy for trauma-induced irreversible intestinal failure. Transplant Proc. 2001;33:3581–2.
53. Barr MI, Beighiti J, Villamii PC, Pomfret EA, Sutherland DS, Gruessner RW, et al. A report of the Vancouver forum on the care of the live organ donor: lung, liver, pancreas and intestine: data and medical guidelines. Transplantation. 2006;81:1373–85.
54. Abu-Elmagd K, Reyes J, Bond G, Mazariegos G, Wu T, Murase N, et al. Clinical intestinal transplantation: a decade of experience at a single center. Ann Surg. 2001;234:404–16.
55. Gangemi A, Tzvetanov IG, Beatty E, et al. Lessons learned in pediatric small bowel and liver transplantation from living-related donors. Transplantation. 2009;87:1027–30.
56. Pirenne J, Kawai M. Intestinal transplantation: evolution in immunosuppression protocols. Curr Opin Organ Transplant. 2009;14:250–55.
57. Quintini C, Kato T, Gaynor JJ, Ueno T, Selvaggi G, Gordon P, et al. Analysis of risk factors for the development of posttransplant lymphoproliferative disorder among 119 children who received primary intestinal transplants at a single center. Transplant Proc. 2006;38:1755–8.
58. Calne R, Friend P. Middleton S, Jamieson NV, Watson CJ, Soin A, et al. Intestinal transplant between two of identical triplets. Lancet. 1997;350:1077–8.
59. Jaffe BM, Beck R, Flint L, Gutnisky G, Haque S, Lambiase L, et al. Living-related small bowel transplantation in adults: a report of two patients. Transplant Proc. 1997;29:1851–2.
60. Misra MV, Bhattacharya K, Nompleggi DJ, Uknis ME, Rastellini C, Cicalese L, et al. Magnification endoscopy as a reliable tool for the early diagnosis of rejection in living-related small bowel transplants: a case report. Transplant Proc. 2006;38:1738–9.
61. Howard L, Malone M. Current status of home parenteral nutrition in the United States. Transplant Proc. 1996;28:2691–5.
62. Abu-Elmagd KM, Reyes J, Fung JJ, Mazariegos G, Bueno J, Janov C et al Evolution of clinical intestinal transplantation: improved outcome and cost effectiveness. Transplant Proc. 1999;31:582 584.
63. O'Keefe SJ, Buchman AL, Fishbein TM, Jeejeebhoy KN, Jeppesen PB, Shaffer J, et al. Short bowel syndrome and intestinal failure: consensus definitions and overview. Clin Gastroenterol Hepatol. 2006;4:6–10.
64. Todo S, Reyes J, Furukawa H, Abu-Elmagd K, Lee RG, Tzakis A, et al. Outcome analysis of 71 clinical intestinal transplantations. Ann Surg. 1995;222:270–80.
65. Rovera GM, Sileri P, Rastellini C, Knight P, Benedetti E, Cicalese L, et al. Quality of life after living-related small bowel transplantation. Transplant Proc. 2002;34:967–8.
66. DiMartini A, Rovera GM, Graham TO, Furukawa H, Todo S, Funovits M, et al. Quality of life after small intestinal transplantation and among home parenteral nutrition patients. JPEN J Parenter Enteral Nutr. 1998;22:357–62.

67. Abu-Elmagd KM. Intestinal transplantation for short bowel syndrome and gastrointestinal failUIV current consensus, rewarding outcomes, and practical guidelines. Gastroenterology. 2006;130(2 suppl 1):S132–7.
68. Rovera GM, DiMartini A, Graham TO, Hutson WR, Furukawa H, Todo S, et al. Quality of life after intestinal transplantation and on toi, il parenteral nutrition. Transplant Proc. 1998;30:2513–4.
69. DiMartini A, Rovera GM, Graham TO, Furukawa H, Todo S, Funovits M, et al. Quality of life after small intestinal transplantation and among home parenteral nutrition patients. JPEN J Parenter Enteral Nutr. 1998;22:357–62.
70. Rovera GM, DiMartini A, Schoen RE, Rakela J, Abu-Elmagd K, Graham TO, et al. Quality of life of patienI after intestinal transplantation. Transplantation. 1998;66:1141–5.
71. Murray JE. Organ transplantation: the practical possibilities. In: Wostenholme GEW, O'Connors M, Editors. Law, ethics of transplantation. London:JA Churchill, Ltd; 1966.
72. Cunningham B. The morality of organic transplantation. Studies Sacred Theol. 1944;86:63.
73. Thomas Aquinas. III Sententiae, d. 29, a. 5, "when one gives one's life for one's friend, he does not love the friend more than himself, but rather prefers one's own "good of virtue" to a physical good."
74. Daube D. Transplantation: acceptability of procedures and the required legal sanctions. In: Wolsenholme GEW, O'Connors M, Editors. Ethics in Medical Progress. Boston: Little, Brown & Company; 1966.193.
75. Caocci G, La Nasa G, d'Aloja, Vacca A, Piras E, Pintor M, Demontis R, Pisu S, et al. Ethical issues of unrelated hematopoietic stem cell transplantation in adult thalassemia patients. BMC Medical Ethics. 2011;12: 4.

Chapter 5
Living Donor Lung Transplantation

Robbin G. Cohen, Mark L. Barr and Vaughn A. Starnes

Introduction

Living donor lobar lung transplantation (LDLLT) was originally developed in the early 1990s, in response to the growing number of patients who were dying while awaiting suitable cadaveric donors for lung transplantation [1]. The procedure involves bilateral lung transplantation using the right lower lobe from one living donor to replace the right lung of the recipient, and the left lower lobe from another living donor to replace the left lung (Fig. 5.1). Because both of the patient's lungs are replaced by lobes from healthy donors, our early experience was confined to children and young adults with cystic fibrosis who, by virtue of their small size, were predicted to receive adequate pulmonary reserve after receiving only two pulmonary lobes. In order to minimize ethical issues regarding the risks of subjecting two healthy donors to a lobectomy for each transplant, only parents or siblings were originally considered as potential donors. Once successful recipient and donor outcomes and safety were established, the use of living lobar lung transplantation

---

R. G. Cohen (✉)
Department of Cardiothoracic Surgery, Keck/USC University Hospital,
USC Healthcare Consultation Center II, Los Angeles, CA 90033, USA
e-mail: rcohen@usc.edu

M. L. Barr
Department of Cardiothoracic Surgery, USC Transplantation Institute,
University of Southern California, Los Angeles, CA 90033, USA
e-mail: mbarr@surgery.usc.edu

V. A. Starnes
Department of Surgery, H. Russell Smith Foundation, Keck School of Medicine of the University of Southern California, Keck Medical Center of USC, Los Angeles, CA 90033, USA

Department of Surgery, CardioVascular Thoracic Institute,
Keck School of Medicine of the University of Southern California,
Keck Medical Center of USC, Los Angeles, CA 90033, USA
e-mail: starnes@usc.edu

J. Steel (ed.), *Living Donor Advocacy*, DOI 10.1007/978-1-4614-9143-9_5,
© Springer Science+Business Media New York 2014

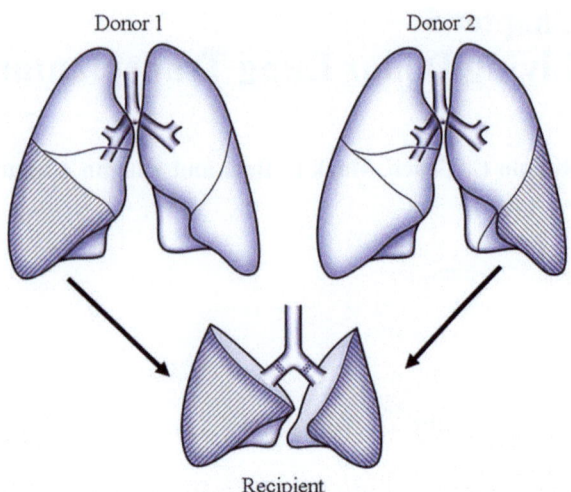

Fig. 5.1 Bilateral living donor lobar lung transplantation. Right and left lower lobes from two healthy donors are implanted in the recipient in place of whole right and left lungs, respectively. (Reprinted from [4], by permission of Oxford University Press)

expanded to include recipients with a wide range of pulmonary diseases, including other suppurative diseases of the lung, as well as pulmonary hypertension, pulmonary fibrosis, and pulmonary obstructive disease. Criteria for lung donation have expanded as well. Whereas the number of living donor lung transplants has decreased in the U.S. due to the success of the lung allocation scoring system implemented by the Organ Procurement and Transplantation Network in 2005, its use has expanded in countries like Japan, where waiting times for cadaveric lungs remain exceptionally long [2, 3].

Patient Selection

The recipient and donor selection process for LDLLT shares much in common with that of cadaveric lung transplantation. The goal is to transplant disease-free lungs that are as immunologically, anatomically, and physiologically compatible as possible in order to ensure the best possible recipient result. Because LDLLT requires that recipient pulmonary function be entirely dependent on two lobes instead of two whole lungs, a more extensive respiratory and anatomical evaluation of both donors and recipients is usually required. The fact that LDLLT utilizes live donors brings psychological and ethical issues into play. These must be carefully considered prior to subjecting healthy volunteers to the risks of major pulmonary surgery.

Recipient Selection

Recipient candidates for LDLLT should meet the criteria for cadaveric lung transplantation, and in the U.S. should be listed on the Organ Procurement and

Transplantation Network lung transplantation waiting list [5, 6]. Given that cadaveric whole lungs are preferable to lobes from living donors, most candidates for living donor lung transplantation should be expected to die or become too ill for transplantation while waiting to receive cadaveric lungs from the waiting list. Approximately 80% of our recipients of living donor lungs, both adult and pediatric, have been transplanted for end-stage pulmonary failure secondary to cystic fibrosis. Other diagnoses include pulmonary hypertension, idiopathic pulmonary fibrosis, bronchopulmonary dysplasia, and obliterative bronchiolitis [7]. Seventy-five percent of adults and 50% of children were hospitalized, and 18% of patients were ventilator dependent at the time of transplantation. In Japan, where cystic fibrosis is rare, interstitial pneumonia is the most common diagnosis, followed by bronchiolitis obliterans, pulmonary artery hypertension, bronchiectasis, and lymphangioleiomyomatosis [3].

Donor Selection

Though living donor kidney and liver transplantation had been performed for some time prior to the first living donor lung transplant, the potential risks associated with pulmonary lobectomy, as well as the need for two healthy donors for each recipient, raised potential ethical issues not previously seen in organ transplantation. In their discussion of the ethics of living donor lung transplantation, Wells and Barr pointed out that donation of a pulmonary lobe by a living volunteer was incompatible with the pillar of medical ethics as established by the Hippocratic maxim "primum non nocere" (first do no harm) [8]. The absence of physical benefit to the donors, coupled with the potential for pain, surgical complications, and long-term pulmonary compromise, required a more complex set of moral theories. These were provided by Beauchamp and Childress [9], who put these issues into the perspective of four basic principles of biomedical ethics:

1. Respect for autonomy: respecting and accepting the decision-making capacity of the autonomous individual.
2. Nonmaleficence (non nocere): minimizing the causation of harm.
3. Beneficence: providing a benefit and balancing this against risk and cost.
4. Justice: fairly distributing benefits, risks, and costs.

Using this framework, it becomes ethically possible to identify healthy donors with adequate pulmonary reserve, appropriate motivation, and an understanding and willingness to accept the risks of donation. Our criteria for donation are as follows:

- Age ≤55 years
- No significant past medical history
- No recent viral infections
- Normal echocardiogram
- Normal electrocardiogram
- Oxygen tension >80 mmHg on room air
- Forced expiratory volume in 1 s and forced vital capacity >85% predicted

- No significant pulmonary pathology on computed tomography (completely normal on donor side)
- No previous thoracic operation on donor side

Whereas we originally considered only parents as appropriate potential donors, we have expanded our criteria to include siblings, extended family members, and occasionally unrelated individuals who can demonstrate an appropriate nonfinancial relationship to the recipient. Potential donors are carefully interviewed and analyzed from a psychological and social standpoint to determine their relationship with the recipient, motivation for donation, ability to withstand the pain and recovery from the operation, and their understanding and ability to withstand a potentially poor recipient outcome. They are also interviewed independently in order to identify potential evidence of coercion or other emotional issues that might exclude them from participating.

After determination of ABO blood group compatibility with the potential recipient, potential donors undergo an anatomic and physiologic evaluation to determine their suitability for donation, and to choose one donor to donate the right lower lobe, and another for the left lower lobe. The evaluation includes a room air arterial blood gas, spirometry, echocardiography, ventilation-perfusion (VQ) scan, and computed tomography (CT) scan of the chest to exclude pulmonary pathology and to allow volumetric assessment of the lobes being considered [10]. Considerable attention must be paid to matching a given recipient with donor lobes that provide adequate function and fit. Undersized lobes run the risk of providing inadequate pulmonary reserve, as well as pleural space problems such as persistent air leaks, pleural effusions, and empyema. Oversized lungs run the risk of atelectasis with subsequent pneumonia, decreased diaphragmatic excursion with poor ventilation, or compression of the contralateral side. Some centers use three-dimensional CT to determine size compatibility of donor lobes and to predict post-transplant graft forced vital capacity [11, 12]. The chest CT scan can also be used to identify anatomic features that can be used to assist in choosing a donor for one side over another. These features might include variations in pulmonary arterial or venous anatomy, or the degree of completeness of the pulmonary fissures. Unilateral pathology, such as small granulomas or blebs, or a history of previous thoracic surgery on one side does not necessarily exclude individuals from donating a lower lobe from the contralateral side.

Operative Description

Bilateral living donor lung transplantation requires the simultaneous use of three operating rooms and operative teams. The recipient operation is performed using cardiopulmonary bypass. In order to minimize both cardiopulmonary bypass time in the recipient as well as ischemic time of the donor lobes, the timing of the three operations is coordinated so that the donor lobes become available when needed by the recipient team. Unlike cadaveric transplantation, the donor teams are responsible for the safety and well-being of the donors, who are both healthy and heroic, as well as for providing grafts that are anatomically and functionally transplantable. Thus, the mindset of the living donor pulmonary surgeon must be one of balance between donor safety and recipient outcome.

Donor Lobectomies

The technical aspects of donor lobectomies are significantly different from lobectomies performed for cancer or other pathology. The donor surgeons must provide the recipient surgeon with grafts containing bronchial and vascular cuffs that are sufficient for surgical implantation using standard surgical anastomotic techniques. At the same time, an adequate margin must be left on each donor side in order to close the lobar bronchus, pulmonary artery, and pulmonary vein without compromising the remaining lungs. Variations in pulmonary vascular and bronchial anatomy, combined with varying degrees of completeness of the pulmonary fissures, can make these procedures challenging. Great care is taken to handle and manipulate the donor lobes as little as possible in order to avoid parenchymal injury that might translate into pulmonary damage or dysfunction in the recipient.

After placement of an epidural catheter for postoperative analgesia, general anesthesia is induced and fiber-optic bronchoscopy performed to exclude bronchial pathology or identify variations in bronchial anatomy. After placement of a double-lumen endotracheal tube, donors are placed in the lateral decubitus position with the operative side up. An intravenous drip of prostaglandin E_1 is initiated and titrated to a systolic blood pressure of 90–100 mmHg in order to dilate the pulmonary vascular bed. A lateral thoracotomy incision is made and the pleural space entered through the fifth interspace. Though we usually start with a relatively small muscle-sparing incision, it is sometimes necessary to enlarge the incision in order to minimize handling of the lobe, as well as maximize safety when dissecting, transecting, and repairing the pulmonary artery and vein. After deflating the lung with the double-lumen endotracheal tube, the lung and pleural space are examined, and a time estimate forwarded to the recipient operating room. Using an atraumatic clamp on the lung for retraction, the inferior pulmonary ligament is incised up to the inferior pulmonary vein. The posterior mediastinal pleura is then incised from the inferior hilum to just below the takeoff of the upper lobe bronchus. After making sure that there are no branches draining either the middle or upper lobes into the inferior pulmonary vein, the inferior vein is circumferentially dissected. Care is taken not to manipulate or injure the phrenic nerve. The pericardium is then opened over the anterior aspect of the inferior pulmonary vein, and then incised circumferentially around the vein in order to maximize the amount of pulmonary venous cuff on the donor lobe. In fact, providing a donor graft with a small amount of left atrial cuff facilitates the venous anastomosis for the implanting surgeon. The pericardium will frequently be adherent to the inferior aspect of the inferior pulmonary vein, making dissection slightly more hazardous in that area. After this point, the dissections of the donor right and left lower lobes differ enough as to require that they be described separately.

Donor Right Lower Lobectomy

After dissecting the inferior pulmonary vein, the pulmonary artery is identified in the fissure between the middle and lower lobes. When the fissure between the middle and lower lobes is incomplete, the dissection is carried out on the middle lobe side of the fissure in order to minimize postoperative air leaks in the recipient. The pulmonary arterial trunk to the lower lobe is circumferentially dissected, identifying the middle lobe arteries as well as the artery to the superior segment of the lower lobe. The ideal anatomic configuration allows placement of a vascular clamp below the middle lobe arteries and above the superior segment artery, with sufficient margin to both close the donor artery as well as provide an adequate arterial cuff for implantation. Early in our experience, we removed and discarded the middle lobe in order to optimize the length of donor arterial cuff. This turned out to result not only in postoperative pleural space problems but also in a waste of donor pulmonary function. Since there are usually two arteries to the middle lobe, one of them can frequently be ligated and transected without significant consequences. We have also occasionally used either pericardial patch extension of the donor pulmonary artery or reimplantation of the middle lobe arteries with good results in order to preserve the middle lobe. It should be noted that the superior segment artery of the lower lobe provides pulmonary arterial flow to a significant portion of the donor lobe, and should be carefully identified and preserved when completing the fissure between the right lower and right upper lobes.

Once the lobar dissection has been completed and it has been determined that the recipient team is ready to receive the lobe, 10,000 units of heparin and 500 mg of methylprednisolone are administered intravenously, and the lung is reinflated and ventilated for 5–10 min to permit the drugs to circulate throughout the lung. During this time, a separate sterile table is set up to receive and perfuse the lobe with preservation solution prior to transporting it into the recipient operating room.

The right lung is then deflated once again so that explantation of the donor lobe can proceed. Once the pulmonary arterial and venous clamps are placed, initiating the graft ischemic time, the lobe is excised expeditiously but carefully and accurately. A difference of as little as a millimeter in vascular or bronchial cuffs can make a significant difference when implanting the donor lobe or closing the vascular and bronchial cuffs on the donor. In order to avoid vascular congestion, an angled vascular clamp is first placed across the donor pulmonary artery before clamping the pulmonary vein. A larger vascular clamp is then placed across the inferior pulmonary vein at the level of the left atrium. The inferior pulmonary vein is then transected, leaving a 2-mm cuff on the donor side that can be safely sutured once the lobe has been removed. Suction should be readily available to keep the blood coming from the partially transected pulmonary vein from obscuring the exposure, so that neither side of the transected vessel will be compromised. The pulmonary artery is then transected in the same fashion, exposing the underlying lobar bronchus.

After identifying the bronchus to the middle lobe, the bronchus to the lower lobe is carefully divided (Fig. 5.2). A no. 15 scalpel is used to open the bronchus just

5 Living Donor Lung Transplantation

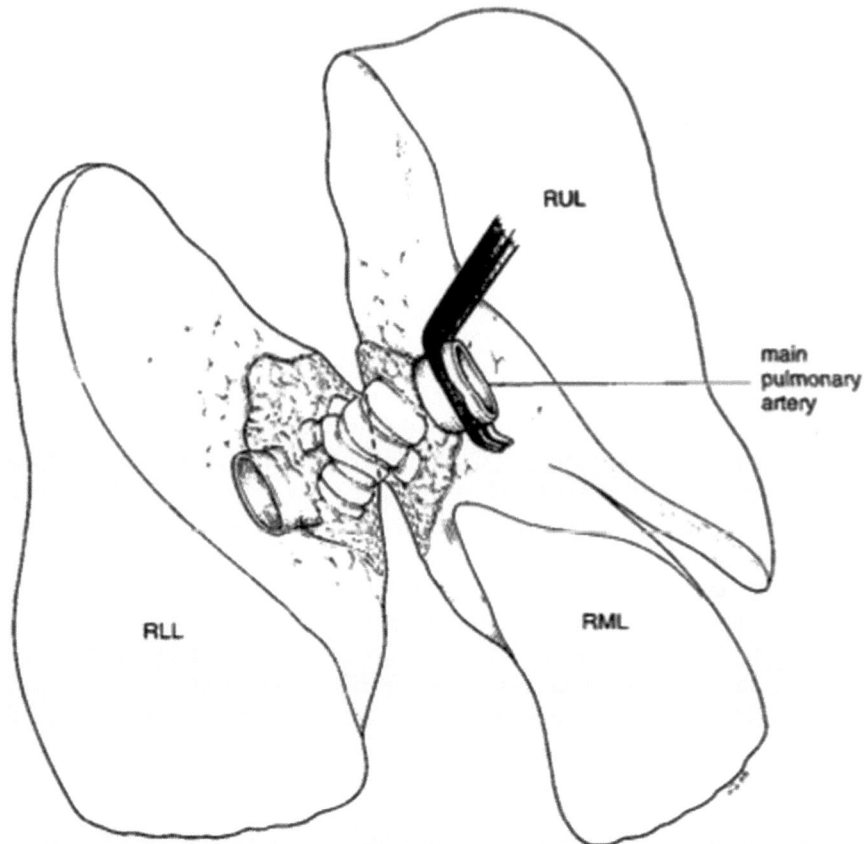

Fig. 5.2 Dissection for donor right lower lobectomy. After transecting the pulmonary artery, a diagonal incision is made across the bronchus to the right lower lobe, being careful not to compromise the right middle lobe bronchus. *RUL* right upper lobe, *RML* right middle lobe, *RLL* right lower lobe. (Reprinted from [13], Copyright 1994)

enough to visualize the inside of the airway, including the takeoff of the bronchus to the superior segment. The remainder of the bronchus is then incised. The angle of the bronchial incision is critical, providing enough bronchial cuff for implantation without compromising the bronchus to the middle lobe. The lobe is then quickly moved to the preservation table for perfusion and then transported to the recipient operating room.

The stump of the donor pulmonary vein is repaired with a double running oversew stitch of 4-0 polypropylene. The pulmonary artery is repaired with a similar double suture using 6-0 polypropylene. Recently, instead of clamping the pulmonary artery and vein, we have had good results with occluding them with the TA-30 vascular stapler (Ethicon Inc.), and transecting those vessels on the graft side of the staple line. This eliminates the need for suture closure of the vascular stumps once the graft has been removed.

After excising the cartilaginous spur at the takeoff of the middle lobe bronchus, the donor bronchus is closed with interrupted 5-0 polypropylene sutures. Excising the cartilaginous spur allows the bronchus to be closed without any tension on the suture line. The pleural space is then irrigated with saline solution and the bronchial stump tested to 30 mmHg with positive pressure ventilation. Two chest tubes are closed and the chest closed in multiple layers.

Donor Left Lower Lobectomy

The initial steps of the donor left lower lobectomy, from positioning and incision through the dissection of the inferior pulmonary vein, are similar as for the right side. Whereas we have seen a more anatomical variation in pulmonary arterial anatomy on the right side, the left donor lobectomy can be challenging due to an incomplete fissure between the left upper and lower lobes, making the separation of the lobes and the identification of the pulmonary artery more difficult. Once the pulmonary artery is identified in the fissure, the superior segmental artery to the lower lobe and anteriorly positioned lingular artery to the upper lobe are identified. The lingular artery may be ligated and divided if it is relatively small and if its location would preclude creating an adequate pulmonary arterial cuff on the donor graft.

After completing the vascular dissection and completing the fissures with staplers, the lung is reinflated and heparin and methylprednisolone are administered. The lung is then deflated, and the pulmonary artery to the lower lobe and inferior pulmonary vein are then occluded with vascular clamps and divided in a fashion similar to the right side (Fig. 5.3). Once the pulmonary artery is divided, the bronchus is exposed and followed superiorly in order to identify the lingular bronchus. The incision on the bronchus begins at the base of the upper lobe bronchus and is carried in a tangential fashion to a spot just superior to the bronchus of the superior segment of the lower lobe. The donor left lower lobe graft is then immediately taken to the preservation table and then either briefly stored in an ice-filled cooler or taken to the recipient operating room for immediate implantation.

Donor Lobe Preservation

Because the donor lobes are harvested simultaneously with the recipient operation at the same institution, ischemic times are shorter for living related lung transplantation when compared with cadaveric lung transplants where the donor is harvested at a distant site. However, in situ flushing of the donor lobes with cold preservation solutions is not possible. This required a separate strategy for post-explantation preservation of the donor lobes. As previously mentioned, a continuous intravenous prostaglandin infusion is initiated at the beginning of the donor lobectomy operation. Once a donor lobe is excised, it is immediately taken to a separate sterile table where it is immersed in a cold crystalloid solution. Care is taken to protect the solution from entering the lobar bronchus. The pulmonary artery, vein, and bronchus are

5 Living Donor Lung Transplantation

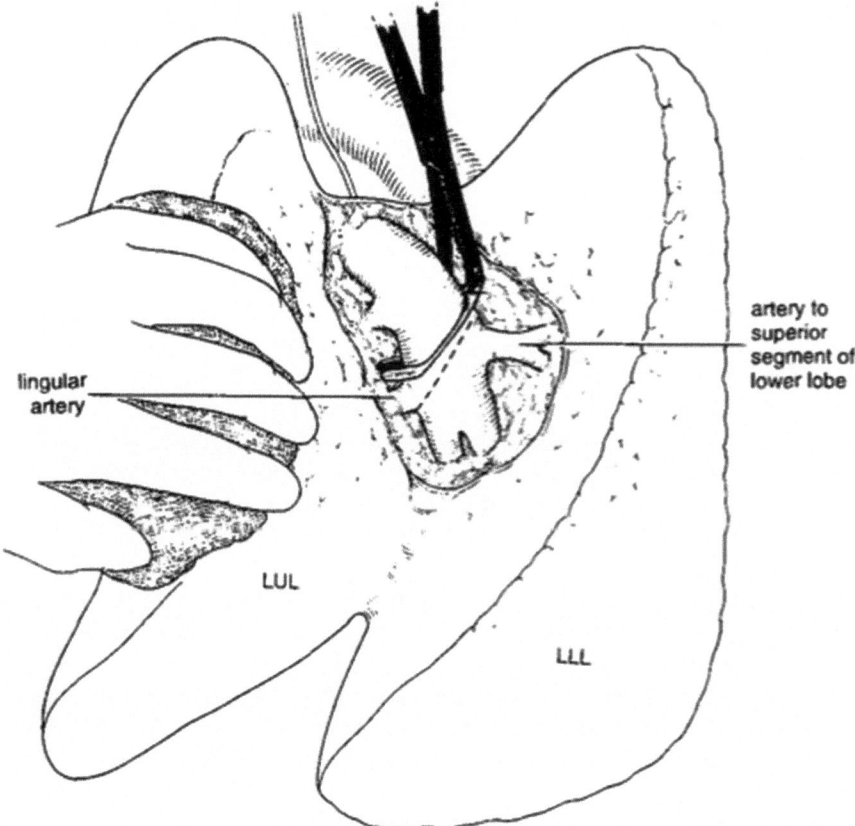

Fig. 5.3 Clamp placement for transection of pulmonary artery on donor left lower lobectomy. *LUL* left upper lobe, *LLL* left lower lobe. (Reprinted from [13], Copyright 1994)

handled with care. The lobar pulmonary artery trunk, which is short and branches early, is cannulated and gently perfused with cold Perfadex (low potassium, dextran, and glucose) solution. The bronchus is simultaneously cannulated and the lobe ventilated, using a manometer to inflate the lobe to a pressure of 20–25 mmHg. The lobe should quickly turn from pink to white and the pulmonary venous effluent from bloody to clear as the lobe is flushed. Selective cannulation of a branch pulmonary artery with a preservation solution or of a branch bronchus with a smaller cannula may be necessary to ensure that all segments of the lobe are both ventilated and perfused. We also routinely perfuse the lobe retrograde through the pulmonary venous stump with 200–300 cc of Perfadex to assure that all parts of the lobe are adequately preserved. Once approximately 1 L of Perfadex has been infused and the entire lobe is homogeneously white, it is approximately 75 % inflated with the endobronchial cannula. A small vascular clamp is then gently placed across the bronchus as the cannula is quickly removed, and the partially inflated graft is placed in a sterile bag filled with cold storage solution. The lobe is then transported to the recipient operation room in an ice-filled cooler for implantation.

Recipient Operation

The recipient operation takes place in a third operating room with the patient in the supine position. The arms are carefully padded, extended, and abducted, and secured to a frame over the face. A bilateral submammary incision (clamshell) is made in the fourth interspace, and the sternum transected in a transverse fashion with an oscillating saw. The internal mammary arteries and veins are identified and carefully clipped or ligated. All recipient operations are performed on cardiopulmonary bypass without cooling. This facilitates and expedites the recipient pneumonectomies, optimizes surgical exposure, and allows for simultaneous reperfusion of both donor lobes. The pulmonary artery and veins are dissected and, if possible, transected at the level of the lobar branches in the hilum of the lungs. This allows the recipient surgeon the option of performing the vascular and bronchial anastomoses between the donor and lobar grafts, using donor structures that more closely approximate the size of the donor lobes. After the recipient pneumonectomies are completed, the pleural spaces are carefully inspected to achieve hemostasis, and then copiously irrigated with antibacterial and antifungal solutions.

It is usually not important which donor lobe is implanted first. The lobe is wrapped in iced, saline-soaked sponges and placed in the recipient pleural space with its hilum aligned with the hilum of the recipient. The bronchial anastomosis is performed using running 4-0 polypropylene sutures, aligning both donor and recipient cartilaginous and membranous bronchi as much as possible (Fig. 5.4). The lobar donor vein is then anastomosed to the superior pulmonary vein of the recipient using a 5-0 polypropylene suture. The suture on the pulmonary venous anastomosis is not tied so that the preservation perfusate can be allowed to escape when initially reperfusing the grafts. The pulmonary artery anastomosis is then performed, also with a 5-0 polypropylene suture. The first lobe to be implanted is then rewrapped in iced sponges and the contralateral implantation performed in a similar fashion.

After completing the bilateral implants, attention is focused on gently reperfusing the grafts. Continuous nitric oxide is initiated at 20 ppm via the anesthesia circuit, as are intermittent doses of aerosolized bronchodilators. The pulmonary venous clamps are removed, followed by the pulmonary arterial clamps. As the lobes begin to reperfuse, the remaining perfusate is allowed to escape from the pulmonary venous anastomoses before tying the sutures. The lungs are then gently inflated by hand bagging, and cardiopulmonary bypass weaned to half flow for approximately 10 min. This regulates the amount of systemic and pulmonary blood flow as the donor grafts are gently reperfused. The recipient is then weaned from cardiopulmonary bypass, and the pulmonary venous flow evaluated with transesophageal echocardiography to assure patency of the venous anastomoses. Bronchoscopy is then performed to remove secretions and to evaluate the patency of the bronchial anastomoses. The recipient is decannulated and the chest closed.

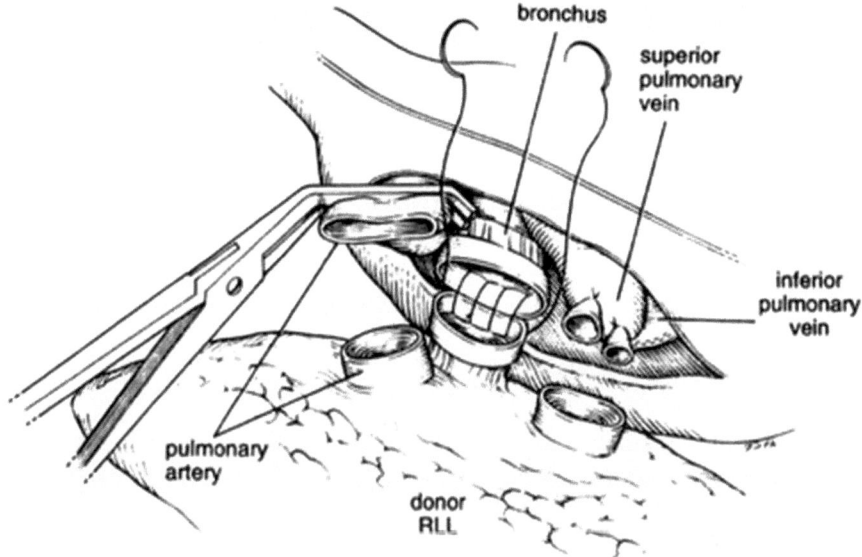

Fig. 5.4 The recipient bronchial anastomosis. (Reprinted with permission from [1])

Postoperative Management

Donor Management

For the most part, donor management is focused on pain control, management of the pleural space on the operative side, prevention of postoperative complications including pulmonary emboli and wound infections, and emotional support. Continuous epidural infusions under the supervision of the anesthesia pain service are the mainstay of pain control. The epidural can be supplemented with nonsteroidal anti-inflammatory agents or oral narcotics as necessary. Epidural catheters are usually removed when a donor's pain is well controlled and the chest tubes have been removed.

Pleural tubes are initially maintained on a suction apparatus but are placed on water seal and then removed when there is no air leak and daily drainage falls below 200 cc/day. Early in our experience, prolonged air leaks (> 7 days) and pleural space problems presented a challenge, especially when both the right middle and lower lobes were removed due to anatomical issues. Prolonged air leaks have become uncommon as we learned to identify potential donors with complete fissures on chest CT, and as we gained more experience with the donor operation.

Emotional support for donors is an important and potentially complicated aspect of living donor lung transplantation. Though significant attention is focused on the preoperative evaluation and education of donors, there is no sufficient way to describe the physical and potential emotional pain that can ensue. This is particularly true when the recipient has a complicated postoperative course, or when a donor's lobe functions poorly, gets infected, or develops rejection in the recipient. When this occurs, a donor's sense of altruism can easily be replaced by guilt. The most dreaded scenario is when a recipient dies in the peri- or postoperative period, leaving the donors to potentially feel as if they have endured significant pain and inconvenience in vain. It is extremely important that a living donor lung transplant program be staffed with social workers, psychologists, and psychiatrists who are prepared for the unique emotional aspects of living donor transplantation. Furthermore, the entire transplant team should be trained to be particularly sensitive to the potential for these issues.

Recipient Management

The pulmonary physiology and early postoperative management of living donor lung transplant recipients is significantly different than for recipients who receive bilateral whole lung cadaveric grafts. Because the pulmonary volumes and vascular beds of the combined transplanted lobes are significantly less than cadaveric lungs, care must be taken to carefully control both ventilation and perfusion of the transplanted lobes. Recipients remain sedated and on the ventilator for at least 48 h, with positive end-expiratory pressures maintained at no more than 5–10 cm H_2O. Because of the potential size mismatch between the donor lungs and recipient pleural space, we have found that conventional chest tube suction at 20 cm H_2O can impair deflation of the transplanted lobes during expiration. This can result in air trapping, increased airway pressures, and increased pulmonary vascular resistance. These phenomena can be prevented by applying what is known at our institution as the "chest tube dance" for the first 24 postoperative hours. Low-level suction (10 cm H_2O) is applied sequentially to each tube, rotating at 1-h intervals. When suction is not being applied to a chest tube, it is placed to water seal. After 24 h, all tubes are placed to suction that is gradually increased to 20 cm H_2O over the subsequent 48 h. Because the transplanted lobes may not completely fill the pleural spaces, chest tube output and the need for prolonged drainage are not uncommon. It is not unusual for chest tube drain to be maintained for 2–3 weeks.

The pulmonary vascular bed of the transplanted lobes is limited when compared with cadaveric lungs. In order to prevent pulmonary edema secondary to overperfusion, recipients are managed in a relatively hypovolemic state, with systemic blood pressures in the range of 90 mmHg. An intravenous nitroglycerin infusion as well as continuous aerosolized nitric oxide are administered for the first 48–72 h of the postoperative period.

Immunosuppression, antibiotic therapy and prophylaxis, and follow-up in our transplant clinic with imaging and pulmonary function testing are similar as for standard cadaveric lung transplant recipients. Bronchoscopy is performed only when clinically indicated by symptoms, changes on imaging, or a decrease in spirometry. Because of the danger of significant parenchymal bleeding, we are reluctant to do transbronchial biopsies unless absolutely necessary.

Clinical Results

Since introducing bilateral living donor lung transplantation in 1992, we have accumulated the largest experience with this procedure in the U.S. at the University of Southern California and Children's Hospital Los Angeles, followed by Washington University in St. Louis. The primary indication for transplantation in the great majority of the patients in the U.S. has been cystic fibrosis, with the remaining recipients having a variety of other diagnoses, including primary pulmonary hypertension and pulmonary fibrosis. At the time of transplantation, many of the patients were critically ill, with most being hospital bound and a significant number being ventilator dependent. Overall, recipient survival in the US cohort has matched that of the International Society for Heart and Lung Transplantation (ISHLT) registry data. Deaths occurring within 30 days of transplantation have been largely due to infection or primary graft failure. Deaths occurring between 30 days and 1 year after transplantation have usually been due to infectious etiologies. Deaths greater than 1 year after transplantation have been predominantly due to infection or bronchiolitis obliterans syndrome. As opposed to cadaveric double lung transplantation in which rejection almost always presents in a bilateral fashion, rejection episodes in the lobar recipients have been predominantly unilateral. There has been no clear pattern with regard to which lobe will be rejected based on the preoperative human leukocyte antigen (HLA) donor–recipient match. Those patients on ventilators preoperatively had significantly worse outcomes [7].

A study of postoperative pulmonary function testing has demonstrated a steady improvement in pulmonary function in those recipients surviving greater than 3 months during the first 12 months post-transplant, which is comparable to cadaveric lung transplant recipients. Maximum workloads at peak exercise, maximum heart rates, peak VO_2, and the ability to maintain oxygen saturation were also similar between living lobar and cadaveric lung transplant recipients. Hemodynamic assessment at 1-year follow-up in a subset of patients demonstrated normal pulmonary arterial pressure and pulmonary vascular resistance, confirming the ability of two lobes to accept a normal cardiac output [14].

With the adoption of the lung allocation score (LAS) system in the U.S. that was instituted in the spring of 2005, the number of lung transplants utilizing living donors steadily decreased over the ensuing 8 years to the point that this operation is now performed only once or twice per year at our institution. However, during the past 10 years, outside of the U.S., this procedure has played a significant role in countries in which there are low rates of deceased donation due to cultural, religious, or legislative barriers to organ availability. Increasing numbers of centers are performing the procedure, with Japan having the greatest annual volumes and smaller activity in Brazil, Canada, China, and parts of Europe. The most recent reports from Japan in a cohort of 100 transplants have yielded an excellent 5-year recipient survival of 81 %, which equals or exceeds any other published survival rates in the field of lung transplantation, regardless of the donor source [15].

With regard to the donors, short-term outcomes were studied by the Lung Working Group of the Vancouver Forum which compiled and published a retrospective review of 550 live lung donors, which constituted 98% of the global experience at that time. In that study, there was no reported perioperative mortality of a lung donor. There were life-threatening complications in 0.5% including intraoperative ventricular fibrillation arrest and postoperative pulmonary artery thrombosis. The mean length of the initial hospitalization following the lung lobectomy was 8.5 days. Approximately 4% experienced an intraoperative complication that included ventricular fibrillation arrest, the necessity for right middle lobe sacrifice, the necessity for right middle lobe reimplantation, the necessity of nonautologous packed red blood cell transfusion, and permanent phrenic nerve injury. Approximately 5% experienced complications requiring surgical or bronchoscopic intervention. These complications included bleeding, bronchopleural fistula, pleural effusion, empyema, bronchial stricture, pericarditis requiring pericardiectomy, arrhythmias requiring ablation, and chylothorax. As much as 2.6% of the live lung donors were readmitted to the hospital because of pneumothorax, arrhythmia, empyema, pericarditis, dyspnea, pleural effusion, bronchial stricture, bronchopleural fistula, pneumonia, hemoptysis, or dehydration. The long-term (defined as greater than 1 year) donor complaints, which were not qualified or quantitated in that study, included chronic incisional pain, dyspnea, pericarditis, and nonproductive cough [16].

In response to the lack of high-quality follow-up information, the National Institute of Allergy and Infectious Diseases (NIAID) is funding an ongoing study of the majority of those individuals who were living lung donors in the U.S. from 1993 to 2006. Preliminary results were recently reported for the retrospective cohort study that assessed short-term morbidity and mortality utilizing the Social Security Death Master File and Scientific Registry of Transplant Recipients databases in 369 lobar donors. A total of 15.7% had in-hospital postoperative complications and 6.5% had a related rehospitalization within 30 days after the donation hospitalization day of discharge. There were no mortalities with a minimal follow-up of 4 years and a maximum of 17 years [17]. The prospective cross-sectional study is currently underway to assess the long-term lung function and psychosocial outcomes [18].

Conclusion

Bilateral living donor lung transplantation has evolved into an alternative to cadaveric lung transplantation for selected patients with end-stage pulmonary diseases, and has been potentially lifesaving for hundreds who might have died while waiting for transplantation with cadaveric donor lungs. The process of evaluating both potential donors and recipients requires a multidisciplinary team with the capacity to address ethical and psychosocial issues, in addition to the medical and surgical issues commonly associated with lung transplantation. Though recipients receive significantly less pulmonary reserve than with cadaveric whole lung transplantation, current results have proven to be adequate for most recipients. The living donor lobectomy has proven to be safe and well tolerated by most donors, though the truly long-term sequelae of being a living lung donor are currently being examined.

References

1. Starnes VA, Barr ML, Cohen RG. Lobar transplantation: indications, technique, and outcome. J Thorac Cardiovasc Surg. 1994;108:403.
2. Egan TM, Murray S, Bustami RT, Shearon TH, McCullough KP, Edwards LB, et al. Development of the new lung allocation system in the United States. Am J Transplant. 2006;6:1212.
3. Date H. Update on living-donor lobar lung transplantation. Curr Opin Organ Transplant. 2011;16:453–7.
4. Date H, Aoe M, Sano Y, Goto K, Kawada M, Shimizu N. Bilateral living-donor lobar lung transplantation. Multimedia manual of cardio-thoracic surgery. 2005 Jan 1;2005(0809).
5. Orens JB, Estenne M, Arcasoy S, Conte JV, Corris P, Egan JJ, et al. International guidelines for the selection of lung transplant candidates: 2006 update—a consensus report from the Pulmonary Scientific Council of the International Society for Heart and Lung Transplantation. J Heart Lung Transplant. 2006;25:745.
6. Barr ML, Starnes VA. Living Lobar Lung Transplantation. In: Sugarbaker DJ, Bueno R, Krasna MJ, Mentzer SJ, Zellos L, editors. Adult Chest Surgery. 2nd ed. New York: McGraw Hill; 2013.
7. Starnes VA, Bowdish ME, Woo MS, Barbers RG, Schenkel FA, Horn MV, et al. A decade of living lobar lung transplantation: recipient outcomes. J Thorac Cardiovascu Surg. 2004;127:114.
8. Wells WJ, Barr ML. The ethics of living donor lung transplantation. Thorac Surg Clin. 2005;15:519.
9. Beauchamp TL, Childress JF. Principles of biomedical ethics. 5th ed. New York: Oxford University Press; 2001.
10. Cohen RG, Barr ML, Starnes VA. . In: Shumway SJ, Shumway NE, editors. Lobar Pulmonary Transplantation. Thoracic Transplantation. Cambridge, MA: Blackwell Science; 1995.
11. Kojimma K, Kato K, Oto T, Mitsuhashi T, Shinya T, Sei T, Okumura Y, et al. Preoperative graft volume assessment with 3D-CT volumetry in living-donor lobar lung transplantations. Acta Med Okayama. 2011;65(4):265–8.
12. Camargo JJP, Irion KL, Marchiori E, Hochhegger B, Hochhegger B, Porto NS, Moraes BG, et al. Computed tomography measurement of lung volume in preoperative assessment for living donor lung transplantation: Volume calculation using 3D surface rendering in the determination of size compatibility. Pediatr Transplantation. 2009;13:429–39.
13. Cohen RG, Barr ML, Schenkel FA, DeMeester TR, Wells WJ, Starnes VA. Living-related donor lobectomy for bilateral lobar transplantation in patients with cystic fibrosis. Ann Thorac Surg. 57:1423–8.
14. Bowdish ME, Pessotto R, Barbers RG, Schenkel FA, Starnes VA, Barr ML. Long-term pulmonary function after living-donor lobar lung transplantation in adults. Ann Thorac Surg. 2005;79:418–25.
15. Egawa H, Tanabe K, Fukushima N, Date H, Sugitani A, Haga H. Current status of organ transplantation in Japan. Am J Transplant. 2012;12:523.
16. Barr ML, Belghiti J, Villamil FG, Pomfret EA, Sutherland DS, Gruessner RW, et al. A report of the Vancouver Forum on the care of the live organ donor: lung, liver, pancreas, and intestine data and medical guidelines. Transplantation. 2006;81:1373–85.
17. Yusen RD, Hong B, Murray SK, et al. Morbidity and mortality of 369 Live Lung Donors. Am J Transplant. 2011;11 Suppl 2:49.
18. Barr ML. 5UO1AI069545-05. http://projectreporter.nih.gov/project_info_description.cfm?aid=7899950&icde=11981871& ddparam=&ddvalue=&ddsub=&cr=1&csb=default&cs=ASC.

Chapter 6
Live Donor Pancreas Transplantation

Miguel Tan

Introduction

The purpose of pancreas transplantation is to restore insulin independence in diabetic patients. Insulin independence allows for a radically improved lifestyle, particularly in those with life-threatening hypoglycemic unawareness. A properly functioning pancreas transplant not only prevents further deterioration of native renal function but can have a protective effect on a concurrent kidney transplant. In some cases, secondary complications of diabetes, such as neuropathy and retinopathy, can be arrested [1].

The pancreas was the first extrarenal organ to be transplanted from a living donor (LD) in 1979 [2]. However, of the more than 20,000 pancreas transplants performed since the advent of the procedure in the 1960s, less than 1% have come from live donors [3, 4].

The lack of popularity of living pancreas donation can be attributed to the potential morbidity of a distal pancreatectomy in an otherwise healthy donor, and the higher technical failure rate compared to deceased donor transplants. In addition, there is the fear of rendering the donor diabetic by reducing their pancreatic mass [5]. In selected cases, however, LD pancreas transplantation may be an appropriate option for highly sensitized recipients who are unlikely to receive a deceased donor organ or uremic diabetics on the simultaneous pancreas–kidney (SPK) waiting list with a particularly long expected waiting time.

Extended waiting time can be a significant issue for uremic diabetics. Diabetic patients on dialysis have increased morbidity and mortality rates compared to non-diabetics on dialysis. The 2- and 3-year mortality rates of diabetics on dialysis are 17 and 27%, respectively, compared to 7 to 8% and 11 to 14% for nondiabetics over the same period of time [6]. Four-year mortality of diabetics on dialysis exceeds 50%.

M. Tan (✉)
Kidney and Pancreas Transplantation, Piedmont Transplant Institute, Piedmont Hospital, 1968 Peachtree Rd. NW 77 Bldg. 6th floor, Atlanta, GA 30309, USA
e-mail: Miguel.Tan@piedmont.org

A rarity today, only a handful of LD pancreas transplants have been performed in the last decade [7]. Historically, LD pancreas transplantation was seen as a way to improve on the high rate of immunologic rejection seen in deceased donor pancreas transplant during the early era of the procedure. However, deceased donor transplantation has improved so significantly over the last 20 years that there is little need to resort to living donation in most cases. Nonetheless, the occasion does arise when living pancreas donation should be considered. The remainder of this chapter will focus on the indications, contraindications, workup, and outcomes of the potential living pancreas donor.

Donor Considerations

The donor operation is a major consideration in performing LD pancreas transplants. The pancreas procurement can be performed using open or laparoscopic techniques. Although open donor distal pancreatectomy can be done safely and is the more established procedure, it is associated with potentially significant postoperative morbidity associated with the bilateral subcostal incision. With the advent of laparoscopic technology, there is an alternative. This has been demonstrated most clearly with laparoscopic donor nephrectomy, which has rapidly become the procedure of choice for kidney donation because of reduced hospital stay and more rapid convalescence [7–9]. Cosmetically, it is more appealing to potential donors compared to the traditional flank incision required for open nephrectomy. It is equivalent to the open procedure in terms of donor safety and quality of allografts [9]. Consequently, laparoscopic techniques have rapidly been applied to other organ systems including the pancreas. Laparoscopic distal pancreatectomies have been described for the treatment of a variety of pathologic states and appear to be safe, with the additional benefits of reduced hospital costs, decreased pain, and accelerated postoperative recovery [10, 11].

Preoperative Donor Evaluation

Metabolic Workup

Because of the potential harm to an otherwise healthy donor, an extensive preoperative workup is essential. The goal is to ensure that the donor can safely undergo donation as well as to ensure that the pancreatic remnant is sufficient to maintain normal metabolic functions. All donors undergo an extensive multidisciplinary evaluation that includes endocrinology, nephrology, cardiology, social services, psychiatry, as well as transplant surgery consultation.

Standard preoperative testing is performed to ensure the medical fitness of the potential donor. This includes electrocardiography (EKG), chest radiography (CXR), as well as biochemical profiles (hemogram, electrolytes, renal function, liver function tests, coagulation profile, and lipid profile) and viral serologies (hepatitis B and C, human immunodeficiency virus (HIV), and cytomegalovirus (CMV)). Panel reactive antibody (PRA) testing and ABO typing are also performed.

In addition, potential pancreas donors are considered only if they fit the following biochemical criteria: body mass index (BMI) <27 kg/m^2, insulin response to glucose or arginine >300% of basal insulin, HbA1C <6%, basal insulin fasting levels <20 μmol/L, plasma glucose <150 mg/L during a 75-g oral glucose tolerance test, and a glucose disposal rate >1% during an intravenous glucose tolerance test. In related donors, no other family members other than the recipient can be diabetic. A genetically related donor (i.e., first-degree relative) should be at least 10 years older than the time of onset of diabetes in the recipient. A history of pancreatic surgery or other pancreatic disorders are also contraindicated. Furthermore, a history of gestational diabetes and BMI greater than 27 kg/m^2 are considered contraindications to donation.

Radiologic Evaluation

Evaluation of the donor's vascular anatomy is undertaken to determine suitability for donation. Magnetic resonance angiography (MRA) is the modality of choice, although computed tomography angiogram (CTA) is also acceptable. MRA appears to be as sensitive as angiography in detecting vascular abnormalities [9]. It is noninvasive in nature, parenchymal details can be visualized, and details of venous anatomy can be seen (Figs. 6.1 and 6.2) [12]. Although angiography may be better at detecting small luminal abnormalities, such as fibromuscular dysplasia, it is associated with complications such as dye allergy, false aneurysms and hematomas at the puncture site, and femoral artery thrombosis [13]. Although the anatomy of the splenic vessels is less variable than the renal vessels, one should try to visualize the takeoff of the splenic artery and the location of the confluence of the splenic vein, inferior mesenteric vein (IMV), and superior mesenteric vein (SMV), since the IMV can sometimes join the splenic vein very close to the portal vein (PV). MRA also allows evaluation of the location and number of renal vessels in the event that a simultaneous nephrectomy is to be done. The decision to procure the left or right kidney is taken on a case-by-case basis and determined by the number and location of accessory renal arteries. Our preference is to procure the left kidney when possible because of the longer renal vein and subsequent ease of dissection of the inferior margin of the pancreas once the upper pole of the left kidney is dissected.

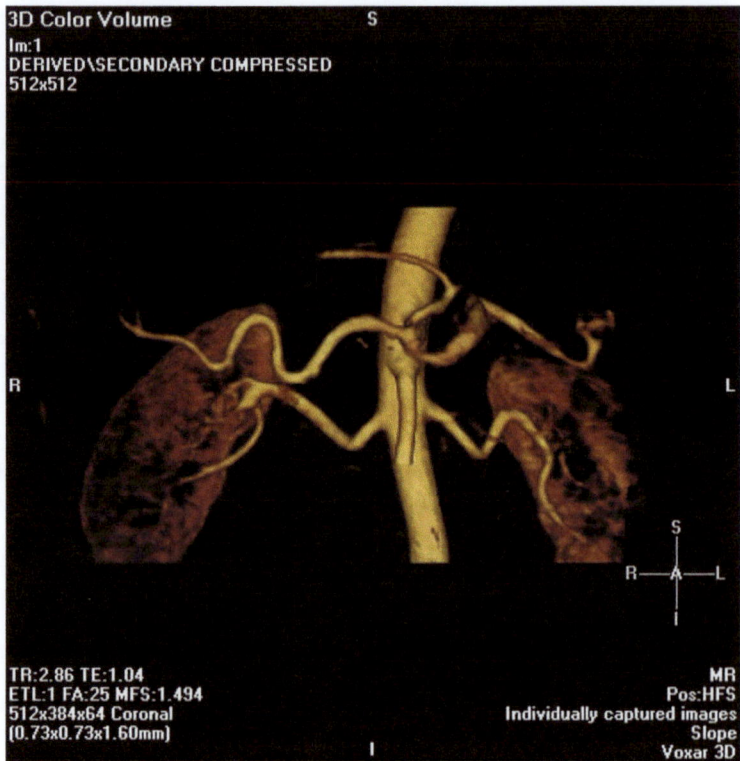

Fig. 6.1 Magnetic resonance angiogram showing anatomy of the splenic and renal arteries. (Reproduced with permission from Humar A, Khwaja KO, Sutherland DER. Pancreas transplantation. In: Humar A, Matus AJ, Payne WD, eds. Atlas of organ transplantation. New York; Springer; 2006)

Operative Considerations

The Donor Operation

Detailed discussion of the operative technique is beyond the scope of this discussion. Procurement of the pancreas (and kidney, in the case of combined kidney–pancreas transplant) may be performed using open or laparoscopic techniques. The decision to perform one or the other is dependent on the surgical experience of the center. Generally, the laparoscopic approach is preferred due to the superior cosmetic outcome and more rapid convalescence of the donor.

In general, we try to preserve the spleen in order to prevent the potential immunologic sequelae associated with a splenectomy, such as overwhelming postsplenectomy sepsis (OPSS). In a series of five laparoscopic donors at the University of Minnesota [14], splenectomy was performed because of a nonviable spleen that was recognized at the time of surgery. Based on the open donor pancreatectomy

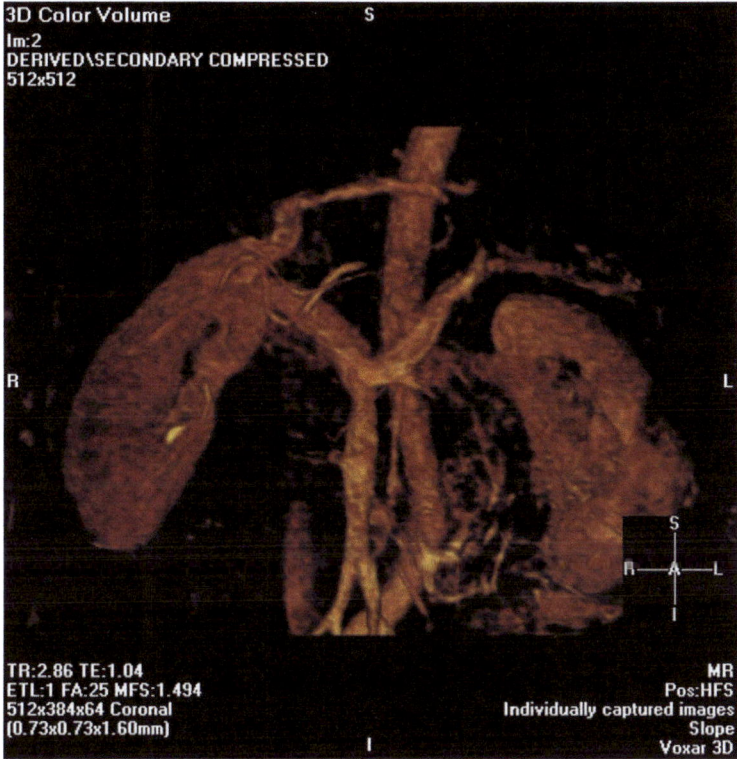

Fig. 6.2 Magnetic resonance angiogram showing anatomy of splenic vein and portal confluence. (Reproduced with permission from Humar A, Khwaja KO, Sutherland DER. Pancreas transplantation. In: Humar A, Matus AJ, Payne WD, eds. Atlas of organ transplantation. New York; Springer; 2006)

data, there is an 8.5–25% rate of splenectomy [15, 16]. At the current stage of evolution of this technique, we prefer the hand-assisted approach, because having tactile feedback greatly facilitates safe dissection and partially overcomes the lack of three-dimensional visualization inherent in laparoscopy.

Postoperative Care of the Donor

Postoperative care of the donor is similar to that of any patient undergoing major abdominal surgery. A nasogastric tube is left in place until return of bowel function. Hemoglobin, serum amylase, lipase, and glucose levels are followed serially. Persistently elevated amylase and lipase levels suggest pancreatitis, a leak, or pseudocyst formation. Persistent or severe left upper quadrant or left shoulder pain should be evaluated with CT and ^{99m}Tc-sulfur-colloid scan of the spleen to assess splenic viability. If the spleen appears infarcted, a splenectomy should be performed.

Donor Outcomes

Open Donor Pancreatectomy

A retrospective study from the University of Minnesota from January 1978 to August 2000 reviewed 115 open LD pancreas transplants: 51 pancreas transplant alone (PTA), 32 pancreas after kidney (PAK), and 32 SPK [16]. There were no donor mortalities. Donor complications can include hemorrhage, splenic infarct, abscess, pancreatitis, and pseudocyst formation. Splenectomy was required in 8% of donors. A recent review documents a rate of splenectomy of 5–15% [17]. Pseudocysts occurred in 10% and percutaneous drainage was necessary in 60%. Within the subset of SPK donors, 20% required perioperative blood transfusions. Two donors required percutaneous drainage of a noninfected peripancreatic fluid collection [18]. The median donor age was 44 years (range 26–49). The median operative time was 6.9 hours with a median length of stay of 8 days (range 6–24) [16].

Long-term follow-up was possible in 67 patients. The remaining 48 could not be located, refused to participate, lived outside of the U.S., or were deceased. Ten donors had abnormal HbA1c levels. Three of them required insulin > 6 years postoperatively. One of these donors had a history of gestational diabetes. The other two had predonation BMI > 27 kg/m^2. Consequently, gestational diabetes and elevated BMI are now considered contraindications to donation. Hyperglycemia, however, may have occurred secondary to development of type 2 diabetes. Since 1996, all donors have maintained normal HbA1c levels (4.9–6.2%) following these guidelines [16].

Laparoscopic Donor Pancreatectomy

From March 1999 to August 2003, five laparoscopic pancreatectomies were performed at the University of Minnesota [14]. The mean donor age was 48.4 years ± 8.7 with a BMI of 23.7 kg/m^2 ± 3.0. The mean length of surgery for PTA donors was 4.5 ± 0.13 hours and for SPK donors, 7.9 ± 0.38 hours. Mean blood loss was 330 mL ± 228. Once the learning curve has been overcome, however, the laparoscopic approach may actually have shorter operative times, as less dissection is required compared to the open technique. In two of the SPK cases, the donor surgical team had to wait 1.5–2 hours for the recipient team to receive the organs, thus prolonging the operative time for the donor. One splenectomy had to be performed at the time of the donor surgery for a nonviable spleen. No pancreatic leaks or pancreatitis was observed. The average serum glucose was 112 mg/dL ± 11.7 upon discharge. The amylase and lipase on discharge were 72.2 U/L ± 26.3 and 67.2 U/L ± 34.0, respectively. None of the donors have required oral antidiabetic medications or insulin. At 3 years follow-up, the mean postoperative HbA1c was 5.7% ± 0.2. One donor refused biochemical follow-up. Postoperative stay for the laparoscopic donors was 8 days ± 2. No obvious statistical advantage was observed in terms of decreased

Fig. 6.3 Surgical incisions 3 weeks post laparoscopic distal pancreatectomy and left nephrectomy. **a** Gelport site; **b** 12-mm camera port site; **c** 12-mm instrument port site. (Reproduced with permission from Humar A, Khwaja KO, Sutherland DER. Pancreas transplantation. In: Humar A, Matus AJ, Payne WD, eds. Atlas of organ transplantation. New York; Springer; 2006)

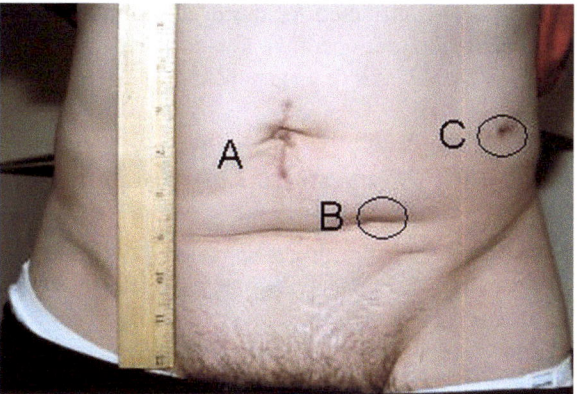

hospital stay. However, based on the first handful of laparoscopic cases performed, this may be a function of over-vigilance on the part of the treating team as tends to occur with new procedures. Certainly, in laparoscopic nephrectomy, the advantages of reduced hospital stay and earlier postoperative recovery have been demonstrated [19, 20]. All the donors have reported that they are back to their preoperative state of health and working. Satisfaction was high in terms of cosmetic result because the donor operation can be performed through a relatively small midline incision and only two trocar sites (Fig. 6.3).

Recipient Outcomes

LD pancreas recipient survival rates were 93 and 90 % at 1 and 5 years, respectively. In the pretacrolimus epoch, technically successful PTA and PAK recipients had a graft survival rate of 68 and 50 %, respectively. The immunologic advantage of LD pancreas transplants, at that time, was clear. Only 13 % of LD pancreas recipients had graft loss secondary to rejection, whereas 41 % of cadaver organ recipients lost their grafts from rejection [16]. In the current immunosuppressive era, this difference hardly exists owing to modern drug regimens (tacrolimus, mycophenolate mofetil), improved operative techniques, and aggressive postoperative anticoagulation. Consequently, although solitary LD pancreas transplants are still performed, the focus is primarily on SPK donors in order to address the shortage of cadaver organs in this subset of pancreas transplant recipients.

Thirty-two open LD SPK transplants were performed at the University of Minnesota from 1994 to 2000 [16]. Patient and kidney graft survival was 100 % at 1 year. Pancreas allograft survival was 87 %. This compares favorably to current cadaver SPK transplant data that demonstrates 84 % 1-year survival for pancreas grafts and 90 % kidney allograft survival [21]. This marked improvement in patient and graft survival, compared to our series of LD PTA and PAK transplants before

1994, may be attributed to improved immunosuppression, routine postoperative anticoagulation (perioperative low-dose heparin and long-term aspirin), and better infection prophylaxis (e.g., gancyclovir) [16].

Recipient Outcomes with Laparoscopic Donor Pancreatectomy

With laparoscopically procured pancreases, patient and kidney graft survival is 100%, with 100% pancreas graft survival at 3-year follow-up [14]. One patient required intermittent subcutaneous insulin postoperatively due to steroids. Once steroids were weaned, insulin requirements ceased. One of five recipients had three episodes of acute rejection that was reversed with steroids and antibody therapy. Four recipients had exocrine bladder drainage; one had enteric drainage. Two recipients had a leak at the duodenocystostomy, and three of five recipients had an intra-abdominal infection.

Conclusion

Although rarely performed, LD pancreas transplantation should be considered in certain difficult-to-transplant diabetic patients and should be in the armamentarium of high-volume pancreas transplant centers with the appropriate expertise.

While the number of available cadaver pancreases currently exceeds the number of pancreas transplants performed each year [22], the waiting list for diabetics awaiting transplantation is growing by more than 15% annually [16]. In the subset of patients awaiting both a pancreas and kidney transplant, the wait time can be lengthy depending on the region of the country. Approximately 6% of these patients die while waiting for an SPK [23]. Compared to patients with nondiabetes-related end-stage renal disease (ESRD), fewer diabetics receive kidney transplants, with a 2- and 3-year mortality rate of dialyzed diabetics at 17 and 27%, respectively [6]. The rationale, therefore, of LD pancreas transplantation, especially LD SPK transplants, is to allow for timely transplantation of high PRA recipients who are unlikely to receive a cadaver graft and to decrease the morbidity and mortality of diabetics on the waiting list.

Although the morbidity and prolonged postoperative recovery on the part of a potential pancreas donor have been a hindrance toward wider acceptance of LD pancreas transplants, use of laparoscopic techniques may make this procedure more appealing. Laparoscopic pancreatectomy appears to be safe, with minimal morbidity and recipient outcomes equivalent or better compared to open techniques of distal donor pancreatectomy. Donor satisfaction is also high in terms of postoperative cosmetic results.

Future Trends

Currently, more institutions are performing robotic-assisted laparoscopic donor nephrectomy. The viability and safety of this modality have been demonstrated in this context [24, 25]. In the future, this may represent the next step in the evolution of laparoscopic donor pancreatectomy because of its advantages over traditional laparoscopic equipment, including better control of fine movements afforded by articulating instruments, as well as elimination of tremor and three-dimensional visualization, which overcomes the lack of depth perception inherent in standard laparoscopic monitors.

References

1. Kennedy WR, Navarro X, Sutherland DE, et al. Neuropathy profile of diabetic patients in a pancreas transplantation program. Neurology. 1995;45(4):773–80.
2. Sharara AI, Dandan IS, Khalifeh M et al. Living-related donor transplantation other than kidney. Transplant Proc. 2001;33:2745–6.
3. Gruessner AC, Sutherland DE. Pancreas transplant outcomes for United States (US) and non-US cases as reported to the United Network for Organ Sharing (UNOS) and the International Pancreas Transplant Registry (IPTR) as of October 2002. Clin Transpl. 2002:41–77.
4. Gruessner RW, Leone JP, Sutherland DE, et al. Combined kidney and pancreas transplants from living donors. Transplant Proc. 1998;30:282.
5. Gruessner RW, Sutherland DE. Simultaneous kidney and segmental pancreas transplants from living related donors—the first two successful cases. Transplantation. 1996;61:1265–8.
6. Gruessner RW. Should priority on the waiting list be given to patients with diabetes: pro. Transplant Proc. 2002;34:1575–6.
7. Tan M, Kandaswamy R, Sutherland DE, Gruessner RW, et al. Laparoscopic donor distal pancreatectomy for living donor pancreas and pancreas-kidney transplantation. Am J Transplant. 2005;5(8):1966–70.
8. Schweitzer EJ, Wilson J, Jacobs S, Machan CH, Philosophe B, Farney A, et al. Increased rates of donation with laparoscopic donor nephrectomy. Ann Surg. 2000;232(3):392–400.
9. Leventhal JR, Deeik RK, Joehl RJ, Rege RV, Herman CH, Fryer JP, et al. Laparoscopic live donor nephrectomy–is it safe? Transplantation. 2000;70(4):602–6.
10. Ueno T, Oka M, Nishihara K, Yamamoto K, Nakamura M, Yahara N, et al. Laparoscopic distal pancreatectomy with preservation of the spleen. Surg Laparosc Endosc Percutan Tech. 1999;9(4):290–3.
11. Vezakis A, Davides D, Larvin M, McMahon MJ, et al. Laparoscopic surgery combined with preservation of the spleen for distal pancreatic tumors. Surg Endosc. 1999;13(1):26–9.
12. Kandaswamy R, Stillman AE, Granger DK, Sutherland DE, Gruessner RW, et al. MRI is superior to angiography for evaluation of living-related simultaneous pancreas and kidney donors. Transplant Proc. 1999;31:604–5.
13. Gruessner RW. Living donor pancreas transplantation. In: Gruessner RW, Sutherland DE, Editors. Transplantation of the pancreas. New York:Springer-Verlag; 2004. 423–40.
14. Tan M, Kandaswamy R, Sutherland DE, Gruessner RW, et al. Laparoscopic donor distal pancreatectomy for living donor pancreas transplantation. Am J Transplant. 2005;5(8):1966–70.
15. Troppmann C, Grussner AC, Sutherland DE, Grussner RW, et al. Organ donation by living donors in isolated pancreas and simultaneous pancreas-kidney transplantation. Zentralbl Chir. 1999;124(8):734–8.

16. Gruessner RW, Sutherland DE, Drangstveit MB, Bland BJ, Gruessner AC, et al. Pancreas transplants from living donors: short- and-long-term outcome. Transplant Proc. 2001;33(1–2):819–20.
17. Reynoso JF, Gruessner CE, Sutherland DE, Gruessner RW, et al. Short- and long-term outcome for living pancreas donors. J Hepatobiliary Pancreat Sci. 2010;17(2):92–6.
18. Humar A, Gruessner RW, Sutherland DE, et al. Living related donor pancreas and pancreas-kidney transplantation. Br Med Bull. 1997;53(4):879–91.
19. Kercher KW, Heniford BT, Matthews BD, Smith TI, Lincourt AE, Hayes DH, et al. Laparoscopic versus open nephrectomy in 210 consecutive patients: outcomes, cost, and changes in practice patterns. Surg Endosc. 2003;17(12):1889–95.
20. Jacobs SC, Cho E, Foster C, Liao P, Bartlett ST, et al. Laparoscopic donor nephrectomy: the University of Maryland 6-year experience. J Urol. 2004;171(1):47–51.
21. International Pancreas Transplant Registry Annual Report. 2002.
22. Sutherland DE, Najarian JS, Gruessner R, et al. Living versus cadaver pancreas transplants. Transplant Proc. 1998;30:2264–6.
23. Gruessner RW, Kendall DM, Drangstveit MB, Gruessner AC, Sutherland DE, et al. Simultaneous pancreas-kidney transplantation from live donors. Ann Surg. 1997;226(4):471–82.
24. Horgan S, Vanuno D, Benedetti E, et al. Early experience with robotically assisted laparoscopic donor nephrectomy. Surg Laparosc Endosc Percutan Tech. 2002;12(1):64–70.
25. Horgan S, Vanuno D, Sileri P, Cicalese L, Benedetti E, et al. Robotic-assisted laparoscopic donor nephrectomy for kidney transplantation. Transplantation. 2002;73(9):1474–9.

Part II
Living Donor Advocacy

Chapter 7
The History of Living Donor Advocacy in Living Donor Transplantation

Talia B. Baker and Helen G. Spicer

> People need to be reminded more often than they need to be instructed.
> Samuel Johnson, English Poet (1709–1784)

In this chapter, we will provide a historical review of the dynamics that have formed the concept of advocacy for living donors. Webster's definition of an advocate is one who pleads the cause of another and it has its roots in the Latin word advocatus, *to summon for counsel* [1]. We use the terms "donor advocate" and "advocacy process" interchangeably. These terms include the tasks of ensuring that the donor is able to understand the information and also include exploring the issues by questioning the understanding of information to test the validity of a decision in an effort to improve the quality of the decision made. These concepts are relevant to kidney as well as extrarenal donation (including living donor liver, lung, intestinal, and pancreas transplants).

We will discuss the landmarks that shaped the past and current thinking in efforts to develop organ transplantation. The major challenges were rejection and suitable organ availability. Transplantation was an unprecedented and unique field in that it depended entirely on the availability of human organs for replacement.

In 1954, the successful transplant of identical twins in Boston proved the feasibility of the surgical procedure for kidney transplant. The ability to find a genetically identical living donor provided the basis for understanding and modulating the immunology of the transplant. It also began to set up the standards for informed consent for living donors and the necessity for a multidisciplinary team with specific

---

T. B. Baker (✉)
Department of Transplant Surgery, Northwestern Memorial Hospital,
676 N. St. Clair Street Suite 1900, Chicago, IL 60611, USA
e-mail: tabaker@nmh.org

H. G. Spicer
Kidney Transplant Services, Henrico Doctors' Hospital,
1602 Skipwith Road, Richmond, VA 23229, USA
e-mail: helen.spicer@hcahealthcare.com

J. Steel (ed.), *Living Donor Advocacy*, DOI 10.1007/978-1-4614-9143-9_7,
© Springer Science+Business Media New York 2014

members assigned to the donor's care. The ethical psychosocial review in this case set the framework for the discussions that would ultimately be developed into the process of donor advocacy. This included discussions of workup, perioperative and after care of any potential living donor [2].

The decade of the 1960s was remarkable for the development of the tools needed to support the expansion of kidney transplantation from identical twins as donor sources to include human leukocyte antigen (HLA)-mismatched living donors and deceased donors. These efforts included advances in organ preservation, tissue typing, medication discoveries, and organizational efforts to allocate deceased donor organs. It also began to consider measures to improve the collection and review of clinical information that would lead to improving and prolonging human life.

The decade of the 1970s was marked by the development and expansion of deceased donor kidney transplants, specifically. There were legislative efforts to promote organ donation and use in all types of organ replacements. The ultimate goal, many believed, was to not depend on living donors who would have to be exposed to excessive risk. Unfortunately, however, at the end of the decade there was a view that this may not be a reasonable endeavor, as living donor kidneys seemed to have significantly superior long-term graft survival as compared to matched deceased donors.

The decade of the 1980s started with a major scientific discovery of the drug cyclosporine. The discovery of this novel immunosuppressant changed the landscape of transplantation, both of renal and of extrarenal organs [3]. Deceased donor kidney transplant 1-year success rates improved from 50 to 89% [4]. With this improved graft survival, however, the transplant community was suddenly faced with a shortage of deceased donor organs. This, in turn, created a need for a central distribution system for the available organs. Living donation emerged as an important and essential means to provide the needed organs.

The decade of the 1990s brought an increase in the general understanding and distribution of knowledge for improving organ survival and patient survival. There were many efforts to increase the use of all deceased donor organs, including expanding the acceptance criteria for both donors and candidates for organ transplant. The gap in the need for organs continued to be filled with living donation, now including living donor transplantation of liver, lung, and intestines. There were concomitant developments in novel complex protocols to reduce the incidence of rejection in highly sensitized patients. By the end of the decade, one in five organs transplanted were from living donors. In 1999, the National Kidney Foundation launched their End the Wait campaign. One goal was to increase the use of living donors in a preemptive kidney transplant scenario [5].

The last decade was a time to take stock of the current status of living donor care. The transplant societies published many consensus papers indentifying best practices in the care of the living donor. The concept of living donor teams and an independent living donor advocate was emerging. The living donor care provider is identified among multiple disciplines and is in the process of developing into a subspecialty. In 2010, the American Foundation for Donation and Transplantation (former South-Eastern Organ Procurement Foundation, SEOPF) began offering training programs for living donor team members. In 2012, The American Society of Transplantation organized a community of practice for the living donor team members. Furthermore, several unfortunate and highly publicized donor deaths attracted the attention of the regulatory agencies. This resulted in regulations at the federal level and, in some cases, at the state level that mandated the inclusion of living donor advocates and living donor teams.

Currently, the role of the living donor advocate is coded into Centers for Medicare & Medicaid Services (CMS) regulations. The Department of Health and Human Services Centers for Medicare and Medicaid Services issued the Conditions of Participation for Organ Transplant programs to be in effect from June, 2007.

The regulations that define the role and responsibility of the living donor advocate are listed in Appendix 7.1, at the end of this chapter.

Kidney transplant from a living donor was first performed successfully in 1954, marking the beginning of the modern era for transplantation. It is instructive to review in detail the social and political contexts that preceded and followed this event. This is a story of the American entrepreneurial spirit that fosters innovation. Once the processes mature, they are recommended for standardization as the best practices and from there they are brought forward to be codified by regulators for compliance. This is clearly the direction that health care is taking as we move to develop accountable care organizations in an effort to define appropriate care for specific disease states and the limits to this care. Transplantation as a discipline, therefore, offers a 50-year history that can help inform our current health care debates.

1947–1959

To fully understand the unique set of forces that led to the development of transplantation in America, it is necessary to begin in the years after World War II. There were many medical discoveries that were seeds to medical advances that occurred in the next two decades. The American cultural changes were rapid and equally dramatic. The role of the physician, the entrepreneurial spirit that was encouraged in the use of public funds for medical research, the coverage of medical care, the right to the understanding of medical procedures—risks and benefits—and the concept of right to health care in the midst of national political debate on the role of government regulations provide a uniquely American story [6].

At the end of World War II, several clinical discoveries were influential in developing kidney transplantation. Dr. Wilhelm Kolff developed the hemodialysis technology during his confinement by the Germans during World War II [2]. Dr. Peter Medawar worked out details on first and second set reactive antibodies that began the science of immunology and the pharmacology of immunosuppressant medications.

In the book, *Surgery of the Soul: Reflections on a Curious Career,* Dr. Joseph Murray details the issues that were addressed in the early days of the experimental years of developing the clinical reality of kidney transplantation. The success of the deceased donor transplant was not possible. This had been demonstrated by the understanding of the body's innate ability to reject foreign protein. It had been known that skin grafts from identical twins would not reject. Therefore, it made sense that the beginning of the experiment of kidney transplantation would require an identical twin pair.

This created the immediate ethical dilemma: "First, do no harm." The balance between doing well and having to outweigh the potential harm was at the core of medical ethics. The only way to perform a living donor kidney transplant was to obtain a kidney from a suitable living person. There was clearly no medical gain for the donor while the potential for harm was significant.

The story of the living donor transplant at the Brigham and Women's Hospital is an appropriate starting point for the understanding of the origins of donor advocacy in transplant care.

Ronald and Richard Herrick were twins. Ronald's brother was diagnosed with glomerulonephritis at age 21. He was admitted to Peter Bent Brigham Hospital in October, 1954. He was disoriented and extremely uncooperative. The psychiatrist noted in the chart "Impression: toxic psychosis reaction superimposed on paranoid personality....I feel the patient will recover from his psychosis with the use of medications and the removal of toxic agents by dialysis" [2].

Dr. Murray relates the processes required to ensure that they were indeed identical twins. This included fingerprinting, genetic testing, and, finally, reciprocal skin grafting. The skin grafts showed no signs of rejection after 4 weeks. This was proof of the genetic identity [2].

Before offering the option of transplantation to Richard, Ronald, and their family, the medical and surgical team consulted experienced physicians inside and outside the University, clergy of all denominations, and legal counsel. Dr. Murray describes several meetings with the family to review the details of preparations for surgery, anesthesia, surgical procedure, possible complications, and anticipated results of the transplant. There were several meetings over time. The family was encouraged to ask any question [2].

Ronald, the identical twin donor, relates: "I had heard of such things, but they seemed to be in the realm of science fiction." He describes feeling excitement as well as fear. The thought of being cut open and having an organ removed was, in his words, "shocking" [2]. Henry Fox, Chief of Psychiatry, noted, "I think we have to be careful not to be too much swayed by our eagerness to carry out a kidney transplant successfully for the first time…seems to be whether we as physicians have the right to put the healthy twin under the pressure of being asked whether he is willing to make this sacrifice. I do not feel that we have this right in view of the potential danger to the healthy twin as well as the uncertainty of the outcome for this patient" [2].

At the last preoperative family conference, Ronald asked whether the hospital would assume responsibility for his health care for the rest of his life. Dr. Harrison (the donor surgeon) replied, "Of course not." However, he immediately followed this declaration with a question: "Ronald, do you think anyone in this room would ever refuse you care if you needed help?" Ronald paused, and then realized that his future health care depended upon our own sense of professional responsibility rather than on legal assurances [2].

The processes described within the account by Dr. Murray set up the professional standards that represent the donor advocacy functions that have been coded into regulations today.

1. There was a team approach to the care of the donor and the recipient.
2. There were multiple meetings with the entire family to outline in detail the procedures and potential outcomes. The donor was present to hear about the reality of the success of this procedure for the recipient.
3. There were psychiatric evaluations for both the donor and the recipient.
4. There were ethical discussions related to the risk to the donor and whether it was right to ask him to take this risk.
5. The donor was able to seek counsel from team members, some of whom agreed and some who did not.
6. There was a separate medical and surgical team for the donor and the recipient. The donor and recipient surgeons were in communication in the operating room. They viewed this process as a continuum: from the donor removal to the recipient implantation, a well-orchestrated procedure that would ensure the success of the procedure. Every detail was important.
7. The final note is the long-term follow-up of the living donor: Who would not be willing to care for the donor if he needed care?

This account of the deliberations and the issue of long-term care for the donor are relevant to our 2013 professional and regulatory debates.

1960–1969

This decade's theme song could be Bob Dylan's "the times they are a changing." The election of John F. Kennedy signaled a country embarking on changes in every aspect of American life. Under the Kennedy and later under the Johnson administrations, there was an array of political and social changes. The passage of Medicare health care coverage in 1965 for those over 65 provided the first steps toward greater access to health care coverage for all citizens.

The success of the identical twin transplants and the public support of the autonomy for medical research set the stage for the remarkable acceleration of key advances in the necessary components for the treatment of end-stage kidney disease in the decade of the 1960s.

At the beginning of this decade, kidney failure was a terminal disease. By the end of the decade, there was the demonstrated ability to provide chronic dialysis, success with living donor and deceased donor transplants, kidney preservation pumps, beginning of immunology, use of cytotoxic crossmatching to identify donors, and use of medications to control rejection. However, there was no way to take this from research to routine practice without a way to pay for the care. Health care financing was provided in several ways. There was care provided by public health research grants given to specific centers involved in research projects. Labor unions, other fraternal organizations, charitable organizations that assisted in initial funding, and the rise of Blue Cross and Blue Shield provided care for those employed. The Veterans Benefits Administration provided care for those who had military service [6].

1970–1979

The major achievement in this decade was funding a system to support kidney dialysis and transplantation. Nixon was elected president in 1968. America was a divided nation. The war in Vietnam had taken center stage as a major issue to be resolved. In addition, the cost of health care was continuing to rise.

Professional organizations were developed in support of dialysis and transplantation. The Southeastern Regional Organ Procurement Program (SEROPP) was founded in 1969 by Dr. David Hume, Chief of Surgery at Medical College of Virginia in Richmond, and Dr. Bernard Amos, Director of Immunology Laboratory at Duke University. Their interest in testing the utility of tissue typing in conjunction with organ allocation attracted other centers to join. Johns Hopkins and the University of Virginia were followed by five other centers from Washington, DC, to Georgia. The organization became SEOPF. The initial funding was provided by a grant from the Public Health Service [7].

At the national level, hearings were convened by the Department of Health, Education and Welfare to obtain input from transplant surgeons concerning the Social Security Act of 1972. This act, later signed into law, established the End-Stage Renal Disease (ESRD) Program. The hearings offered a way to provide the care required for ESRD. Shep Glazer's testimony while receiving hemodialysis noted issues of lack of funding, which resulted in the death of individuals because they had to stop dialysis. Patients' request was for payment to cover the cost of dialysis, kidney transplantation, and organ procurement for deceased donors and live donation [3].

Public financing was proposed via Medicare entitlement. The inclusion of kidney transplant offered a way to reduce the cost of this chronic disease, as the kidney transplant would allow the recipient to recover and return to gainful employment and therefore not require Medicare funding for the treatment [8].

This funding was approved and became available in 1973. It supported the continued growth of the ESRD care. This reinforced the belief that lobbying for a specific disease had more opportunity for success [6].

The American Society of Transplant Surgeons had their first meeting in 1974. At the fourth annual meeting in 1978, there were 29 transplant programs with fellowship training. There were five pharmaceutical companies acknowledged as supporting the meeting. Two presentations of interest noted the difficulties faced in this decade.

In a single-center study from the University of Minnesota, a review of the 2-year patient and graft survival in 767 kidney transplants performed between January 1, 1968 and September 1, 1977 clearly demonstrated the superior results of HLA-identical sibling into a nondiabetic recipient at 98% patient survival and 92% graft survival compared to the diabetic sibling at 87 and 86%, respectively. The living donor organs were noted as being from related donors. The data demonstrated that the better the HLA matching the better the outcome. The cadaveric transplants had graft function noted from a high of 60% to a low of 36%. It was noted that in a nondiabetic recipient of age 50 years or greater, the survival can be increased from 47% with a cadaveric graft to 90% if the kidney is from a living related child [9].

The second paper was an analysis of the cost of renal transplant. This was a response to a paper in the *New England Journal of Medicine* that suggested that the cost reduction from dialysis might be at the expense of decreased life expectancy. The paper reviewed 446 transplants performed at the University of California, San Francisco, between September 1972 and August 1976. The outcomes for the living related donor were 100% at 1 year and 98% at 2 years. The average length of hospital stay was 21 days for a living donor recipient and 23 days for a cadaveric recipient. The costs were US$6,340 for cadaveric and US$7,495 for living donor, respectively. The conclusion was that the patient survival and the actual cost of care clearly constitute a way to reduce the cost of the medical expenditures [10].

This decade has the recipient of a living donor as the patient with the most promise of success. The donors were selected from within family units. The many eligible patients without a living donor felt they were better off on dialysis [3].

At the end of the decade, in a paper published in *Transplant Proceeding*, March 1979, Dr. Melvin Williams noted the discouraging survival rates in kidney transplantation. He noted that, in the field of transplant, there was a unique situation in which the technical prowess of the surgeon had no relationship to graft survival. He outlined the lessons learned during the decade and noted that HLA testing held the key to success with living donors. The key was to find out the immunological processes that would improve cadaveric transplants. An additional goal was to improve patient and graft survival beyond 3 years [11].

1980–1989

The discovery of cyclosporine ushered in the modern era of transplantation. The researchers at Sandoz were on a routine review for antibiotics and anti-cancer agents [3]. In the beginning of 1970, they increased this effort, investigating 20 new agents per week. A fungus sample was brought in by a Sandoz researcher from a holiday visit to Scandinavia in 1970. By the end of 1973, the immunosuppressant effects of the sample were demonstrated. Sandoz was hoping to develop drugs to assist in the treatment of inflammatory diseases. They named the drug cyclosporine, as it was found in a spore and contained a cyclical peptide. The drug was approved by the Food and Drug Administration (FDA) in 1983 and was rapidly adopted by transplant centers [3]. There was a learning curve in the use of this drug. There was a rapid development of protocols that allowed for the decrease in the amount of drug by combining previous immunosuppression agents, including prednisone and Imuran.

The success rates also were evident in the extrarenal organ transplants. The liver and heart transplant programs were able to provide more patients with a successful transplant. However, there was no organized system for organ allocation or payment for these "experimental" procedures [3, 12].

The Department of Health and Human Services (DHHS) expressed concern over the lack of a system to evaluate emerging medical technologies. During this hearing, the kidney transplant community noted that the lack of suitable kidneys for transplantation had not gotten this attention because the kidney was not viewed as a life-saving organ: "However this is the plight of many thousands of patients waiting at 150 transplant hospitals over the past decade..." [13].

Mel Williams, MD, noted that the shortage was likely to be based on lack of adequate systems for organ procurement as well as negative public attitudes to organ donation [14].

Transplant procurement coordinators noted the never-ending struggle to educate the hospital nursing staff and physicians in the care of potential donors. There did not seem to be an understanding of the plight of those awaiting a transplant [14].

C. Everett Koop, MD, Surgeon General, representing the view of President Ronald Reagan, stated that the DHHS would assist a private sector in organizing systems to address the problem: "I would like to keep away from regulatory suggestions and offer an educational alternative to improve organ donation" [14, 15].

Public Law 98-507, "The National Transplantation Act" (1984), provided the basis for the Organ Procurement Transplant Network (OPTN). The SEOPF was awarded the bid as a private vendor to supply the requirements of the government contract, what is known today as the United Network for Organ Sharing (UNOS). This created the structure for rapid development of the organ allocation systems for each organ based on established principles and clinical research.

In the era of improved graft survival with deceased donor transplants, there were statements by some programs that the use of living donation would decline. There were centers that would only use living donors if there was a decided advantage in long-term results such as HLA-identical siblings. In a paper published in 1986 entitled, "The Living Kidney Donor Alive and Well," Aaron Spital, MD, noted that improvement in the access to dialysis and the results of cadaveric transplants had changed the view of risk vs. benefit for living donation. In a report of a survey of 52% of the transplant programs in the U.S., all centers reported the use of living donors. Sixteen percent used unrelated donors, and 40% stated that they would allow spouses to donate. In their report, they noted there were other advantages to the use of the living donor, including immunological conditioning and logistical planning. The review of reasons for a willing donor to be disqualified included a large percentage of reasons of immunological incompatibility. This could be remedied by a living donor exchange program. In conclusion, there was support of the continued

7 The History of Living Donor Advocacy in Living Donor Transplantation 111

use of living donors as the data continued to endorse the long-term success obtained by their use [16].

The decade ended with living donors supplying 20% of the total kidney transplants. Liver transplant noted 2 out of 2,202 transplants from living donor sources (UNOS/OPTN data).

1990–1999

Bill Clinton was elected president in 1993 and served until 2001. The implementation of the landmark legislation that created the OPTN proved controversial, especially among the liver transplant centers. As the work groups strived to create objective measures to allocate the available livers, there were changes in access to the organs. Local interests were evident in the arguments to allow the allocation to remain in the local area before being shared beyond the local boundaries. There was further lobby from the federal government. Al Gore, then Vice President, had disagreed with the original plan to keep control in the private sector [17]. The outcome of this discussion became known as the Final Rule. This gave guidance to the efforts to improve allocation to a larger geographical area [18].

The effort to increase the organ donation rate resulted in impressive gains. The rate of donation rose from 13,140 at the end of 1989 to 22,026 at the end of 1999. This was a 67.6% increase. The living donor number increased as well: kidney, from 1,903 at the beginning of 1990 to 4,721 in 1999; a 148% increase. This proved to be an answer to the organ shortage for this life-saving surgery.

The use of living donors to supplement the need for transplant was growing. The acceptance of spousal and nonrelated donation increased based on data from the Terasaki registry, noting that living unrelated donors had graft survivals equal to one haplotype siblings. This was an improvement over the cadaveric donor [19].

The search to improve the morbidity of postoperative recovery for the living donor resulted in the development of the laparoscopic approach to donor nephrectomy pioneered by Dr. Lloyd Ratner [20]. This approach was adopted by centers with expertise in minimally invasive surgical techniques and it eventually replaced open nephrectomy as standard of care. This dramatically improved the recovery time and length of stay for the donor.

2000–2013

The use of living donors was increasing. In 1998, there were 4,545 living kidney donors. This represented one out of five donors for all transplants [21]. A consensus conference sponsored by grants from the National Kidney Foundation, American Society of Transplantation, American Society of Transplant Surgeons, American Society of Nephrology, the UNOS, and the National Institutes of Health was organized in June

2000. The notice on the National Kidney Foundation's website remarked that living donor transplants are a fast-growing trend in the U.S., which raises serious medical and psychosocial questions and concerns. The conference featured analysis, debate, and consensus development, with the goal of maximizing the opportunity for successful transplantation. A consensus statement on the live organ donor was published in the *Journal of the American Medical Association*, December 2000. In the introduction to the paper, the authors noted the increase in the use of live donors for renal and extrarenal organs. This need was based on the continued shortage of cadaver organs. As part of the recommendations to ensure informed consent and voluntary decision, an "independent advocate whose only focus is the best interest of the patient" was deemed a necessary member of the evaluation team. In addition, there was a recommendation for a separate medical team for the donors [22]. This report has been the basis of many subsequent consensus reports as well as being encoded into regulations.

On the political front, "HHS Secretary Donna E. Shalala announced creation of an Advisory Committee on Organ Transplantation (ACOT) to strengthen scientific, medical and public involvement in the department's oversight of transplantation policy. In particular, the new committee will provide independent review and advice to HHS concerning revised organ allocation policies being developed by the nation's transplantation network. It was noted that the new committee, to be formed this fall, was recommended by the Institute of Medicine (IOM) in a report mandated by Congress in 1998" [23].

In 2002, ACOT made the following recommendations to the HHS related to living donation to improve safety:

Recommendation 1 That the following ethical principles and informed consent standards be implemented for all living donors.

The person who gives consent to becoming a live organ donor must be:

- Competent (possessing decision making capacity)
- Willing to donate
- Free from coercion
- Medically and psychosocially suitable
- Fully informed of the risks and benefits as a donor
- Fully informed of the risks, benefits, and alternative treatment available to the recipient

Recommendation 2 Each institution that performs living donor transplantation should provide an independent donor advocate to ensure that the informed consent standards and ethical principles described above are applied to the practice of all live organ donor transplantation.

Recommendation 3 A database of health outcomes for all live donors should be established and funded through and under the auspices of the U.S. Department of Health and Human Services.

Recommendation 4 A serious consideration should be given to the establishment of a separate resource center for living donors and their families.

Recommendation 5 The present preference in OPTN allocation policy—given to prior living organ donors who subsequently need a kidney—should be extended so that any living organ donor would be given preference as a candidate for any organ transplant, should one be needed [24].

In 2002, a tragic death of a living liver donor at Mt. Sinai Hospital in New York heralded a change in the public attitude toward living donation and the postoperative care.

This resulted in a detailed report entitled "New York State Committee on Quality Improvement in Living Liver Donation, A Report to: New York State Transplant Council and New York State Department of Health December 2002." This document outlined the role of an independent living donor team [25].

There were additional consensus conferences organized with a different focus on the evaluation and management of the living donor:

2004—The Consensus Statement of the Amsterdam Forum on the Care of the Live Kidney Donor. This report detailed the medical evaluation of the living kidney donor. The goal was to have this adopted as an international standard [26].

2006—The Ethics Statement of the Vancouver Forum on the Live Lung, Liver, Pancreas, and Intestine Donor [27].

2008—The Declaration of Istanbul was published in response to the World Health Assembly urging that member states take measures to protect the poor and vulnerable from transplant tourism and to address the wider problem of international trafficking of human organs and tissues. The inclusion of these issues as pertains to donor protection and donor rights has certainly added to and broadened the role of the independent donor advocate [14].

Conclusion

We believe that it is essential to develop a living donor team that uniquely serves the needs of the living donors through all phases of the donation experience. There is an increasing necessity to identify testing, follow-up care, and long-term monitoring of every living donor. The requirement of a transplant center where living donations are performed to provide a donor advocate as an integral part of the care in selection as well as after care is unquestionable. The role of the living donor will certainly continue to evolve and requires active and ongoing commitment and research

Appendix 7.1

Center for Medicare and Medicaid

Standard: living donor selection
The living donor selection criteria must be consistent with the general principles of medical ethics. Transplant centers must carry out the following procedures.

Ensure That a Prospective Living Donor Receives a Medical and Psychosocial Evaluation Prior to Donation

Instructions to the surveyor:

For a center that performs living donor transplants, verify that the transplant program's policy requires that prior to donation the prospective living donor receives a medical and psychosocial evaluation that is completely independent of the recipient evaluation. An *independent evaluation* requires that the transplant recipient (or other individuals vested in the recipient's transplant) may not be present during the donor's psychosocial and medical evaluation. The donor and recipient evaluations must be filed in respective individual medical records and must not be dually documented in both medical records.

The transplant program's policy is expected to: (1) indicate the length of time in which the medical and psychosocial evaluations are deemed to be current; (2) identify the type of qualified health care professional(s) who may complete these evaluations; and (3) include the follow-up and referral procedures if a living donor requires such activities.

The post-June 28, 2007, sample of living donor medical records to verify that the psychosocial and medical evaluations were completed independently from the evaluations of the transplant recipient: were done within the time frame established by the program's policy; completed prior to the donation; and performed by the person(s) identified in the transplant program's policy as qualified to conduct such evaluations.

The medical evaluation is expected to address not only the living donor's medical suitability for donation, but also any of the donor's health issues that would be affected by the donation: for example, if the donor were taking any medications treating an existing condition and this medication regimen would have to be stopped or altered for any period of time following the donation.

While the transplant program has flexibility in the specific psychosocial tool to be used, the psychosocial evaluation is expected to be completed and to be focused on the individual's suitability for donation. It is expected that a psychosocial evaluation of this nature would address the following:

1. Social, personal, housing, vocational, financial, and environmental supports
2. Coping abilities and strategies
3. Understanding of the risks of donation
4. Ability to adhere to a therapeutic regimen
5. Mental health history, including substance or alcohol use or abuse and how it may impact the donor following the donation

Document in the Living Donor's Medical Records the Living Donor's Suitability for Donation

Instructions to the surveyor:

Review the sample of living donor medical records to verify that each donor's suitability for donation is documented. At a minimum, the surveyor will verify that there was a discussion by the multidisciplinary team (which would include the independent living donor advocate) of the relevant findings of the medical and psychosocial evaluations and the impact of those findings on the donor's suitability for donation.

If the multidisciplinary team has a meeting to discuss the donor's suitability for donation, this would comply with the requirements of the regulation. If there is not an actual meeting by the multidisciplinary team, then there must be evidence in the medical record and/or other documentation that there is a formal process for all members of the multidisciplinary team to raise concerns and discuss any issues that they may have regarding the donor's suitability.

This process must be managed such that:

1. There is clear written evidence that multidisciplinary team members have reviewed, discussed, and are aware of one another's concerns about the donor's suitability.
2. There is a process for the members of the multidisciplinary team to register their agreement/disagreement regarding the donor's suitability.

Document that the Living Donor has Given Informed Consent, as Required Under § 482.102

Instructions to the surveyor:
The medical record should provide evidence that the living donor has provided consent and that it is informed consent. "Informed consent" generally means the individual participates in his or her health care decision-making through a process which: (1) provides information about the decision and procedures, alternatives, risks, relevant uncertainties, benefits, and other pertinent information; (2) is provided to the individual in a manner suitable for comprehension; (3) includes an assessment by the informing practitioner that the person understands and can articulate this understanding; and (4) that there is voluntary consent by the living donor.

The surveyor should review the documentation in the medical record that describes the completed informed consent process and review all dated and witnessed forms signed by the living donor.

Regulations Developed by the OPTN

In bylaw Appendix B attachment 1. XIII, D.,2, a, vi related to staff required for the transplant program that performs living donor surgery:
… the center has an independent donor advocate (IDA) who is not involved with the potential recipient evaluation, is independent of the decision to transplant

the potential recipient and, consistent with the IDA protocol referred to below, is a knowledgeable advocate for the potential living donor. The goals of the IDA are:

1. To promote the best interests of the potential living donor
2. To advocate the rights of the potential living donor
3. To assist the potential living donor in obtaining and understanding information regarding the:

(a) Consent process
(b) Evaluation process
(c) Surgical procedure
(d) Benefit and need for follow-up

References

1. Mckechnie JL. Webster's new twentieth century dictionary unabridged (2nd ed.). Cleveland: The World Publishing Company; 1956. p. 29.
2. Murray JE. Surgery of the soul: reflections on a curious career. Sagamore Beach: Science History Publications; 2001. p. 61, 62, pp. 73–78.
3. Hamilton D. A history transplantation. Pittsburgh: University of Pittsburg Press; 2012. p. 304, 386, pp. 337, 380–384.
4. Rosenthal J, Hakala T, Iwatsuki S, Shaw B, Starzl T, et al. Cadaveric renal transplantation under cyclosporine-steriod therapy. Surg Gynecol Obstet. 1983 Oct;157:4.
5. National Kidney Foundation. www.kidney.org. Accessed 15 May 2013.
6. Starr P. The social transformation of American medicine. New York: Basic; 1982. p. 291, pp. 334–339.
7. Terasaki PI. History of transplantation: thirty five recollections. Los Angeles: UCLA Tissue Typing Laboratory; 1991. pp. 277–278.
8. Rettig RA. Implementing the end-stage renal disease program of medicare. Santa Monica: Rand Corporation; 1980. p. 31.
9. Sommer BG, Sutherland ER, Simmons RL, Howard RJ, Najarian JS et al. Prognosis after renal transplantation: Cumulative influence of combined risk factors. American Society of Transplant Surgeons, Fourth Annual Meeting, 1978 June 1–3.
10. Salvatierra O Jr, Feduska NJ, Vincenti F, Duca R, Potter D, Nolan J, et al. Analysis of cost and outcomes of renal transplantation at one center. American Society of Transplant Surgeons, Fourth Annual Meeting, 1978 June 1–3.
11. Williams AM. Progress in clinical renal transplantation. Transplant Proc. 1979 March;11(1):4–10.
12. National Organ Transplantation Act of 1984, Pub L. 98-507, 98 Stat. 2339–2348 (Oct. 19, 1984).
13. Iglehart JK. Transplantation: the problem of limited resources. N Engl J Med. 1983;309:124–6.
14. Steering Committee of the Istanbul Summit. Organ trafficking and transplant tourism and commercialism: the declaration of Istanbul. Lancet (London, England). 2008;372(9632):5–6.
15. Koop CE. Increasing the supply of solid organs for transplantation. Public Health Rep. 1983 Nov-Dec;98(6):572.
16. Spital A, Spital M, Spital R, et al. The living kidney donor alive and well. Arch Intern Med. 1986;146:1993–5.
17. National Organ Transplant Act. Reprint from collections of Michigan Library. p. 111.
18. Cecka M. Clinical Transplants 2003. UCLA Immunogentics Center; 2003. p. 3.

19. Final Rule Federal Register. (Vol. 63, No. 63/Thursday, April 2, Rules and Regulations; 1998, p. 16302.
20. Ratner LE. Laparoscopic assisted live donor nephrectomy—a comparison with the open approach. Transplantation. 1997 Jan 27;63(2):229–33.
21. OPTN website data analysis. http://optn.transplant.hrsa.gov/. Accessed 17 June 2013.
22. The Authors for the Live Organ Donor Consensus Group. Consensus statement on the live organ donor. JAMA. 2000;284(22):2919–26.
23. www.Organdonor.gov ACOT website HHS Archive. Accessed 15 May 2013.
24. www.Organdonor.gov ACOT website HHS Archive. Accessed 15 May 2013.
25. New York State Committee on Quality Improvement in Living Liver Donation. A report to: New York state transplant council and New York state department of health. (Dec 2002). http://www.health.ny.gov/professionals/patients/donation/organ/liver/. Accessed 3 Oct 2013.
26. Delmonico FL. A report of the Amsterdam forum on the care of the live kidney donor: data and medical guidelines. Transplantation. 2005;79(6 Suppl): S53.
27. Pruett TL, Tibell A, Alabdulkareem A; Bhandari M, Cronin, DC, Dew MA, et al. The ethics statement of the Vancouver Forum on the live lung, liver, pancreas, and intestine donor, transplantation. 2006 May 27;81(10):1386–7.

Chapter 8
Findings from a National Survey of Living Donor Advocates

Jennifer L. Steel, Andrea Dunlavy, Maranda Friday, Mark Unruh, Chanelle Labash, Kendal Kingsley, Henkie P. Tan, Ron Shapiro and Abhinav Humar

---

J. L. Steel (✉)
Department of Surgery, Psychiatry, and Psychology,
University of Pittsburgh Medical Center, 3459 Fifth Avenue,
MUH 7S, Pittsburgh, PA 15213, USA
e-mail: steeljl@upmc.edu

A. Dunlavy
Department of Surgery,
University of Pittsburgh School of Medicine, 3459 Fifth Avenue,
Montefiore 7S, Pittsburgh, PA 15213, USA
e-mail: adunlavy@gmail.com

M. Friday
Department of Surgery, Starzl Transplant Institute and Liver Cancer Center,
Montefiore Hospital, University of Pittsburgh, 7S, 3459 Fifth Avenue,
Pittsburgh, PA 15213, USA
e-mail: fridaymn@upmc.edu

M. Unruh
Department of Internal Medicine, Department of Nephrology, MSC 10-5550,
University of New Mexico, Albuquerque, NM 87131-0001, USA
e-mail: mlunruh@salud.unm.edu

C. Labash
Department of Surgery, University of Pittsburgh Medical Center,
Kaufman Building, Suite 601, 3471 Fifth Avenue,
Pittsburgh, PA 15213, USA
e-mail: labashcr@upmc.edu

K. Kingsley
Department of Surgery, UPMC Montefiore Hospital,
3459 Fifth Avenue, Pittsburgh, PA 15213, USA
e-mail: kingsleyka@upmc.edu

H. P. Tan
Department of Transplant Surgery, Veterans Hospital of Pittsburgh,
University of Pittsburgh Medical Center/Starzl Transplant Institute,
3459 Fifth Avenue, UPMC/MUH N725 Starzl Transplant Institute,
Pittsburgh, PA 15213, USA
e-mail: tanhp@upmc.edu

J. Steel (ed.), *Living Donor Advocacy*, DOI 10.1007/978-1-4614-9143-9_8,
© Springer Science+Business Media New York 2014

Introduction

The inadequate supply of organs in the U.S. and other countries continues to drive the need for living donor transplantation [1]. Although living donor surgeries have been performed since the 1950s, it was not until 2000 that representatives from the transplant community convened for a meeting on living donation to develop a consensus statement to promote the welfare of living donors [2]. As a part of the consensus statement, it was recommended that transplant centers retain an independent living donor advocate (ILDA) whose primary focus be on the best interest of the donor [2].

The two primary governing bodies of transplantation include the Department of Health and Human Services (DHHS) and the United Network for Organ Sharing (UNOS). After the consensus statement was published in 2000, the DHHS and UNOS began to develop guidelines for the qualifications, professional boundaries, and practices of the ILDA [3, 4]. Similar to other medical specialties who evaluate transplant candidates and living donors, the guidelines developed by these organizations provided a broad interpretation of the role of the ILDA.

Although the DHHS and UNOS have similar guidelines for the ILDA, the organizations emphasized different aspects of the role. For example, the DHHS included guidelines that ILDAs' responsibilities were to (1) ensure the protection of current and prospective living donors; (2) be knowledgeable about living organ donation, transplantation, medical ethics, and the informed consent process; (3) not be involved in transplantation activities on a routine basis; and (4) represent and advise the donor, protect and promote the interests of the donor, respect the donor's decision, and ensure that the donor's decision is informed and free of coercion [3].

Similarly, the UNOS included in their bylaws, the same year that all transplant centers must have, an ILDA who is (1) not involved with potential recipient evaluation on a routine basis; (2) independent of the decision to transplant the potential recipient; and (3) a knowledgeable advocate for the potential living donor [4]. According to the UNOS, the responsibilities of the ILDA are to advocate for potential living donors; promote their best interests; and to assist the potential living donor in obtaining and understanding the consent and evaluation process, surgical procedures, and the benefit and need for postsurgical follow-up [4].

Despite the requirements set forth by the DHHS and the UNOS, and the costs of ILDAs to medical centers (approximately US$ 9 million annually) [3], the so-

---

R. Shapiro
Department of Surgery, Division of Transplantation,
Starzl Translpant Institute, University of Pittsburgh Medical Center,
3459 Fifth Avenue, UPMC Montefiore 7S, Pittsburgh, PA 15213, USA
e-mail: shapiror@upmc.edu

A. Humar
Department of Surgery, University of Pittsburgh, Room 725,
3459 Fifth Avenue,
Pittsburgh, PA 15213, USA
e-mail: humara2@upmc.edu

ciodemographic characteristics, selection and training, and clinical practices of ILDAs are not well understood. As a result, our team aimed to better understand the ILDAs' background, professional boundaries, clinical responsibilities, and how ethical challenges encountered by ILDAs are managed.

The study that was conducted was a survey of ILDAs across transplant centers performing living donor surgeries in the U.S.. Each of the 201 transplant centers in the U.S. that perform living donor surgeries was contacted to identify the ILDA at their center. The survey included 63 quantitative and qualitative items that queried the ILDA with regard to sociodemographic information (e.g., age, gender, and education), roles and responsibilities (e.g., number of hours worked and timing of contact with donors), and ethical challenges associated with living donor advocacy (e.g., descriptions of when the ILDA felt as though the donor was being pressured or coerced). For greater details regarding the design and methods of the study, please refer to the original paper [5].

The findings of this study suggest that there is a marked variability in the sociodemographic characteristics, definition of the role of the ILDA, the clinical practice of ILDAs, and how ILDAs manage ethically challenging issues associated with living donation. A wide range of educational backgrounds, including those with less than high school diploma to professional degrees (MDs/PhDs), were reported; however, the majority of ILDAs reported having a Bachelor's or Master's degree and were trained as either nurses or social workers. A small percentage of ILDAs (2%) were from ethnic or racial minority backgrounds, which reflects the disparity also observed of transplant candidates and donors.

The position of the ILDA is quite recent, and many of the ILDAs were appointed by the transplant team and were often someone whom the team worked with in some capacity prior to becoming the ILDA (e.g., social worker or nurse; Fig. 8.1). Depending on the size of the transplant center, the ILDA role is sometimes combined with another role of the living donor team, most often a social worker or nurse. Approximately 53% of ILDAs perform a second role within transplant.

The definition of the "independent" living donor advocate has been previously debated [6]. The findings of this survey suggested that ILDAs themselves may have many definitions regarding the term "independent" as it refers to their role as an ILDA. Figure 8.2 depicts the responses the ILDAs reported when queried about the definition of "independence" as it refers to their role as the ILDA.

According to the governing bodies of Center for Medicare and Medicaid services (CMS) and UNOS, the role of the ILDA includes both "advocating" and "protecting" the donor. It is unclear at this time if an ILDA can necessarily perform both of these tasks. With regard to the ILDA advocating and protecting the donor, the ILDAs were queried about how they would proceed with regard to the following scenario:

> How would you proceed if you felt that the donor having surgery would be detrimental to their physical or psychological well-being, but (1) this had been explained to the donor in detail and the donor understood the potential consequences; (2) the donor has been approved to proceed with surgery by the medical and psychosocial team members; and (3) the donor wants to proceed with surgery despite the potential risks?

We found that 29% of ILDAs responded that they would document their concerns but would "approve" the donor for surgery ("advocate" for the donor). However,

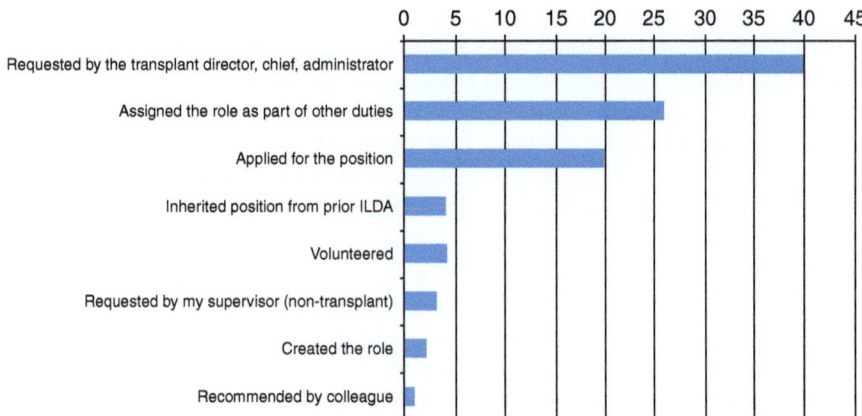

Fig. 8.1 Percentage of ILDAs reporting how they were selected as an ILDA at their transplant center

the majority of ILDAs reported that they would document their concerns and "not approve" the donor for surgery (51%; "protect" the donor). The remaining ILDAs (20%) had a variety of responses, including not being aware they were involved in the selection process (see Chap. 22 for further discussion regarding the dilemma of advocating versus protecting).

Most would agree that the primary responsibilities of the ILDA are to confirm that the donor (1) is willing to donate; (2) is competent to donate; (3) is not under any undue pressure or coercion to donate; (4) is not being compensated to donate; and (5) understands the informed consent process including the medical, psychosocial, and financial risks of donation. Further, the ILDAs were queried about any issues they have had when evaluating the potential donors for competency. The ILDA

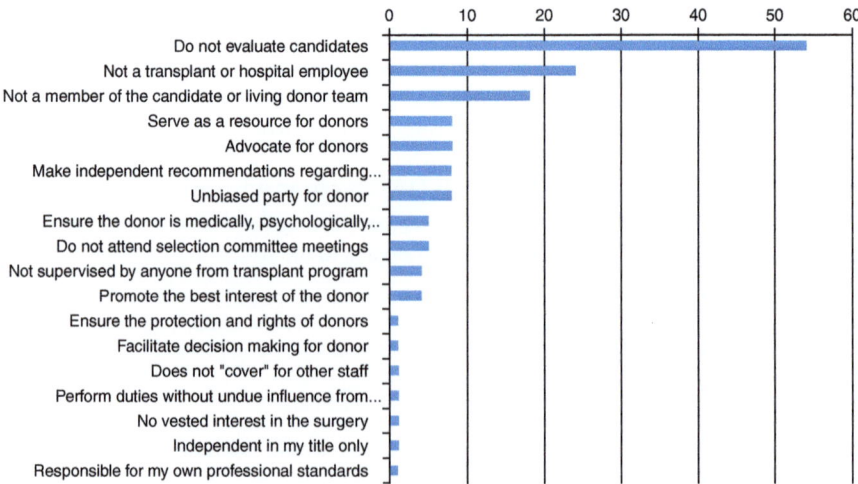

Fig. 8.2 Percentage of ILDAs reporting their definition of "independent"

Table 8.1 Examples when the ILDA declined a donor for issues concerning competency to donate

A belief that risks did not apply to the donor because of God protecting him absolutely

A donor who had a ninth-grade education, unstable home life, although temporarily living with a girlfriend, wanted to donate to a friend. It was not clear if the donor was just trying to please his friend and if he totally understood informed consent process

Donor with an extensive alcohol abuse history and who had served a prison sentence. Poor historian, her stories did not match up between the team members. She did not seem to understand the process and we excluded her from donation

A donor who stated that he had not read any of the donation education information but he had signed and returned an agreement of understanding. My assessment was that I was not sure he could read and/or he lacked ability to understand the material. Patient was ruled out for medical reasons but I would have recommended neuropsychological assessment if he had been able to proceed with evaluation

We had a donor who was a relative and had suffered traumatic brain injury in a motor vehicle accident. We did the regular evaluation with a complete psychiatric evaluation as to cognition and competency. It was determined that this person was capable of making decision regarding surgery

I had one case where a potential donor was a foreign national visiting the recipient and my initial interview needed to be interpreted by the donor's wife on the spot due to time being limited. I had no way of knowing if the translation was accurate or not. I did get the sense that the donor truly wanted to help his friend and understood there were some risks always involved with surgery

Donor was donating to his cousin, with whom he resided and who was providing financial support to the donor (who was not working at the time). Donor reported a history of special education courses in school. Donor did not appear to understand any of the medical aspects of surgery or the long-term implications of his decision. He had limited knowledge of his own personal finances (e.g., did not know if he had health insurance) and appeared generally cognitively impaired. Donation was advised against. The cousin later called and yelled at the coordinators, who subsequently requested a reevaluation. A more in-depth psychological and cognitive evaluation was completed, which revealed borderline intellectual functioning of the donor

I evaluated a donor under 20 years of age developmentally disabled man who wanted to donate a kidney to his sister. His family was in full support, and I believe that he was quite close to his sister. Although he was fairly high functioning in some ways, I did not fully believe that he understood all of the risks and benefits or that he could make a decision without the influence of his very involved family

Younger sibling was to donate to older, more successful sibling. Donor was on a very low developmental level and was not able to articulate or describe the risks that would be faced. This donor just kept repeating again and again, "I am not being pressured, I am not being paid." The donor was not even able to understand the evaluation or results or the work-up process

A woman once called me and wanted to be a donor for her mother. During the entire telephone interview, the potential donor's mother was in the background responding to questions. When I asked a question, the mother would answer and she would repeat that answer to me. The donor was on disability, but could not explain to me why donor was disabled. She said that it was from "when I was a little girl" but could not name the disorder. When I asked her who her MD was, she gave me a name and told me she took "little black and yellow pills"

may not formally assess the donor's competency but may refer a donor for further neuropsychological or psychiatric evaluation for concerns regarding competency. The ILDAs described several examples in which they may decline a donor for surgery due to issues of competency and understanding of the information consent process (Table 8.1).

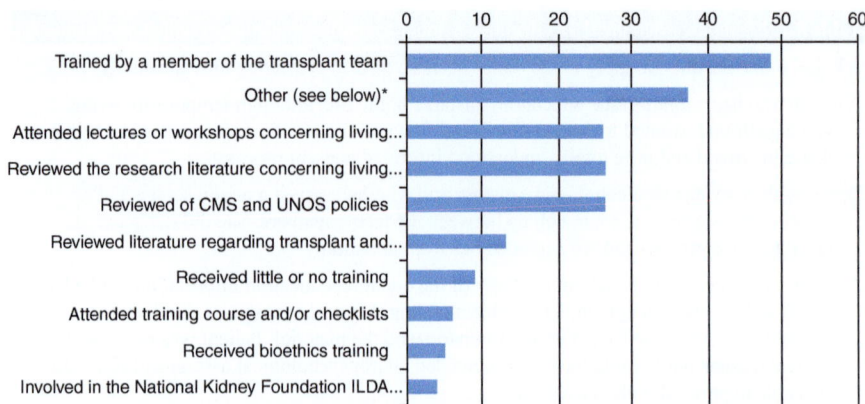

Fig. 8.3 Percentage of ILDAs reporting how they were trained as an ILDA. *Other* ILDAs serve on ethics or selection committee, own research and writing, consult with other health care professionals, learned from patients and families

Since the inception of this position in 2007, no formal training for ILDAs has existed. Many of the ILDAs, when queried as a part of this survey, stated that they had received training from a variety of sources and the type and duration of training varied greatly among ILDAs (Fig. 8.3).

As the field of living donation and the guidelines and requirements set forth by the DHHS and UNOS continue to evolve, formal training and continuing education are recommended. Because of the diversity of professional backgrounds of ILDAs, it may be a challenge to identify a common forum (e.g., professional meeting) for training and continuing education. The development of written and/or web-based educational materials for ILDAs could be an approach that would facilitate consistency in knowledge and practices of ILDAs.

With regard to ILDA practices, approximately half of the ILDAs combined the ILDA evaluation with other responsibilities (e.g., psychosocial, medical, or nursing evaluation). The advantages of combining the ILDA evaluation include a more comprehensive understanding of the donor and family dynamics, which in turn can facilitate the decision-making process regarding the donors' suitability for surgery. Disadvantages may include the ILDA's role becoming diffuse and unable to "advocate" for the donor if she/he believes that there is a psychosocial, financial, or medical contraindication for surgery secondary to their other role.

The educational information the donor receives may be important in his or her decision to proceed with surgery and therefore materials developed by and vetted through health care professionals should be provided to donors rather than information developed by individuals including ILDAs. The ILDAs who provided educational information to donors reported that only a small percentage (20%) of materials were developed by UNOS or other national organizations related to transplantation and vetted through health care professionals working in transplantation.

With regard to the ILDA's practices, the majority of ILDAs reported attending multidisciplinary selection committee meetings in which donor, and sometimes transplant, candidates were discussed. The consensus statement published in 2000 suggested that the ILDA should have the power to "veto" the surgery [1]. It is clear from the findings of this study that a minority of ILDAs have the power to "veto" the surgery, while some ILDAs were not even aware that this was an option for them. If the ILDA is a part of the selection process, the ILDA may be obligated to disclose to the medical team(s), the reasons for recommending against surgery, both verbally and as part of the donor's medical record. It is unlikely that the donor candidates are aware that information disclosed to the ILDA will be shared with the transplant team(s) and possibly with other health care professionals who may have access to their medical records. If ILDAs are involved in the selection process, this should be included in the informed consent process so that the donors are aware that the information disclosed to the ILDA may be shared with other health care professionals. If members of both the donor and candidate transplant teams are present at the selection committee meetings, and the ILDA discloses information discussed with the donor, there may be an increased risk of the donor's confidentiality being breached to family members and/or recipients through members of the candidate team.

As part of the survey, we queried ILDAs regarding reasons provided for declining donors for surgery (Fig. 8.4). Although declining donors for surgery with regard to specific ILDA-related reasons was rare, it was observed that some ILDAs would decline a donor for reasons that may not be associated with the role of the ILDA (e.g., psychiatric diagnosis and medical reasons).

LaPointe Rudow and colleagues suggested that ILDAs be involved in both the short- and long-term follow-up of living donors; however, this may have fiscal implications for the transplant and/or medical center supporting the ILDAs [7]. At least for some donors, long-term follow-up by the ILDA may be recommended, particularly for those who experienced medical, psychosocial, or financial complications surrounding donation; loss of their loved one during or shortly after the

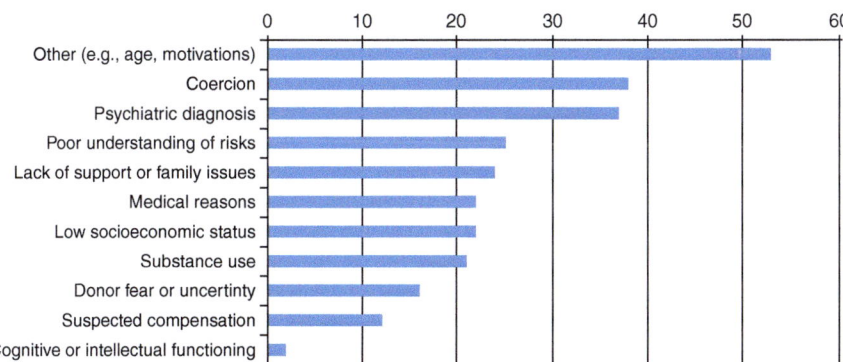

Fig. 8.4 Percentage of ILDAs reporting the reasons for declining donors for surgery

transplant; or when the donor may be facing a new medical diagnosis as a result of the donor evaluation process (e.g., cancer and Hepatitis C).

One of the most controversial areas in living donation is "valuable consideration" [8–10]. The role of the ILDA is to ascertain if a donor is receiving compensation for their organ and to inform the donor of the law associated with valuable consideration. The National Organ Transplantation Act (NOTA, P.L. 98–507) permits living and deceased organ donation but prohibits the sale of organs. Section 301 of NOTA specifically prohibits the exchange of v*aluable consideration* (money or the equivalent) for organs [11]. Valuable consideration "does not include the reasonable payments associated with the removal, transportation, implantation, processing, preservation, quality control, and storage of a human organ or the expenses of travel, housing, and lost wages incurred by the donor of a human organ in connection with the donation of the organ." [10] The penalty for such a violation is "a fine not more than $50,000 or imprisonment not more than five years, or both." [11] Because of the potential consequences to the donor for being compensated for the donation of their organ, the ILDA's understanding of this law is important to help guide the donor. However, before the donor can understand this law, the ILDA must also understand this law to be able to appropriately inform donors. As part of the survey, we queried ILDA with regard to how they would respond to hypothetical scenarios that may or may not involve valuable consideration (Table 8.2).

The ILDAs were also asked to describe some of the problems or controversies that they experienced in their role as the ILDA (Fig. 8.5). As the field of living donation continues to evolve as well as the role of the ILDA, attention should be given to the difficulties ILDAs may encounter in their positions. Development of methods to resolve such disagreements between the ILDAs and the transplant team would provide the ILDAs with autonomy and the ability to protect and advocate for the living donors (See Chap. 15 for further details). A national ombudsman appointed through the DHHS or UNOS could be available for ILDAs who are not able to resolve conflicts at their transplant center.

The ILDA were also asked to provide examples where they had observed pressure and/or coercion of the donor by the candidate or the medical team. The ILDAs provided the examples presented in Table 8.3. Although the donor likely experiences a degree of pressure or obligation as a family member or friend, the role of the ILDA is to ascertain if the donor is experiencing undue pressure or coercion from the candidate, candidate's family, or medical team.

By nature of the position, the ILDA experiences not only ethical challenges as described earlier (e.g., compensation for donation and advocate versus protection of donor) but also other ethical issues such as the examples described in Table 8.4.

This survey identified marked variability in the position and practice of the ILDA in transplant centers. Although practice variability exists in all disciplines, many professions have practice guidelines to provide a minimum standard. Practice guidelines are often recommended for legal and regulatory issues, consumer and/or public benefit (e.g., improved service delivery, avoiding harm to the patient, and decreasing disparities in underserved or vulnerable populations), and for professional guidance (e.g., risk management issues and advances in practice).

Table 8.2 ILDA responses to hypothetical scenarios

Scenarios considered "acceptable" by the ILDAs	Percentage
Receiving financial assistance from the transplant candidate (or candidate's family) for the flight, to be evaluated for donation or for the surgery	7.1
Receiving financial assistance from the transplant candidate (or candidate's family) for unemployment benefits lost while recovering from surgery	47.1
Receiving financial assistance from the transplant candidate (or candidate's family) for wages lost while recovering from surgery	64.7
If the transplant candidate is an employer and the donor is the employee, the donor receives from the candidate, time off for the surgery and recovery with pay	35.3
Receiving financial assistance from the transplant candidate (or candidate's family) for a vacation with the candidate's family	2.9
Receiving financial assistance from the transplant candidate (or candidate's family) for the expenses for lodging and food while being evaluated for donation or surgery	85.3
Receiving financial assistance from the transplant candidate (or candidate's family) to cover the mortgage/rent, car payment, and utilities while recovering from surgery	41.2
Receiving financial assistance up to US$ 5,000 from the transplant candidate (or candidate's family) for expenses related to the donation	25.3
Receiving financial assistance from the transplant candidate (or candidate's family) for the donor's discretion	2.9

ILDA independent living donor advocate

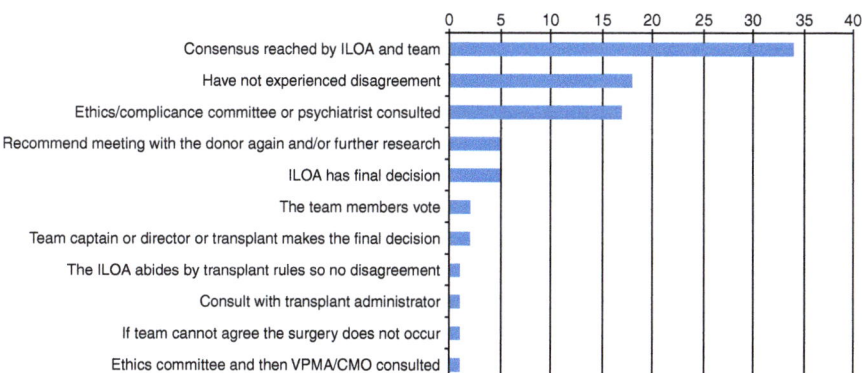

Fig. 8.5 Percentage of ILDAs reporting the methods used to resolve disagreements between the transplant team and ILDA

Table 8.3 Examples that the ILDA provided with regard to instances of pressure/coercion from the candidate or medical teams

Pressure from the transplant candidate
Donor came forward to donate a kidney to an immediate family member. Before surgery took place, donor reported that the recipient was calling her everyday demanding that donor donate a kidney. Recipient also lied to donor about risks and recovery time
A woman who had known her boss for a long time, were friends, and she felt obligated to give her kidney. He gave her a bonus out the blue, gave her all time off whenever she wanted and treated her differently from the team
A donor candidate who was under the age of 25 and a veteran with PTSD whose father expects him to donate, cannot let his father down. The father got very angry when we turned down his son's application to donate
I had the donor tell me that the recipient was forcing him to do it. He did not want to proceed. "How could we get him out of this?" We told the recipient that he was not a suitable candidate without giving any details
Younger sibling was pushed to donate when the older sibling was screened as unsuitable. Donor was told by the family that she was the only one who could donate
Pressure from the medical team
The transplant team tells the donor that this was the recipients' only option
Not emphasizing "opt outs" or "medical outs"
When the health of the recipient or the wait on the list for a cadaveric donor is mentioned regularly
Donor is unwilling but feels responsible or guilty if he/she did not agree to proceed
Demanding the left kidney when the donor team only approves the right kidney secondary to risk and or complexity
Team not listening to donor's verbal and/or nonverbal cues
I do not really ever see any pressure on the donor from the medical team(s); just pressure on me detected by frequent calls to reverse my decision
Either subtle or direct suggestions about which family or friends would be the most ideal donors
If the team is making multiple phone calls to a potential donor who has not continued the evaluation. If a recipient physician urges the potential donor team to expedite the evaluation
Pressing forward with donation in the face of objections from team members. Suggesting to someone directly that he/she would make a good donor
When there is a need for a specific type of blood/tissue or if it has been a long time since we have had approvals.
When deep concerns from living donor advocate or social worker are overlooked by the transplant team

PTSD post-traumatic stress disorder

Without such practice guidelines, there is a possibility that donors (and indirectly, candidates) may be negatively affected through the screening and/or selection process. The ILDA's decisions can have a significant impact on a donor (e.g., felony charge for valuable consideration) and/or the transplant candidate (e.g., candidate death). Even though the evaluation of living donors is a multidisciplinary process, the development of uniform practice guidelines for ILDAs is critical for decreasing potential disparities, particularly if the ILDA has "veto" power, as was evidenced by some ILDAs.

Table 8.4 Examples of ethical challenges reported by the LDAs

Donor with developmental disorders, the family wants the donor to proceed although donor advocate is concerned if the donor can provide informed consent
Donor with drug and alcohol issues but the medical committee wants to proceed with surgery
Donor who recently attempted suicide but the transplant candidate and team wanted donor to proceed with surgery
A donor who is under 18 years of age donating to her child
Donor wanting other surgical interventions (hernia repair) during donation surgery
Donors found candidate on the Internet/Facebook
Transplant candidate was HIV positive but had not disclosed HIV status to donor
Donors who do not have health insurance coverage
Donors diagnosed with serious illness such as pancreatic or breast cancer and have no insurance
Misattributed paternity
Physician with end-stage organ disease soliciting his patients for organ donation
An ILDA being pressured by the team to approve someone who the he/she strongly believes is not acceptable. This is usually in the form of pressure from the surgeon that is handed down to the coordinators, which is then passed on to the ILDA
Protecting privacy of donors when recipients try to insert themselves into donor evaluations/care
Supporting and educating donors who know that their recipients are not eligible for deceased donor transplants and are deemed "living" donor only candidates
Supporting and educating donors who suspect that their recipients are not being truthful about the progression of their disease, nonadherence, or other treatment options
Introduction/facilitation of meetings between nondirected donors and their recipients
Transplant candidate paying third party to find a donor
Foreign immigrant with citizenship, returned to native country, found a wife willing to donate organ, brought her back to the U.S. to be tested (prior to getting married)
Donors who come from other countries and admit they have no access to follow-up care in their country of origin
Unemployed and no source of income
Donor with a diagnosis of bipolar disorder, which was untreated and the desire to donate was likely related to symptoms of grandiosity
Need for ongoing psychotropic medications
Responded to an ad in a bar for a donor. Donor was an unemployed drifter with no visible plan for after care
Young donor to older candidate (60-year difference between donor and candidate)
Convicted of felony, wanting to donate without job or insurance

References

1. Pomfret EA, Sung RS, Allan J, Kinkhabwala M, Melancon JK, Roberts JP. Solving the organ shortage crisis: the 7th Annual American Society of Transplant Surgeons' State-of-the-Art Winter Symposium. Am J Transplant. 2008;8(4):745–52.

2. Abecassis M, Adams M, Adams P, Arnold RM, Atkins CR, Barr ML, et al. Consensus statement on the live organ donor. JAMA. 2000;284:2919–26.
3. Department of Health and Human Services, Part II. Centers for Medicare & Medicaid Services 42 CFR Parts 405, 482, 488, and 498 Medicare Program; Hospital Conditions of Participation: Requirements for Approval and Re-Approval of Transplant Centers To Perform Organ Transplants; Final Rule Federal Register/ Vol. 72, No. 61/ Friday, March 30, 2007/ Rules and Regulations, 15198–15280.
4. United Network for Organ Sharing Bylaw. Appendix B, Section XIII, 2007.
5. Steel JL, Dunlavy A, Friday M, Kingsley K, Brower D, Unruh M, et al. A national survey of independent living donor advocates: the need for practice guidelines. Am J Transplant. 2012;12(8):2141–9.
6. Boyatzis R. Transforming qualitative information: thematic analysis and code development. Thousand Oaks:Sage; 1998.
7. LaPointe Rudow D. Living donor advocate: a team approach to educate, evaluate, and manage donors across the continuum. Prog Transplant. 2009;9(1):64–70.
8. Gaston RS, Danovitch GM, Epstein RA, Kahn JP, Schnitzler MA. Must all living donor compensation be viewed as valuable consideration? Am J Transplant. 2007;7:1309–10.
9. Gaston RS, Danovitch GM, Epstein RA, Kahn JP, Schnitzler MA. Reducing the financial disincentives to living kidney donation: will compensation help the way it is supposed to? Nat Clin Pract Nephrol. 2007;3(3):132–3.
10. International Forum on the Care of Live Kidney Donors. A report of the Amsterdam forum on the care of live kidney donor: data and medical guidelines. Transplantation. 2005;79(S2):S53–66.
11. The National Organ Transplant Act (1984; 98–507), approved October 19, 1984 and amended in 1988 and 1990.

Chapter 9
The Independent Donor Advocate and the Independent Donor Advocate Team

Dianne LaPointe Rudow

Introduction

Critical shortages of deceased organ donors have resulted in the need for living donors to be utilized for solid organ transplant. Federal regulations require transplant programs to appoint an independent living donor advocate (ILDA) to ensure safe evaluation and care of live donors [1]. The Organ Procurement and Transplant Network (OPTN) requires that the living kidney donor recovery hospital provides an ILDA who is not involved with the potential recipient evaluation and is independent of the decision to transplant the potential recipient [2]. Operationalizing the role of the ILDA varies across transplant programs. This includes debates regarding whether the ILDA should be an individual or a team of advocates.

Individual ILDA Versus the Team Approach

Commonly, a transplant program will appoint one person to serve in the role of the ILDA. This person can be someone from the transplant team already involved in the donor care but relieved of recipient care, such as the live donor social worker or physician, or it can be a person outside the transplant team whose sole role is to advocate for the donor. Steel et al. found significant variation in types of professionals functioning as advocates among programs across the U.S. [3] (Table 9.1). Additionally, when the ILDA intervened, how integrated they are within the donor team, the role, and how much autonomy vary and can result in different levels of advocacy. The professional background of a specific ILDA may also affect the scope and implementation of the role for that advocate. According to OPTN, the ILDA

D. L. Rudow (✉)
Recanati Miller Transplantation Institute, Mount Sinai Medical Center,
One Gustave L. Levy Place,
Box 1104, New York, NY 10029, USA
e-mail: Dianne.LaPointeRudow@mountsinai.org

Table 9.1 Professions performing the role of independent live donor advocate (ILDA) in the U.S. Adapted from [3]	Nurse Social worker Clergy Psychology Other

Table 9.2 Pros and cons of the independent live donor advocate team	*Benefits of the team approach* Expertise in different aspects of donation Discussion may ensure sound reasoning Improves education through repetition and questions Increased resource for improved care *Benefits of the individual approach* Minimizes donor time during evaluation Team appointments may be difficult to coordinate Team has added expense, smaller programs may not be able to justify expense

must promote the best interests of the potential living donor, advocate for the rights of the potential donor, and assist the potential donor in obtaining and understanding information [2]. This may be difficult to achieve if an ILDA has one interview at one instance in time during the evaluation period and is not involved in discussions regarding the donor candidacy. In practice, this should be done by all hospital personnel evaluating and caring for the potential live donor; hence, the concept of the independent live donor advocate team (ILDT). Live donor specialists acknowledge that a donor matures through the process and his or her understanding and desire to donate can change over time [4]. Additionally, risks and benefits of donation vary from individual donor to donor. An ILDT working together to evaluate, educate, and advocate for a potential donor may ultimately result in an informed choice to proceed or not.

Benefits of an ILDT

With a team approach to the ILDA role, all who are involved in the evaluation and management of potential and actual live donors have a primary role to care for the donor. They are "independent" of recipient care (or intended recipient care) and decisions are not influenced by recipient needs. Table 9.2 summarizes the benefits of a team approach to advocacy. A significant benefit of an ILDT is that each member comes from different disciplines and brings his/her own area of expertise and personal experiences to the team and may interpret a donor's questions and responses differently. Their interactions with the donor vary based on these variables, and a potential donor may be more candid or bond more with one advocate versus another. The roles and responsibilities of each team member should be delineated ahead of time to maintain appropriate boundaries, avoid conflict, and send a consistent message to the potential donor. The ILDT has expertise in different aspects of donation and transplant; however, to be successful, it is crucial that all understand the end-stage organ disease and the transplant process so that they can accurately depict the process. At a minimum, each member should possess the knowledge expected of the donor at the completion of the evaluation. Each advocate is responsible for education and reinforcing key concepts. Repetition and time for questions can improve the education process.

At the completion of the potential donor's comprehensive evaluation, the ILDT should formally meet to review each donor evaluation results and discuss the impression of each individual meeting. Discussion within the team in order to reconcile any differences in views about a donor's suitability to donate can help to ensure sound reasoning regarding candidacy recommendations. Additionally, as donors mature through the process, their feelings, thoughts, and concerns about donation may change, and a team—by virtue of its multidisciplinary composition—may identify additional areas to focus interventions. As with all teams, a strategy to handle differences of opinions and managing conflict within the group must be identified ahead of time.

Structure of the Team

The professions that make up a team of advocates may vary at each center; however, critical members include the physician assigned to medically evaluate and assess risk, the transplant nurse coordinator assigned to educate and oversee the process, and the social worker assigned to assess psychosocial risk, competency, and coercion. Other clinicians that add benefit to the team include the donor surgeon, psychiatrist, nutritionist, financial counselor, and ethicist [5]. One may argue that the additional transplant staff, such as nutritionist or financial coordinator, are not involved with donor advocacy; however, their role is crucial with select donors. For instance, a young obese kidney donor may need a nutritionist to educate him/her about weight loss and the need for long-term healthy eating. If a potential donor cannot comply or is not willing to comply with such recommendations, the nutritionist may advocate for the donor choosing not to donate.

Roles and Responsibilities of the ILDT

It is the entire ILDT's responsibility to be involved in the donation process throughout the donation continuum [6]. When and for how long will vary according to the team members' skill sets and an individual donor's needs. The process and

Table 9.3 Roles and responsibility of the ILDT

Regulatory compliance
Policy and protocol development
Evaluation
Education
Informed consent
Determination of donor candidacy
Advocacy
Support before donation, if declines and after surgery
Documentation
QAPI

components of the medical and psychosocial evaluation are prescribed by the Centers for Medicare & Medicaid Services (CMS) and OPTN regulations, policies, and bylaws [1, 2]. It is, however, up to individual transplant programs to determine how they will comply with such rules and develop individual policies and protocols for live donor evaluation, education, and follow-up (Table 9.3). It is important that the input of all ILDT members is considered when developing such policies. Additionally, all members need to have a full understanding of and comply with the regulations and the program's polices for donor care.

The ILDT should have input into the education materials developed for the live donor. Written, video, and oral education need to have a consistent message. Additionally, all team members involved in educating donors should be consistent with the risk projection, process, and post-donation experience. It can be confusing to a potential donor if team members have conflicting messages. For instance, if one member describes a risk of bleeding to be 2 % and another 5 %, a donor may become confused. This all needs to be agreed upon by the ILDT ahead of time, reviewed periodically, and based on the evidence in the literature and the program-specific results.

Depending on the profession of each individual team member, they may or may not be responsible for performing the medical or psychosocial evaluations, but all should understand the outcome of each component of the evaluation. Additionally, all should provide education and assess the donor's understanding of the process and results of such evaluations. Documentation of donor interviews, education, the evaluation results, all correspondence, and team meetings regarding candidacy is critical to maintain team communication and provide evidence of comprehensive donor care.

At the completion of the evaluation, the ILDT should meet face to face and describe the results and impressions of the evaluation in order to advocate for the donor and assist in determining if a donor can be approved for donation. Frank discussion within the team regarding candidacy and the risks and benefits of approval will facilitate sound reasoning and improve outcomes. Conflict management should be resolved within the team with deliberation, team meetings with the donor to clarify issues, and ongoing discussions. Ethics consults may be necessary if unresolved conflict exists.

The ILDT should review and revise the process as needed and examine outcomes through the Quality Assurance and Performance Improvement (QAPI) process existing within the transplant program. CMS requires all transplant programs to have a robust quality program to monitor compliance with regulations and outcomes [1]. It is, however, important for the live donor program to develop their own process and outcome indicators annually to ensure that the evaluation, consent, and follow-up process is adequate and meets the requirements of the programs and the regulatory bodies. It is important to get input from ILDT members. Attendance at meetings to discuss process improvement and determine if changes are needed will help the ILDT to advocate for future donors in the program.

Advocacy Throughout the Process

ILDT members should advocate for the donor and provide support throughout the process, this includes during the decision-making process, if a donor is cleared, is unable to donate, and post donation [6]. The role of each team member during the evaluation is understood and implemented across transplant programs fairly consistently. The role of the advocate/advocate team during the rest of the donor continuum is ill-defined in the transplant community. Most agree that there is a role for the advocate but how, when, and how often are unclear. Clarity exists if one uses a team approach. The team is not one person at one point in time with other responsibilities or distantly related to the issues, but rather a group of health care professionals intimately involved with the donor and their specific candidacy considerations.

When a donor is declined by the team to donate because of medical or psychiatric reasons, it can be devastating to the donor candidate. One often feels like they failed the recipient and can suffer psychologically. The ILDT has responsibility to ensure the well-being of all potential and actual donors, especially a declined donor [7]. A member of the ILDT should provide education, support, and advocacy in order to assist the donor to process the decision and provide supportive counseling as needed to avoid psychological harm to the donor. Follow-up with the donor after a period of time is important to ensure that the donor has accepted the decision after time has been allotted to process the decision. Often giving the declined donor another "role" in the transplant candidate's care can assist them in feeling that they are still helping the person. One may suggest being a live donor champion within the social network of the candidate to promote live donation in hopes that someone else will come forward. If the ILDT feels the donor has suffered ongoing psychological stress, referral for counseling may be indicated. If a donor is declined for medical reasons or because of the diagnosis of a new illness, the ILDT can facilitate understanding of the medical issue, provide counseling and support, and ensure referral for care.

A donor's choice not to donate can be even more devastating to a donor. They may experience feelings of guilt or shame and be unable to vocalize their decision to the recipient. They may request a "medical out." It is the ILDT's role to ensure that a donor truly understands what this means. For instance, they should not take a medical out and then change their mind in the future without admitting to the recipient that they took the "medical out." It is also not advisable to deceive the recipient or the donor's family in such a way that they think the donor is sick when they are not. Often a donor needs the ILDT's help in talking with their family regarding the decision not to proceed and support them through the process.

After donation, the ILDT's role is critical in helping the donor early in recovery and for a long term as needed. Reinforcing the education about the needs for follow-up and long-term health maintenance is critical. Psychological support is also needed at this point. Often donors feel very overwhelmed in the hospital and shortly after discharge because the reality of the donation has occurred. Pain, fear of complications, and returning to a normal routine can provoke stress. Having an advocate to ensure safe discharge and support can be beneficial. Psychological stress may be worse if the recipient has a complication, graft failure, or death. The ILDT can address feelings of grief and disappointment that can occur if expectations with donation were not met. An ILDT can help the donor process the experience and treat/ensure referral for treatment of emerging anxiety/depression if it occurs. In the long term, the ILDT should ensure that a live donor has access to health care and reeducation about long-term health.

Role of Donor Mentors

In addition to a multidisciplinary team of advocates, having a potential live donor communicate with a previous living donor can be an effective part of the education, informed consent process, and recovery [8]. By providing every potential donor the opportunity to meet with a person who has gone through the donor experience, he or she can learn, from a donor's point of view, the donation process. One can have a better understanding of the risks and benefits to live donation, the expectations of the recovery process, and have the ability to ask questions in a nonthreatening environment to someone who has gone through the process. It is important that if a mentor is provided, the donor understands that everyone's donation experience is different and one may have an easier or more difficult time with surgery. However, having an independent advocate outside the medical profession and the donor's social network to call and ask questions when concerns come up can be invaluable to a positive donation experience.

Nontraditional Advocates

The live organ donation experience comprising the comprehensive testing, the education about the process, risk and benefits, the personal disclosure required for the assessment of risk, the decision to proceed or not to proceed with donation, the surgical procedure, and recovery can be a very overwhelming experience for anyone. Having an advocate in the donor's social network, whether this is family or friend, is critical to assisting a donor through the process.

The family of the potential donor is a critical part of the ILDT. It is recommended that a potential donor needs to be willing to have a family member or a support person educated about live donation so that they can listen and discuss the risks and help a donor decide whether donation is right for them [6]. The family/support team needs to agree to be educated and take responsibility to assist the donor. This part of the advocate team assists with the development and implementation of a concrete plan regarding finance, child care, transportation, caregiving, and communication. This team member can facilitate the creation of two teams of caregivers, one for the donor and one for the recipient. During the inpatient stay, the family/support person provides vigilant advocacy and can act as the gatekeeper to provide organized communication with the medical team and other family members and friends. They can be a facilitator of interactions as needed. They accept discharge responsibilities for housing, nutrition, legal matters, and assistance with long-term follow-up.

For those donor candidates with no family advocate, such as a live donor who is donating to their spouse who cannot take on the advocacy role or a donor with a limited social network, it may be necessary to create a "family" advocate with coworkers, church groups, or neighbors. The hospital-appointed ILDT can be a facilitator and assist the potential donor with a family advocate.

The Donor as Part of the ILDT

The ILDT as a group along with the family advocate must create an environment to educate a donor regarding how donation can affect them. They must listen to the donor's concerns, assist in clarifying the risks and benefits, and listen to fears and concerns in a transparent, open relationship [4]. This relationship with the ILDT provides a varied group with different styles of interaction and unique perspectives on the issues. It is this multidisciplinary team approach that will create a partnership in which, ultimately, the donor must advocate for himself or herself [6]. If they do not want to donate they should feel comfortable enough to say so. In fact, if they have a complication, it impacts them the most. Therefore, the ILDT must provide the potential donor the tools to advocate their wishes. This is often difficult because the decision not to donate affects human lives. This is the reason the ILDT partnership is critical in the care of live organ donors and is not one interview with one person at one point in time but rather a detailed process with the maturation of a decision whether to proceed or not. Optimal outcomes begin with prepared, educated, uncoerced, and motivated donors, and it is the ILDT's role to help live donors achieve this.

References

1. Center for Medicare Conditions of Participation for Transplant Centers. http://www.cms.gov/Medicare/Provider-Enrollment-and-Certification/CertificationandComplianc/Transplant.html. Accessed 20 April 2013.
2. Organ Procurement and Transplantation Network (OPTN) Kidney Live Donor Polices. http://optn.transplant.hrsa.gov/PoliciesandBylaws2/policies/pdfs/policy_172.pdf. Accesses 20 April 2013.
3. Steel J, Dunlavy A, Friday M, Kingsley K, Brower D, Unruh M, et.al. A national survey of independent living donor advocates: The need for practice guidelines. Am J Transplant. 2012;12(8):2141–9.
4. Sites AK, Freeman JR, Harper MR, Waters DB, Pruett TL. A multidisciplinary program to educate and advocate for living donors. Prog Transplant. 2008;18(4):284–9.
5. LaPointe Rudow D. Development of the center for living donation: incorporating the role of the nurse practitioner as director. Prog Transplant. 2011;21(4):312–6.
6. LaPointe Rudow D. The living donor advocate: a team approach to educate, evaluate, and mange donors across the continuum. Prog Transplant. 2009;19(1):64–70.
7. Jennings T, Grauer D, LaPointe Rudow D. The role of the independent donor advocate team in the case of the declined living donor candidate. Prog Transplant. 2013;23(2):132–6.
8. Hays R, Gladdy H. Helping helpers: a living donor mentor program. Nephrol News Issues. 2007;5(41):45–7, 51.

Chapter 10
Classification of Living Organ Donors

Andrew W. Webb, RN, BSN, CCTC

Introduction

The kidney used in the first successful transplant came from a living donor. The surgery occurred in 1954 at the Peter Bent Brigham Hospital in Boston, Massachusetts. The kidney came from Ronald Herrick, a living donor, and was transplanted into Richard Herrick, his identical twin brother. Due to their identical genetics, the kidney was spared the risk of acute rejection and gave Richard 8 more years of life, during which he got married and had two children. Ronald lived another 56 years before passing away at the age of 79 while recovering from heart surgery. In the 58 years since this landmark case, living organ donors have continued to be a part of the transplant landscape. Living donors can be categorized by their relation to the recipient and the type of organ they are donating, while some subgroups of donors face unique challenges.

Relation Between Living Donor and Recipient

One way to categorize living donors is by their relation to their intended recipient. Living donors related to their intended recipient include consanguineous relatives such as parents, siblings, grandparents, aunts, uncles, and cousins. Based on the data from the Organ Procurement and Transplantation Network (OPTN), 53.3 % of living donors in 2011 were related to their recipients, with the three most common relationships being full sibling (19.4 %), child (15.7 %), and parent (9.2 %) [1]. Out of the 46.5 % who were unrelated to their recipients, the three most common relationships were other (22.0 %), spouse (11.5 %), and paired donation (7.3 %) [1]. Driven mainly by kidney donors, there has been a steady increase in unrelated living donors

---

A. W. Webb, RN, BSN, CCTC (✉)
Renal Transplant Office, University of Missouri Hospital and Clinics,
DC035.00, One Hospital Drive, Columbia, MO 65212, USA
e-mail: WebbAW@health.missouri.edu

over the last decade both in percentage of the whole and raw number. In 2000, 1,549 unrelated living donors contributed organs, which comprised 26.1% of the living organs donated during that year [1]. By 2011, the number of unrelated living donors was up to 2,801, which accounted for 46.5% of the whole, while the number of related living donors fell from 4,375 (73.8%) in 2000 to 3,209 (53.3%) in 2011 [1]. The factors that may explain this shift include increased emphasis on living donor recruitment as wait list times have increased, evidence that kidney graft survival from unrelated living donors is superior to that of deceased donors, an increased number of altruistic donors, and the growth of kidney paired donation (KPD) programs.

Increasing recipient wait times for kidney transplant has resulted in efforts to increase the number of living donor transplants and created two growing subsets of unrelated donors. The first is the altruistic donor who chooses to donate a kidney to an unknown recipient on the transplant wait list. Although this type of donor was initially met with some skepticism, it has become more accepted and common in the U.S., although many countries still do not accept altruistic and/or unrelated donors. OPTN data reveal that the number of unrelated anonymous donors has increased from 21 in the year 2000 to 161 in 2011 [1]. This subset of living donors best illustrates the collision of two core responsibilities of the independent living donor advocate (ILDA). They must both advocate for the right of the altruistic donor to give their organ while also promoting their best interests, which may not be served by giving an organ to a stranger. Determining how the ILDA should balance the potential tension between these two mandates is arguably the most controversial aspect of their role and will be discussed in more detail later in the book.

The second growing subset of unrelated donors derives from the population of living donors unable to donate to their intended recipient due to blood-type or crossmatch incompatibility. The development of KPD programs gives these incompatible donors a chance to donate to a compatible recipient and have their intended recipient receive a kidney from a compatible living donor. This can take the form of a simple exchange or a more complicated chain of several pairs of donors and recipients. In an exchange, you have two incompatible donor/recipient pairs that are able to donate to each other. For example, donor A is blood type B and thus incompatible with recipient A, who is blood type A. Donor B is blood type A (subgroup A1) and thus incompatible with recipient B, who is blood type B. However, donor A is compatible and can donate to recipient B, while donor B is compatible and can donate to recipient A (Fig. 10.1).

An altruistic donor's kidney can start a sequence of transplants between incompatible donor/recipient pairs. For example, the altruist donates a kidney to recipient A, donor A donates to recipient B, donor B donates to recipient C, donor C donates to recipient D, and so on until the chain reaches its conclusion (Fig. 10.2). The number of KPD transplants has increased from 2 in 2000 to 429 in 2011 [2]. This growth has occurred despite the barriers of increased logistical challenges for geographically distant donor/recipient pairs, the potential for broken chains caused by donors who back out, and the KPD system being fragmented across multiple programs managed by organizations such as the OPTN, the National Kidney Registry (NKR), and Alliance for Paired Donation (APD). The longest KPD chain to date

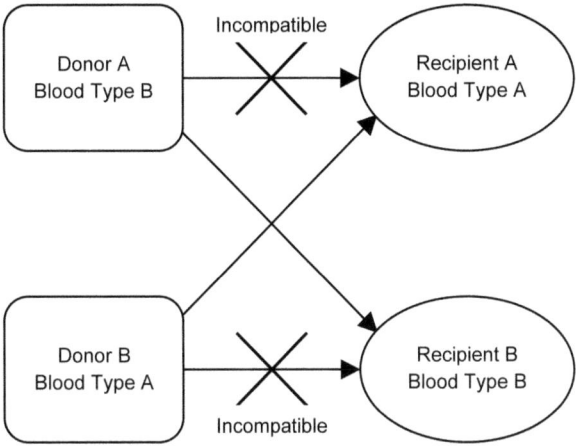

Fig. 10.1 Donor A and donor B are both blood type incompatible with their intended recipients. They are blood type compatible with the other's recipient. In a KPD program, donor A can donate a kidney to recipient B in exchange for donor B donating their kidney to recipient A

was a series of 30 living donor kidney transplants, which took place over 4 months involving 17 hospitals across 11 states and was organized by the NKR [3, 4].

Despite the increased numbers of altruistic and KPD donors, the total number of living donors has decreased by 13.9 % from a high of 6,991 in 2004 to 6,019 in 2011 [2]. While the exact cause of this decrease is unknown, it may be partly attributable to increasing governmental oversight of living donor outcomes. Increased program accountability for living donor outcomes could result in programs declining more marginal candidates. The ILDA can influence the use of these marginal candidates in two distinct ways. In the short term, they can fulfill one aspect of their role through increased advocacy for the donor's right to donate, although this may be at the cost of their mandate to promote the donor's best interests. In the long term, the ILDA can take an active role in monitoring their follow-up to determine if their donation does place them at higher risk for poor outcomes.

What Organs Can a Living Donor Donate?

Living Kidney Donors

Living kidney donors are the most common type of living organ donor and they comprise a significant amount of the kidney transplants performed. Of kidney transplants performed in 2011, 32.7 % came from living donors [2]. This 32.7 % represents 5,768 people stepping forward and voluntarily choosing to have one of their kidneys removed for no personal medical benefit with the intent of improving the recipient's quality of life. The acceptance of living kidney donation by the transplant community and the public is based on studies that have found that the rate of end-stage renal disease in living kidney donors is equal to or better than the rate found in the general population [5–8].

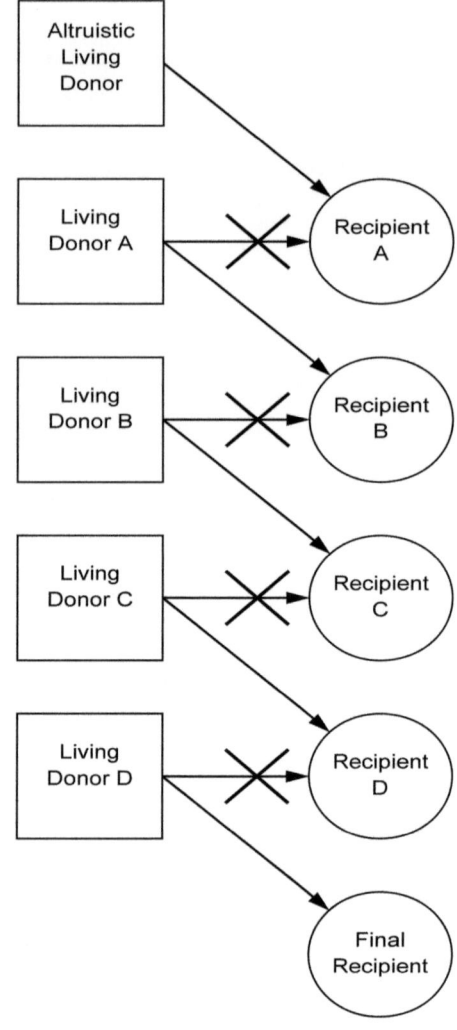

Fig. 10.2 In this example, living donors A–D are incompatible with their intended recipients. An altruistic donor is the catalyst in creating a chain of compatible transplants. The final recipient may be another recipient with an incompatible donor or a recipient listed on the deceased donor wait list

There has been a steady increase in the number of unrelated living kidney donors over the past 11 years [2]. Graft survival rates for kidney transplants from unrelated living kidney donors have been found to be similar to those from related living donors [8, 9], while both types of living donor kidneys have superior outcomes to kidneys from deceased donors [2]. Living donor kidney graft survival compared to deceased donor graft survival is 96.5% versus 91.9% at 1 year, 82.9% versus 70.6% at 5 years, and 60.9% versus 43.4% at 10 years [10]. The differences in these outcomes are often attributed to the scheduled nature of the procedure resulting in decreased cold ischemic time and the living donor evaluation process screening out marginal donors. For example, a transplant program might accept a 55-year-old deceased donor with a 2-year history of diabetes, but it is unlikely they would accept a living donor with these same attributes.

Despite the decline in living donors, they continue to comprise a significant portion of the number of yearly kidney transplants. New OPTN policy implemented in February 2013 should improve collection of follow-up data for the first 2 years post donation. However, it is important that the transplant community continue to engage in long-term tracking and analysis of kidney donor outcomes as it provides essential information to appropriately educate potential living donors of their risk.

Living Liver Donors

While the total number of liver transplants has increased over the past decade, the number of living liver donors has decreased by 52.9% to 247 in 2011 [2]. Livers from living donors have higher rates of graft survival compared to livers from deceased donors [2], with rates of 88.7% versus 85.3% at 1 year, 75.8% versus 68.4% at 5 years, and 59.8% versus 54.4% at 10 years [10]. Accounting for only 3.9% of the liver transplants performed in 2011, it is likely that the decrease in living liver donors over the past decade is the result of donor safety concerns [11].

Living Lung Donors

Lung transplants from living donors have never been widely performed and have become extremely rare in the U.S. since 2005, when the implementation of the lung allocation score (LAS) resulted in a substantial decrease in the waiting time for a deceased lung transplant [2, 12]. The median wait time for a lung transplant in 2004, prior to the implementation of the LAS, was 17.3 months compared to a median wait time of 3.6 months in 2011 [2, 10]. The LAS is designed to provide lungs based on medical urgency, thus providing a transplant quickest to those most in need [13]. It is possible that this quicker access to a deceased donor for those most ill combined with the potential risk to a living donor has contributed to the decreased use of living lung donors in the U.S. While there have been 143 living lung donors since 1998, there have only been 2 since 2008 [2]. Due to the low number of donors, it is difficult to accurately compare outcomes in graft survival.

Other Living Donors

Although extremely rare, it is possible to donate a portion of your intestine or pancreas. According to OPTN data, there have been 39 living intestine donors and 7 living pancreas donors since 1994 with only 4 intestine donors and 1 pancreas donor since 2008 [1]. Due to the low number of donors, it is difficult to accurately compare outcomes in graft survival.

Factors that Impede Living Donation

Donating to Undocumented Recipients

Substantial financial barriers typically arise when a living donor attempts to donate to a recipient who is undocumented. Medicare will not pay for the undocumented recipient's transplant surgery and private insurance for the recipient can be difficult to obtain. The impact of these financial barriers can be seen in the experience of Angel, an undocumented immigrant in need of a kidney transplant whose brother was a willing living donor [14]. It was only after 2 years of negotiating costs with their hospital, high-profile national attention, and fund-raising that they were finally able to overcome this barrier and proceed with the transplant [14].

It is interesting to note that in most states, Medicaid pays for patients to undergo dialysis as an emergency measure regardless of their documentation status. The irony is that a kidney transplant, which lasts 3 years, begins to become a less expensive treatment option than dialysis. Considering that 82.9% of transplanted kidneys from living donors are still working 5 years after the transplant [10], a strong argument can be made that it is financially advantageous to the taxpayer for Medicare to cover the cost for undocumented recipients with living donors [15].

Military Donors

The different branches of the military have service-specific guidelines regarding active-duty personnel being a live organ donor. Those covering the Navy and Marines can be found in the Department of the Navy, Bureau of Medicine and Surgery (BUMED), Instruction 6300.8A [16]. Those covering the Army can be found in Army Regulation (AR) 40-3 [17], and those covering the Air Force can be found in Air Force Instruction (AFI) 44-102 [18].

The guidelines covering the Army and Navy/Marines are extremely similar and can be considered together. They both state that, "Active duty members may serve as living-related or living-unrelated organ donors in the absence of better-matched volunteer donors" [16, p. 6, 17, p. 29]. However, they also mandate that the potential donor be counseled that his or her "qualification for continued service will be contingent upon favorable medical evaluation results following organ donation" [16, p. 6, 17, p. 29].

If the donor is going to donate their organ outside of the Army/Navy Organ Transplant Service located at Walter Reed Medical Center, they need to go through additional approval and documentation [16, 17]. If the donation is going to be performed at an another transplant facility, then the service member will have to obtain prior approval through their chain of command and submit documentation as specified in the appropriate service guidelines [16, 17]. It is also mandated that post donation, when they would normally be discharged from the transplant hospital, they will be instead transferred to a military treatment facility to be, "medically evaluated after the organ donation to determine his or her future profile, assignments, and qualifications for continued service" [16, p. 7, 17, p. 30].

Although the Air Force guidelines use different language and are less specific, they have similar content as AR 40-2 and BUMED 6300.9A. It lists specific steps for a potential living donor to follow to obtain approval through the chain of command but warns that, "complications might limit or prohibit further active duty service" [18, p. 50]. The instructions do not make a distinction based upon whether the donation is performed at a military transplant program or an outside program, nor does it require that the donor be transferred to a military treatment facility for evaluation at the time of discharge from the hospital [18].

Although it is unclear how often it occurs, there are provisions within each branch of the military for active-duty personnel to become living donors, and news stories show that it does occur [19, 20]. It is critical for potential living donors in any branch of the military to obtain proper approval through the chain of command and be educated that their continued military service will be based on their post-donation medical evaluation.

Conclusion

Although the total number of living organ donors in the U.S. has decreased over the past 7 years, there have been increases in the number of unrelated living kidney donors driven by successful outcomes, the flourishing of KPD programs, and increased acceptance of altruists. The use of living donors for pancreas, intestine, and lung transplants has dropped to a negligible amount, while the use of liver donors has decreased by half over the past decade. It should be a priority for the transplant community to identify the causes of this contraction and determine what, if anything, should be done to counteract it.

Acknowledgments This work was supported in part by Health Resources and Services Administration contract 234-2005-37011C. The content is the responsibility of the authors alone and does not necessarily reflect the views or policies of the Department of Health and Human Services, nor does mention of trade names, commercial products, or organizations imply endorsement by the US Government.

The data and analyses reported in the 2010 and 2011 Annual Data Report of the US Organ Procurement and Transplantation Network and the Scientific Registry of Transplant Recipient have been supplied by the United Network of Organ Sharing and the Minneapolis Medical Research Foundation under contract with HHS/HRSA. The authors alone are responsible for reporting and interpreting these data; the views expressed herein are those of the authors and not necessarily those of the US Government.

References

1. Organ Procurement and Transplantation Network Data Reports (US) [Internet]. Rockville (MD): Department of Health and Human Services, Health Resources and Services Administration, Healthcare Systems Bureau, Division of Transplantation. [1988]—[cited 2013 Feb 15]. Available from http://optn.transplant.hrsa.gov/latestData/advancedData.asp.
2. Organ Procurement and Transplantation Network (OPTN) (US) and Scientific Registry of Transplant Recipients (SRTR) (US). OPTN/SRTR 2011 annual data report. Rockville (MD): Department of Health and Human Services, Health Resources and Services Administration, Healthcare Systems Bureau, Division of Transplantation; 2012.
3. Sack K. 60 lives, 30 kidneys, all linked. The New York Times [Internet]. 2012 Feb 18 [cited 2013 January 16];Sect. A1. Available from http://www.nytimes.com/2012/02/19/health/lives-forever-linked-through-kidney-transplant-chain-124.html?pagewanted=all&_r=1&.
4. National Kidney Registry (NKR). NKR paired exchange results quarterly report. Babylon (NY): National Kidney Registry; 2012 Sep 30.
5. Cherikh WS, Young CJ, Kramer BF, Taranto SE, Randall HB, Fan PY. Ethnic and gender related differences in the risk of end-stage renal disease after living kidney donation. Am J Transplant. 2011;11:1650–5.
6. Ibrahim HN, Foley R, Tan L, Rogers T, Bailey RF, Guo H, et al. Long-term consequences of kidney donation. N Engl J Med. 2009;360:459–69.
7. Gossmann J, Wilhelm A, Kachel HG, Jordan J, Sann U, Geiger H, et al. Long-term consequences of live kidney donation follow-up in 93 % of living kidney donors in a single transplant center. Am J Transplant. 2005;5:2417–24.
8. Fuller TF, Feng S, Brennan TV, Tomlanovich S, Bostrom A, Freise CE. Increased rejection in living unrelated versus living related kidney transplants does not affect short-term function and survival. Transplantation. 2004;78(7):1030.
9. Organ Procurement and Transplantation Network (OPTN) (US) and Scientific Registry of Transplant Recipients (SRTR) (US). OPTN/SRTR 2008 annual data report. Rockville (MD): Department of Health and Human Services, Health Resources and Services Administration, Healthcare Systems Bureau, Division of Transplantation; 2008.
10. Organ Procurement and Transplantation Network (OPTN) (US) and Scientific Registry of Transplant Recipients (SRTR) (US). OPTN/SRTR 2010 annual data report. Rockville (MD): Department of Health and Human Services, Health Resources and Services Administration, Healthcare Systems Bureau, Division of Transplantation; 2011.
11. Pomfret EA, Fryer JP, Sima CS, Lake JR, Merion RM. Liver and intestine transplantation in the United States, 1996–2005. Am J Transplant. 2007;7:1376–89.
12. Iribarne A, Russo MJ, Davies RR, Hong, KN, Gelijns AC, Bacchetta MD, et al. Despite decreased wait-list times for lung transplantation, lung allocation scores continue to increase. Chest. 2009;135(4):923–8.
13. Egan TM, Murray S, Bustami RT, Shearon TH, McCullough KP, Edwards LB, et al. Development of the new lung allocation system in the United States. Am J Transplant. 2006;6:1212–27.
14. Bernstein N. From brother to brother, a kidney, and a life. The New York Times [Internet]. 2012 Apr 6 [corrected 2012 Apr 11; cited 2013 January 16];Sect. A15. Available from http://www.nytimes.com/2012/04/07/nyregion/after-years-of-obstacles-an-illegal-immigrant-gets-a-transplant.html.
15. Linden EA, Cano J, Coritsidis GN. Kidney transplantation in undocumented immigrants with ESRD: a policy whose time has come?. Am J Kidney Dis. 2012 Sep;60(3):354–9.
16. Department of the Navy (US). Instruction 6300.8A [Internet]. Falls Church (VA): Department of the Navy (US), Bureau of Medicine and Surgery; 2010 [cited 2013 January 16]. Available from http://www.med.navy.mil/directives/ExternalDirectives/6300.8A.pdf .
17. Department of the Army (US). Army regulation 40-3 medical, dental and veterinary care [Internet]. Falls Church (VA): Department of the Army (US); 2008 [revised 2010 Mar 12; cited 2013 January 16]. Available from http://www.apd.army.mil/pdffiles/r40_3.pdf.

18. Department of the Air Force (US). Air Force instruction 44-102 medical care management [Internet]. Rosslyn (VA): Department of the Air Force (US); 2012 [cited 2013 January 16]. Available from http://www.af.mil/shared/media/epubs/AFI44-102.pdf.
19. Ellis K, Zill R. Soldier gives NCO gift of life at Walter Reed. Army News Service (US) [Internet]. 2009 Apr 27 [cited 2013 Feb 24]. Available from http://www.army.mil/article/20196/.
20. Official Blog of the U.S. Navy Judge Advocate General's Corps [Internet]. Washington Navy Yard (DC): U.S. Navy Judge Advocate General's Corp; [c2011] NLSO EURAFSWA and BUMED assist sailor and family with living donor program. 2012 Feb 23 [cited 2013 Feb 24]. Available from http://usnavyjagcorps.wordpress.com/tag/walter-reed-national-military-medical-center/.

Chapter 11
Unrelated Donors

Mary Amanda Dew, Ginger Boneysteele and Andrea F. DiMartini

Introduction

The traditional solid organ donor is either biologically related (e.g., a parent, child, sibling, or other family member) or emotionally related (e.g., a spouse or partner) to the intended recipient, and the majority of donations are between such donor–recipient pairs. The terms "biologically" or "emotionally" related suggest important and meaningful connections between donor–recipient pairs, and it is commonly assumed that an existing relationship between the donor and recipient confers a special connection that—if not providing some protection against risk for poor psychosocial outcomes—at least makes the offer to donate appear understandable. However, increasing numbers of donors without such biological or emotional connections are coming forward to donate, and transplant teams must be prepared to evaluate and determine their suitability for donation. In addition, as for all donors, teams have an ethical mandate to work to ensure unrelated donors' protection against psychosocial harm secondary to donation.

In this chapter, we address issues relevant to the psychosocial evaluation and informed consent process with unrelated donor candidates, defined as individuals who are neither emotionally nor biologically related to the intended transplant recipient. In addition, we consider the more recent phenomenon of unrelated donors arising from organ exchange programs, and we consider issues in the follow-up of unrelated donors after donation. Beyond the safeguards and assessment consider-

---

M. A. Dew (✉) · A. F. DiMartini
Department of Psychiatry, School of Medicine and Medical Center, University of Pittsburgh, 3811 O'Hara Street, Pittsburgh, PA, USA
e-mail: dewma@upmc.edu

A. F. DiMartini
e-mail: DiMartiniAF@upmc.edu

G. Boneysteele
Department of Psychiatry, University of Pittsburgh Medical Center, 3811 O'Hara Street, Pittsburgh, PA, US
e-mail: boneysteelejg@msn.com

ations that apply to related donors, we describe how special care must be taken to ensure that unrelated donors are carefully evaluated to reduce the likelihood that individuals at high risk for poorer psychosocial outcomes would proceed to donation. In fact, some of their very motivations for donating may place them at risk for poor psychosocial outcomes. For these reasons, donors who are neither biologically nor emotionally related to the intended recipient have been considered with some degree of suspicion by clinicians and transplant programs alike. Clinicians who perform the psychosocial evaluations of unrelated donors (which in some programs, includes the independent living donor advocate (ILDA)) require skills to conduct such a heightened assessment and specific strategies to assess donor motivation, decision making, and the potential for coercion. The ILDA, if not involved in conducting the psychosocial evaluation of unrelated donors, requires similar expertise in order to review the results of the evaluation and advocate for the best interests of the prospective donor.

A Continuum of Relatedness

Several terms are used in the literature for unrelated donors: altruistic donors, Good Samaritan donors, stranger donors, or more recently anonymous directed and anonymous nondirected donors. In this chapter, we will use the term "unrelated donor," and we will include individuals who have no previous relationship with the intended recipient as well as those who may not be complete strangers but do not have a strong emotional connection with the intended recipient. In clinical practice, donor teams will see a wide range of relatedness and relational circumstances between donor–recipient pairs. In fact, emotional relatedness, as with biological relatedness, can be considered along a continuum (Fig. 11.1). Even among biologically related individuals, varying degrees of emotional relatedness can be observed. Consider as an example of this complexity a donor–recipient pair who are coworkers but are more emotionally related than a biologically related pair who are extended family members and may have met only once or twice in their lives.

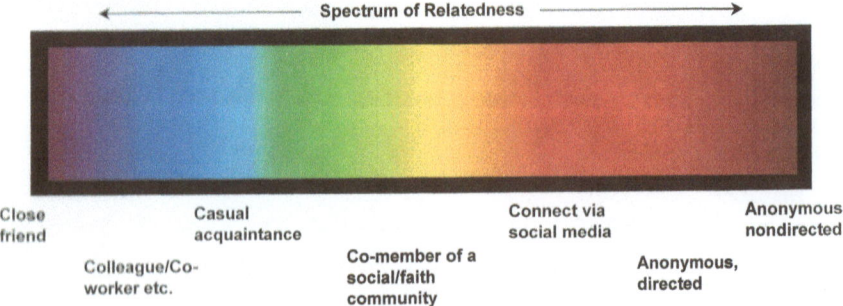

Fig. 11.1 Emotional relatedness: How unrelated are unrelated donors?

Increasing Numbers of Unrelated Donors

In the US, unrelated kidney donations have markedly increased over the past 20 years, with over 2,000 in 2012, or 37% of the total number of living kidney donors [1] (Fig. 11.2). In contrast, unrelated donors constituted only 4% of all donors 20 years earlier. Over the past 20 years, the composition of the pool of unrelated donors has also changed. Since the advent of paired kidney exchange donation in the early 2000s and domino chains later in the decade, the number of kidney donors participating in these programs has increased, and they constituted about 9% of all donors in 2012. The numbers of anonymous nondirected donors have increased as well. There were no such donors in the early 1990s, but they accounted for 3% of all donors by 2012. The situation in living liver donation is somewhat different. The total number of living liver donors is considerably smaller, rising over the past 20 years from just 33 in 1992 to 363 by 2012. The proportion of unrelated donors has increased from 12% to 26% over that time. However, the vast majority of unrelated living liver donors are directed donors (i.e., they have some connection with the intended recipient even if it is not a close connection). In addition, the majority of living liver donors continue to be individuals who are biologically related to the transplant recipient.

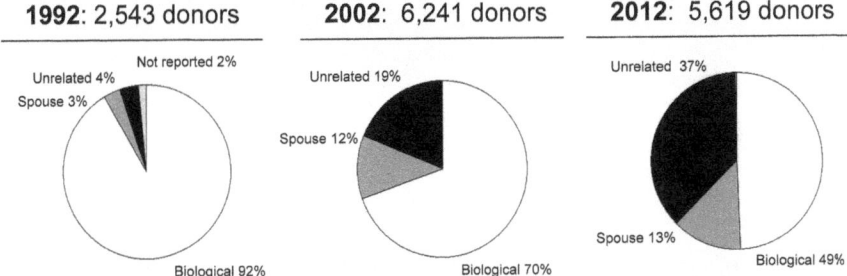

Fig. 11.2 Changing distributions of types of living kidney donors in the US (data from OPTN/UNOS [1]). Unrelated donors include nonbiological directed donors, anonymous donors, and exchange donors

Increasing Acceptance of Unrelated Donors

The increasing number of unrelated donors by itself suggests a trend toward greater acceptance by transplant programs of the idea that these individuals are suitable and appropriate donors. In addition, several surveys of transplant programs over the past 20 years directly show that attitudes toward unrelated donation have become gradually more favorable. In 1999, while almost all surveyed programs responded that they would consider a close friend as a donor, only 38% of programs said they would consider an altruistic/stranger donor (compared to 8% in 1987) [2].

Interestingly, at that same time a public survey of over 1,000 US adults showed that 90% supported the concept of close friend donors and 80% accepted donation by altruistic strangers [3].

A recent survey of 132 US kidney transplant programs (53% of programs listed by the United Network for Organ Sharing (UNOS) revealed that now most programs, but not all, accept donors other than immediate family, close friends, or extended family members with close emotional ties to the intended recipient [4]. For a variety of other types of donor–recipient relationships, the programs' acceptance lies along the continuum of emotional connectedness. Programs had greater concern as the emotional connection between donor and recipient becomes weaker. For example, while 92% said they would find a patient's coworker to be acceptable as a potential donor, 74% felt that acquaintances with no emotional ties to the recipient would be acceptable, 61% thought nondirected donors were acceptable, and only 30% were willing to consider publicly solicited donors [4]. There was some evidence that programs in geographic regions with longer wait times and lower deceased organ donation rates were more likely to consider unrelated donors for their patients [4]. At the time of this survey, while most programs required all donors to undergo a mental health evaluation, 10% of programs required only certain types of donors (e.g., unrelated donors) to be seen for more extensive consideration by a mental health professional [4]. Notably, at the time of this survey only about half of the kidney programs were participating in paired kidney exchange. Even more importantly, although many programs appeared to support the concept of unrelated donors, in practice, these types of transplants remain less common than those with biologically or closely emotionally related donors (i.e., spouses). Thus, while agreeing philosophically with the concept of unrelated donors, when faced with an actual volunteer, programs might be reluctant to proceed, with many programs expressing concerns about the motives of a completely unrelated donor [2, 4].

Ethical and Psychosocial Issues Arising from Increases in Unrelated Donations

The need for and acceptance of unrelated donors has been driven by the continued shortage of donor organs relative to patients who need transplants. Recognition that biologically unrelated donor grafts (e.g., from spouses) did not adversely affect donor medical outcomes [5, 6] set the stage for consideration of a much wider population of potential donors. It also allowed for the development of novel approaches to the use of organs from unrelated kidney donors to increase the numbers of transplants performed, including paired exchanges and domino chains (see Chap. 2). However, the increase in unrelated donors has also prompted concerns at the stages of screening prospective donors and conducting the pre-donation psychosocial evaluation; concerns regarding the informed consent process for these individuals to ensure that they understand what they are volunteering to do; and concerns about whether these donors have unique psychosocial risks and require more careful follow-up after donation [7]. In the remaining sections of the chapter, we address issues in each of these domains, particularly as they pertain to the ILDA's involvement and responsibilities in donor care.

Screening and Evaluation of Prospective Unrelated Donors

Screening and Types of Unrelated Donors that Provoke Heightened Concern

Most donor programs conduct an initial screen with prospective donors before they are asked to come in for a full medical and psychosocial evaluation. This screen is often conducted by telephone. ILDAs may perform screens, but the screens are more typically completed by a living donor coordinator, who may consult with the ILDA if concerns arise. Some types of unrelated donors who come forward for initial screening may indeed raise such concerns, as enumerated in a consensus conference offering guidelines for the screening and evaluation process [7, 8]. Such individuals include those who are:

- Solicited from the internet or other social media appeals,
- In a superior/subordinate relationship with the intended recipient (employers/employees; teachers/students),
- Of very low socioeconomic status,
- Foreign nationals,
- Members of organizations/faith communities,
- Seeking to make an anonymous donation (either directed or nondirected), and
- Involved in paired/list exchange or chain donation.

It is noteworthy that the concern is not that these individuals should automatically be ruled out as donors (although sometimes this may indeed be the case). Instead, these individuals and their circumstances often require more extensive psychosocial evaluation in order to determine whether donation is a realistic possibility for them. Thus, the telephone screen is helpful for identifying initial "red flags" that will require more attention in the full-scale psychosocial evaluation. For example, as we discuss later in the chapter, there are varying ways in which coercion or undue pressure could influence or affect some of these types of donors. In addition, individuals coming forward as unrelated donors may have much less knowledge about the transplantation process than individuals who have seen a loved one become ill and cope with chronic illness. They may have also been influenced by the emotional appeal of a case in the news or an acquaintance who has become ill, without having yet had the time to learn about the range of treatments that might be available to the ill individual or the risks associated with donation. Some persons interested in unrelated donation may not understand even rudimentary aspects of what donation entails.

> **Case Vignette**
>
> A young woman called a donor program to ask if she could be considered as a donor for a coworker. She said that she had not yet talked to her coworker about it, but she had read a considerable amount on the internet about kidney donation and she felt that it was the right thing for her to do. The living donor coordinator, as part of the program's standard screening protocol, began to review the steps that would need to be undertaken in order for the woman to be evaluated for donation, and commented on the surgery and how long the recovery period typically lasted. At that point, the young woman said, "Oh, you mean this requires surgery?" She said that she would have to think more about it and would call back if she wanted to continue to move forward.

The telephone screen allows an initial opportunity for the donor program to begin the process of learning about the prospective donor and also educating him or her about donation. If it is not automatically clear that a prospective donor is medically or psychosocially unsuitable for or uninterested in further evaluation, then the prospective donor is typically scheduled for such evaluation.

Special Considerations in the Psychosocial Evaluation of Unrelated Donors

The psychosocial evaluation that is conducted with prospective unrelated donors who come to the donor program for a full workup is in many ways identical to that conducted for any other prospective donor. Thus, the central goals for the evaluation are to (1) identify and appraise risks for poor psychosocial outcomes, (2) assess donor capacity to understand information and make decisions, and (3) identify factors warranting intervention before donation can occur [7–12]. In order to accomplish these goals, the evaluation includes a variety of components: obtaining standard information on demographic and psychosocial history; determining the individual's cognitive capacity; ascertaining mental health history and current status; examining donor motivation; exploring the nature of the relationship (if any) with the intended recipient; assessing knowledge, preparation, and expectations for donation surgery; assessing available social supports and attitudes of others about the donation; and reviewing financial considerations [7–15]. Although there are no national standards for the exact content or process of conducting the psychosocial evaluation, the domains listed earlier cover the elements currently required by Organ Procurement and Transplantation Network (OPTN) policy [16]. In conjunction with recently approved policy modifications, the OPTN/UNOS Living Kidney Donor Psychosocial Evaluation Checklist provides a useful tool to ensure that essential elements are covered in the evaluation [17].

In some programs, the ILDA may conduct the psychosocial evaluation. In other programs, the ILDA does not conduct the evaluation but must carefully review its results, along with meeting the prospective donor to review and discuss all aspects of the medical and psychosocial evaluation process. For unrelated donors, key components of the psychosocial evaluation require more extended consideration, both during the evaluation itself as well as in any separate meeting the ILDA has with the individual. We have listed several of those components in Table 11.1: those related to motivation, relationship with the intended recipient, knowledge, social supports, and financial issues. We have also enumerated in Table 11.1 important issues and questions to be asked, as well as "red flags" that, if present, could indicate that the individual is not a suitable donor [7, 8, 13–15]. We note that many of these issues could apply to biologically and emotionally related donors as well. Our point is, however, that they are often of heightened importance when evaluating unrelated donors. For example, "red flags" when assessing prospective unrelated donors' motives would include evidence uncovered of a desire to form a relationship with intended recipient even if the donor is going to engage in anonymous nondirected donation, or evidence that the prospective donor is seeking public recognition of their act of donation.

The clinician who conducts the psychosocial evaluation as well as the ILDA during the subsequent review of its results, must bear in mind that prospective donors may not answer all questions truthfully. This is often not to be intentionally untruthful, but rather that they may be attempting to say what they think the evaluator wants to hear or what they hope will be sufficient so that they will be approved as donors [11, 12]. This effort at self-presentation may be heightened to the extent that they are feeling pressured to consider donation. Hence, questioning about motives for coming forward, asked in a nonconfrontational manner, becomes particularly critical in order to help ensure that prospective donors have made their own choice regarding donation. Alternatively, rather than the prospective donor appearing to offer information that is not completely truthful, the evaluator and/or the ILDA may have the impression that the individual is withholding certain information or is particularly wary of providing complete information.

Case Vignette

A middle-aged woman came for a psychosocial evaluation by the donor program because she sought to "donate a kidney to a child." She later changed this request to donate to anyone. She gave an address several hundred miles from the donor program and was noted to be carrying what appeared to be most, if not all, of her possessions. She denied being seen at any other transplant facility, despite the long distance between her home address and the donor program, and the existence of other donor programs closer to her home. She answered most questions appropriately but with very few words and she was unable to elaborate on them or provide any specifics. She denied any mental health history. She refused to allow contact with her family, past treating physicians or friends and so no collateral information was available. She also had no plan for any follow-up care and seemed to assume the recipient and the hospital would bear all responsibility for her and any care needed. It was decided that the woman would not be a suitable donor at the current time.

Table 11.1 Components of the psychosocial evaluation for living organ donors: Issues to cover, examples of questions to ask, and responses suggesting heightened risk

Issues to cover	Types of questions	Red flags
Motives for donation Reasons for coming forward Decision-making process Coercion or inducement Ambivalence If relevant: views and understanding of kidney exchange	How did the prospective donor learn about the possibility of donating? Did someone ask the donor to come forward? Was there pressure to donate from anyone or because the situation appears urgent? What is the primary motivation for donation? Why donate? Why now? What volunteer or helping acts have been most important in the individual's life up to this point? Are there other possible donors? What if someone else could do it instead? Did anyone attempt to influence the individual's decision to come forward? Did anyone state or imply that there could be negative consequences for the individual if they did not come forward? Or that the individual would receive something (tangible or non-tangible goods) if he/she came forward? What does the individual see as the consequences to him/herself if the donation does not occur? How would a donor feel if a deceased donor organ became available? Would not donating to a loved one change their feelings about willingness or desire to donate? If option for kidney exchange is present: Does the option of chain/exchange make the donor feel obligated to donate? Does the donor feel any pressure that many other donors/recipients may be counting on them?	Prospective donor made a blind agreement to donate with no information (e.g., promise to "do anything to help" long before donation was needed) Donor has a history of impulsive decision making, uses poor judgment, and is an excessive risk taker Desire to: Atone for or reduce a sin Form a (closer) relationship with the intended recipient Make up for past problems with others/loss of loved one Serve humanity despite no evidence of past service Gain recognition from others for act of giving Obtain financial rewards/benefits Donor is counting on a deceased donor organ becoming available Donor is hoping someone else will come forward to donate If option for kidney exchange is present: Donor feels less capable of deciding not to donate, or pressured to participate in an exchange Donor feels guilty or as if they would let others down if they did not participate

Table 11.1 (continued)

Issues to cover	Types of questions	Red flags
Relationship with intended recipient		
Nature of any existing relationship Degree of closeness (if any) of relationship Perceived obligations/expectations	How long have the prospective donor and intended recipient known each other? When/how did they meet? What is the relationship like? Does the donor feel any obligation to donate? Will the intended recipient feel indebted? How will the relationship change if the donation takes place? Or if it does not take place? How will the donor view the recipient's behavior after transplant (e.g., if the recipient is not adherent)? How will the donor feel if he/she never meets (or rarely sees) the recipient?	Prospective donor wants to have an upper hand in the relationship; desire for control Donor has a subordinate relationship to the intended recipient (e.g., employee) Relationship has a history of conflict or estrangement Donor is worried about what will happen to the relationship if donation cannot occur
Knowledge about surgery/recovery		
Understanding of risks Understanding of likely outcomes Expectations	If the prospective donor knows the intended recipient, does the donor understand what type of disease the recipient has? Are there treatment alternatives to a living donor transplant? Has the recipient received a transplant before? Why is another transplant needed? What does the donor understand to be the risks/benefits to the recipient? What are the major risks to the donor? How does the donor expect his/her own postoperative recovery to go? How would the donor feel if the donated organ turned out to be of little or no benefit? Or if the recipient died?	Prospective donor cannot articulate recipient risks/benefits Donor cannot articulate his/her own risks Donor expresses no sense of concern in the event that the transplant procedures prematurely end his/her life Donor says that if the recipient does not survive the transplant, then neither should the donor Donor expects no short-term physical impairments after the surgery Donor expects to be able to return to work within days after the surgery

Table 11.1 (continued)

Issues to cover	Types of questions	Red flags
Social supports and others' attitudes		
Nature of existing family, friend, employer networks	Did the prospective donor consult with his/her spouse/partner?	Donor has no emotional support from family or friends for the donation
Emotional and practical support available from family, friends, employer	What was that person's reaction?	Donor has active opposition from family and friends
Pressure or opposition from family or friends about donation	What was the reaction from other family members, friends, peers, coworkers, and boss at work?	Donor says he/she does not care whether there is support because "it's my body and I can do what I want with it."
	Did the donor seek advice from anyone?	Donor does not feel able to tell employer of plans because of expected negative reaction
	Did anyone's reactions or advice affect the donor's decision?	
	If their reactions were negative, how is the donor managing this?	Intended recipient has stated unequivocally that he/she will refuse to accept the donation
Financial status		
Financial stability	Does the prospective donor expect any negative impact on finances due to lost time at work?	Prospective donor has no permanent source of income (unemployed or transient employment)
Insurance coverage	What about potential additional expenses and the possibility of financial hardship?	Donor has no health insurance
Resources for unexpected expenses	Does the donor have life insurance?	Donor has no financial cushion
	What is the donor's understanding of whether donation would change eligibility for health or life insurance?	Others in donor's family depend heavily on donor income for meeting expenses
	Has the donor thoroughly considered the possible economic effects of donating an organ?	

Case Vignette

A young woman presented to the donor program asking to be an anonymous nondirected donor. During her psychosocial evaluation, she revealed that she had been treated for anorexia in the past but had no problem with this presently. The evaluator discussed this condition with her in relation to her well-being and to recovery from surgery. She stated that she understood her nutritional needs and how she would care for herself. The next morning, when she returned to the donor program for addition procedures, she passed out in the waiting area and admitted she had had nothing to eat and had run 3 miles. The evaluator judged that her ability to connect her words and actions put her at risk for poor outcomes should she undergo the surgery. There was additional concern that her history of anorexia and desire to lose weight was contributing to her wish to donate an organ.

Case Vignette

A middle-aged man came to the donor program to be considered as a donor for his employer. He performed maintenance duties at several facilities owned by the employer. He stated that no one had asked him to come forward but that he felt that it was the least he could do. During the course of the evaluation, he revealed that his employer was planning to lay off some of his staff across all departments, including maintenance. He denied that he had been informed of any pending layoff involving his own position. However, he was found to have a number of medical morbidities that would have made him a poor donor candidate. It was determined that he should not go forward with donation secondary to medical contraindications and in light of concerns about his psychosocial circumstances.

Finally, the process and timing of the psychosocial evaluation deserve consideration. Given the donor program's mandate to preserve donor safety and well-being, it is important to ensure (when possible) that the evaluation process is not rushed and that there is time to build enough trust with the prospective donor that he/she will feel able to openly discuss all of the issues raised in the evaluation. While this can sometimes be difficult with related donors due to the urgency of the intended recipient's medical condition, with unrelated donors—particularly anonymous nondirected donors—time pressures are generally lessened or minimal. With all donors, however, it is important to allow some time for the prospective donor to reconsider his/her decision based on all of the information provided by the donor team (i.e., a "cooling-off" period), as well as time to have additional consultation with the ILDA as a follow-up to the completion of the medical and psychosocial evaluation.

The Informed Consent Process: Special Considerations with Unrelated Donors

The informed consent process and the role of the ILDA in this process are discussed in Chap. 18. Here, we focus on issues of particular concern that arise during the informed consent of unrelated living donors [7, 11, 14].

Coercion or Undue Pressure to Donate

Unrelated prospective donors may have come forward due to pressure from others. This pressure may be psychological or financial, and the risk may be accentuated when donors are responding to public solicitation, when they come from very poor socioeconomic circumstances, when they are in a subordinate position relative to the intended recipient, or when they are involved in paired exchange donation. With respect to public solicitation, internet or other media advertising that facilitates strangers learning about the needs of individual transplant candidates may present a compelling case for the need that is couched in desperate and emotion-laden terms which elicit a strong psychological response from readers of the messages. A potential donor has this response in the absence of also receiving other information on alternative treatment for the ill individual, or other risks or benefits of donating an organ. Such solicitation may result in prospective donor feelings of high commitment to donation that may be difficult to modify once additional information is provided by the donor program [7].

Individuals' vulnerability to coercion or pressure may also increase if they come from poor socioeconomic circumstances because they may perceive there could be some personal or financial gain from donating. Indeed, there have been widely publicized cases involving the offering of financial incentives or demands for payment at the time of solicitation [18–20], despite the fact that it is a federal crime for any person to knowingly acquire or otherwise transfer any human organ for anything of value such as money or property. It is not difficult to understand, however, that an individual in desperate economic circumstances would see donation as an option; this in fact is not an uncommon motivation in some other countries where organ vending is accepted [21, 22].

Finally, as we noted earlier, individuals who are in subordinate positions to the intended recipient may perceive or experience external pressure to volunteer to donate. They may worry about losing a job (as implied by a case vignette earlier), or they may feel that it would increase their chances of advantage within their workplace, or advantage within the type of relationship they have with the intended recipient (e.g., between a student and a teacher).

Exchange donation presents additional opportunities for coercion or pressure. Paired exchanges and domino chains are swaps or exchanges between donor–recipients pairs where ABO- or crossmatch incompatibility is a barrier. When an exchange donation is offered to overcome incompatibility, prospective donors who are ambivalent, reluctant, or feel otherwise pressured to donate can no longer rely on a medical reason for not undergoing the surgery [23]. Donors may also feel as if the psychological benefit of donation may be more "diffuse" because their organ will not go to their intended recipient with whom they do have a relationship [23]. This may cause greater psychological pressure on the donor because the donor is now put in the position of being asked to give a kidney to a stranger rather than to a loved one [24]. A survey of donor attitudes toward a very specific type of exchange (altruistic unbalanced paired kidney exchange) showed ambivalence by donors about this type of exchange, with participation in the exchange being more likely if the recipient was known [25]. Most worrisome was the expression of concern by half the donors that the opportunity to participate in the exchange would place unwanted pressure on them [25]. The psychosocial evaluator as well as the ILDA must carefully cover these issues in order to provide potentially vulnerable donors adequate protection from coercion or distress.

Although domino chains are limited by the exchange between two or more donor recipient pairs, a variant is for a nondirected donor to begin an extended chain unrestricted by the requirement for reciprocal matching. This may then facilitate many more transplants at higher compatibility levels. Although nondirected donor-initiated chains are considered a major breakthrough in kidney donation, the high publicity of these chains increases the potential for coercion. As touted by the National Kidney Registry, "chains are a way for one Good Samaritan donor to help many patients get transplants instead of just one person" [26]. The most highly publicized chain to date, "Chain 124," occurred in 2011 and was described as "a selfless action of donating to a total stranger" that "saved 30 lives and forever linked 60 people across the country" [27, 28]. It is not hard to imagine the possible psychological coercion of feeling able to save 30 lives or being revered as such a hero.

At the end of chains that are begun by nondirected donors is the "bridge donor," i.e., an individual who is a member of the last pair in the chain and who could have donated to a transplant candidate on the deceased donor wait list, or who instead may wait and initiate a continuation in the chain. The potential for pressure or subtle coercion of this individual exists as well [29]. For example, the bridge donor's circumstances may change as time passes: When they are finally called to donate, they may feel that they are unable to do so for any number of reasons. Thus, perhaps their family member who received a kidney has not done well and they are the primary family caregiver; perhaps they have now lost their job and their socioeconomic circumstances have become very unstable. Yet, to the extent that others state or imply that they (or any other potential donor in the chain) are "reneging" in their obligation or failing to abide by a moral contract to donate, this could have a powerful coercive effect. These sentiments are also expressed by those involved in orchestrating chain donations. When a prospective donor in Chain 124 withdrew for "personal reasons," it was described that the donor "just put 23 patients at risk" [30].

For all of the scenarios described earlier, the ILDA has a critical role determining whether the prospective donor has freely made the decision to donate. The ILDA's obligation is to put the donor's rights and interests ahead of the wishes of anyone else, including the intended recipient and the intended recipient's transplant team. The presence of coercion means that this obligation to the donor can become challenging to uphold. A prospective unrelated donor experiencing coercion may have already decided on their own that donation is the best (or only) option. This may then put the ILDA in the position of appearing to the donor to *not* be supporting what the donor feels is best. The donor may very well feel that the ILDA is not appearing to act as their advocate at all. In such circumstances, it will be important for the prospective donor to understand that the ILDA must not only advise the individual and serve as a resource, but also uphold the ethical mandate to promote the individual's safety and well-being. Indeed, this mandate is shared by everyone on the donor team.

Benefits vs. Risks of Donation

There are several features of the benefit vs. risk issue that are distinctive for unrelated as opposed to related donors. As we discussed in the context of the psychosocial evaluation, prospective donors must show an understanding of the risks and benefits of the donation surgery, both for themselves and for the intended recipient. This is important in order to determine that they have the psychosocial resources necessary to undergo the process (e.g., availability of supports during the recovery period, and financial resources in the event of unanticipated expenses). It is also important in terms of informed consent. Unrelated prospective donors who are vulnerable to coercion or pressure to donate due to their socioeconomic circumstances, for example, may focus on only the possible benefits but not the risks of donation [21, 22]. Individuals who are seeking to donate because they desire personal psychological gain (e.g., to make up for past wrongs or to achieve recognition from others) may also be driven by a focus on such benefits without recognizing the real risks.

Prospective donors must demonstrate an understanding of the risks, benefits, and alternative treatments available to the recipient. Unrelated donors, particularly those who have no personal connection to the transplant candidate, may have difficulty understanding these elements or feeling personally affected by them: to some extent, they are likely to seem "theoretical" or "hypothetical." The prospective unrelated donor, unlike a related donor, may have not observed a loved one live with the illness leading up to a need for transplantation and will not have experienced the fear of losing the individual to death as a result of surgery (or as a result of not having the surgery). Thus, learning about probabilities associated with recipient outcomes may have limited significance to the unrelated donor.

The benefit-to-risk ratio is also different in unrelated donors compared to biologically or emotionally related donors [7]. Related donors are likely to personally and psychologically benefit from seeing their loved one's health improve with transplantation. However, unrelated donors assume risks to their own health and well-being without necessarily having any opportunity to share in the benefits reaped by the recipient. Lack of a connection to the recipient and the attendant known or direct benefits of contributing to their health therefore lead back to the question of the unrelated donor's motivations. Thus, a complete understanding of motivation is not only a prominent issue in the psychosocial evaluation, but also ultimately will affect the ILDA's determination that the prospective donor can give informed consent.

Confidentiality

Given the ILDA's obligation to the prospective donor, confidentiality is a critical concern. Anonymous donation and donation from individuals with minimal social connections to the intended recipient bring some unique concerns in this area. There must be heightened attention by all members of the donor team and recipient team regarding what information, if any, is transmitted to the intended recipient, as well as what information about the recipient is given to the donor. We noted previously that donors must understand the risks, benefits, and alternative treatment available to the intended recipient. Yet, this information must be provided so as to safeguard the recipient's medical information. In addition, unrelated (and, in particular, anonymous) donors and recipients may ultimately be curious about each other and want to know more or meet each other after donation. In one survey, for example, 85 % of anonymous donors reported that they had met their recipient [31]. Alternatively, some anonymous donors may desire not to meet their recipient. In some exchanges and chains, some donor–recipient pairs may not wish to meet any other pairs; this has been the case in some highly publicized chains, even though the majority of donors and recipients have eventually met. A donor's desire to remain anonymous (or pairs' decisions not to meet other pairs) may not be understood by the recipient(s), or may be misinterpreted as a rejection. Protocols should be in place within donor programs to offer guidelines for the circumstances under which previously anonymous individuals can decide to meet, with strategies available to help ensure that neither donor nor recipient (nor donor–recipient pairs in exchanges) feel pressured or otherwise compelled to do so.

Follow-Up After Donation: Special Considerations with Unrelated Donors

Ability to Follow Up Donors After Donation

The submission of information about living donors to the OPTN is required through the 2 years post donation [16]. With recent policy modifications, submitted information for kidney donors must be complete for the majority of donors (i.e., donors must be reached and assessed and cannot be simply marked as lost to follow-up or not contacted). It is likely that such requirements will go into effect for liver donors within the next several years as well. The purpose of collecting such information is to work to ensure the safety of living donation and to provide data on adverse outcomes post donation. We know of no evidence to date that unrelated donors are more (or less) difficult to follow up post donation. On the one hand, one might suggest that unrelated donors would be more difficult to track because there are fewer potential ways to remain in contact or relocate them; for example, their lack of close (or any) ties with the recipient means that neither the recipient nor their family would necessarily be of any assistance in relocating the donor. On the other hand, unrelated donors have often had to take much greater initiative to be evaluated and to engage in organ donation; their commitment to the process may make them easier to follow up after donation.

Psychosocial Outcomes

Although the literature on unrelated donors post donation is scarce, there is little indication to date that their general medical or psychosocial outcomes differ from those observed in related donors [32]. For example, in a recent study, Rodrigue et al. compared a sample of anonymous kidney donors (including nondirected and directed donors) to a group of related donors [31]. The two groups reported similar levels of psychological benefits and health consequences of donation. The groups also did not differ in quality of life, financial consequences of donation, or general satisfaction with having donated. Massey et al. [33] obtained similar findings. Both reports indicate some evidence, however, that anonymous donors may be more likely than other donors to experience negative reactions by others regarding their decision to donate anonymously, and these reactions may cause distress for the donor. Finally, one small report of kidney exchange participants found no evidence that these individuals required additional psychosocial services or practical or emotional support after donation [34]. No studies have compared outcomes among unrelated vs. related living liver donors.

An important concern is whether recipient outcomes would have similar or varying impact among unrelated vs. related donors. On the one hand, the lack of a close connection between unrelated donors and their recipients might lead to less distress in unrelated donors in the event that the recipient has significant posttransplant morbidity or does not survive. Alternatively, given the lessened likelihood of observing even short-term benefits for the recipients that would be observed by related donors, unrelated donors may feel even more devastated at learning of the death of their recipient because this might be the only specific information they have about the recipient's outcomes. This supposition is supported by recent work by Lentine et al. [35]. Although the donor program would engage in mandated follow-ups with these donors as they do with all donors, the ILDA should consider contacting donors as well; additional contact with unrelated donors, particularly in the wake of the recipient's death, may need to be tailored to recognize how the impact of this death may differ in unrelated vs. related donors.

Conclusion

A living donor's relationship to a transplant recipient falls along a continuum of biological and emotional connection. Although the group we have described as unrelated donors are alike in having no biological link to their recipients, they are heterogeneous in their degree of closeness to their recipient. Despite this heterogeneity, we have delineated certain issues that arise in the screening, psychosocial evaluation, and informed consent process before donation that warrant special consideration in all unrelated donors. Many of these issues are linked to each other: Motives for donation assessed during the psychosocial evaluation are inevitably related to whether prospective donors have been coerced or been pressured to come forward; desire for recognition or expectations of post-donation benefit are related to understanding the benefits and risks of donation. Thus, the psychosocial and informed consent processes are ultimately overlapping and interwoven, and the ILDA will have a key role in interpreting the information collected in both processes and integrating them. Strategies for the inclusion of unrelated donors in living donation continue to expand, with major developments in kidney paired exchange and chain donation. The ILDA must bear in mind the implications of these new strategies for both the evaluation and informed consent of unrelated donors, and consider the challenges that can arise in advocating for donors in these situations. Although we have little information regarding unique issues in unrelated donors post donation, the fact that this segment of the donor population has grown so greatly within organ transplantation in the past 20 years points to the need to carefully monitor their outcomes post donation in order to maximize their safety and well-being.

References

1. U.S. Organ Procurement and Transplantation Network and the Scientific Registry of Transplant Recipients. Living donor transplants by donor relation table for U.S. Transplants performed January 1, 1988-January 31, 2013, kidney, http://www.optn.transplant.hrsa.gov. Department of Health and Human Services, Health Resources and Services Administration, Healthcare Systems Bureau, Division of Transplantation, Rockville, MD; United Network for Organ Sharing, Richmond, VA; Last accessed 21 April 2013.
2. Spital A. Evolution of attitudes at U.S. transplant centers toward kidney donation by friends and altruistic strangers. Transplantation. 2000;69:1728–31.
3. Spital A. Public attitudes toward kidney donation by friends and altruistic strangers in the United States. Transplantation. 2001;71(8):1061–4.
4. Rodrigue JR, Pavlakis M, Danovitch GM, Johnson SR, Karp SJ, Khwaja K, et al. Evaluating living kidney donors: relationship types, psychosocial criteria, and consent processes at US transplant programs. Am J Transplant. 2007;7:2326–32.
5. Terasaki PI, Cecka JM, Gjertson DW, Takemoto S. High survival rates of kidney transplants from spousal and living unrelated donors. N Engl J Med. 1995;333(6):333–6.
6. Lee SG. Living-donor liver transplantation in adults. Br Med Bull. 2010;94:33–48.
7. Dew MA, Jacobs C, Jowsey SG, Hanto R, Miller C, Delmonico FL. Guidelines for the psychosocial evaluation of living unrelated kidney donors in the United States. Am J Transplant. 2007;7:1047–54.
8. Dew MA, Jacobs CL, Jowsey SG, Hanto R, Miller C, Delmonico FL. Psychosocial evaluation of living unrelated kidney donors in the United States: Summary of guidelines from a consensus conference. In: Weimar W, Bos MA, Busschbach JJ, Editors. Organ transplantation: ethical, legal and psychological aspects. Towards a common European policy. Lengerich: Pabst Science Publishers; 2008. pp. 208–215.

9. DiMartini AF, Sotelo JL, Dew MA. Organ transplantation. In: Levenson JL (Editor). The American Psychiatric Publishing textbook of psychosomatic medicine: Psychiatric care of the medically ill. 2nd ed. Washington DC: American Psychiatric Publishing; 2010. pp. 725–58.
10. DiMartini A, Dew MA, Crone C. Organ transplantation. In: Sadock BJ, Sadock VA, Ruiz P, Editors. Kaplan and Sadock's comprehensive textbook of psychiatry, 9th ed. Vol. 2. Philadelphia: Lippincott Williams & Wilkins; 2009. pp. 2441–56.
11. Jowsey SG, Schneekloth TD. Psychosocial factors in living organ donation: clinical and ethical challenges. Transplant Rev. 2008;22(3):192–5.
12. Olbrisch ME, Benedict SM, Haller DL, Levenson JL. Psychosocial assessment of living organ donors: clinical and ethical considerations. Prog Transplant. 2001;11:40–9.
13. Fisher MS. Psychosocial evaluation interview protocol for living related and living unrelated kidney donors. Soc Work Health Care. 2003;38:39–61.
14. Leo RL, Smith BA, Mori DL. Guidelines for conducting a psychiatric evaluation of the unrelated kidney donor. Psychosomatics. 2003;44:452–60.
15. Schroder NM, McDonald LA, Etringer G, Snyders M. Consideration of psychosocial factors in the evaluation of living donors. Prog Transplant. 2008;18:41–9.
16. Organ Procurement and Transplantation Network, Policy 12, Living donation. http://optn.transplant.hrsa.gov/policiesandbylaws2/policies/pdfs/policy_172.pdf. Last accessed 21 April 2013.
17. Organ Procurement and Transplantation Network. Living kidney donor psychosocial evaluation checklist. http://optn.transplant.hrsa.gov/news/newsDetail.asp?id=1590. Last accessed 21 April 2013.
18. Halbfinger DM. 44 charged by U.S. in New Jersey corruption sweep. New York Times. 2009 July 23. http://www.nytimes.com/2009/07/24/nyregion/24jersey.html?_r=0. Last accessed 21 April 2013.
19. Associated Press. Guilty pleas to kidney-selling charges. New York Times. 2011 October 27. http://www.nytimes.com/2011/10/27/nyregion/guilty-plea-to-kidney-selling-charges.html. Last accessed 21 April 2013.
20. Satel S. An internet lifetime: in search of a kidney. New York Times. 2005 November 22. http://www.sallysatelmd.com/html/a-nytimes19.html. Last accessed 21 April 2013.
21. Goyal M, Mehta RL, Schneiderman LJ, Schgal AR. Economic and health consequences of selling a kidney in India. JAMA. 2002;288;1589–93.
22. Zargooshi J. Quality of life of Iranian kidney "donors." J Urol. 2001;166:1790–9.
23. Patel SR, Chadha P, Papalois V. Expanding the live kidney donor pool: ethical considerations regarding altruistic donors, paired and pooled programs. Exper Clinic Transplant. 2011;9(3):181–6.
24. Mazaris E, Papalois VE. Ethical issues in living donor kidney transplantation. Exper Clinic Transplant. 2006;4(2):485–97.
25. Ratner LE, Rana A, Ratner RE, Ernst V, Kelly J, Kornfeld D, et al. The altruistic unbalanced paired kidney exchange: proof of concept and survey of potential donor and recipient attitudes. Transplantation. 2010;89:15–22.
26. National Kidney Registry. Living donors. http://kidneyregistry.org/living_donors.php. Last accessed 21 April 2013.
27. Menon P. Rick Ruzzamenti's donation of kidney to stranger sets off the worlds' longest kidney transplant chain. Cure Talk. 2012 February 24. http://trialx.com/curetalk/2012/02/rickruzzamenti%e2%80%98s-donation-of-kidney-to-stranger-sets-off-the-worlds%e2%80%99-longest-kidney-transplant-chain/. Last accessed 21 April 2013.
28. Linked for life: The incredible story of kidney transplant Chain 124. Everyday Health. 2012 February 21. http://www.everydayhealth.com/healthy-living/0221/linked-for-life-the-incredible-story-of-kidney-transplant-chain-124.aspx. Last accessed 21 April 2013.
29. Woodle ES, Daller JA, Aeder M, Shapiro R, Sandholm T, Casingal V, et al. Ethical considerations for participation of nondirected living donors in kidney exchange programs. Am J Transplant. 2010;10(6):1460–7.

30. Sack K. 60 lives, 30 kidneys, all linked. New York Times. 2012 February 18. http://www.nytimes.com/2012/02/19/health/lives-forever-linked-through-kidney-transplant-chain-124.html. Last accessed 21 April 2013.
31. Rodrigue JR, Schutzer ME, Paek M, Morrissey P. Altruistic kidney donation to a stranger: psychosocial and functional outcomes at two US transplant centers. Transplantation. 2011;91:772–8.
32. Dew MA, Jacobs CL. Psychosocial and socioeconomic issues facing the living kidney donor. Adv Chron Kidney Dis. 2012;19(4):237–43.
33. Massey EK, Kranenburg LW, Zuidema WC, Hak G, Erdman RA, Hilhorst M, et al. Encouraging psychological outcomes after altruistic donation to a stranger. Am J Transplant. 2010;10:1445–52.
34. Kranenburg L, Zuidema W, Vanderkroft P, Duivenvoorden H, Weimar W, Passchier J, et al. The implementation of a kidney exchange program does not induce a need for additional psychosocial support. Transpl Int. 2007;20:432–9.
35. Lentine KL, Schnitzler MA, Xiao H, Axelrod D, Davis CL, McCabe M. Depression diagnoses after living kidney donation: linking U.S. registry data and administrative claims. Transplantation. 2012;94(1):77–83.

Chapter 12
Education of the Donor by the ILDA (Psychosocial Aspects)

Marjorie A. Clay

Primary-care physicians frequently point out that a high percentage of diagnoses can be determined by a careful, thorough interview. Although they disagree about the actual percentage of correct diagnoses based on complete history alone (estimated between 70 and 90%), they accept the view that listening to and eliciting the patient's story is a central part of developing an accurate differential diagnosis and effective problem solving as axiomatic [1–3]. So it is with the psychosocial and educational portions of the evaluation of living donors (LDs): if these early stages of the evaluation are done well, the transplant team's attention can be focused on the candidates most likely to proceed to donation. As the medical literature indicates that nonacceptance of living donors ranges from 13 to 36% [4–6], it is clear that transplant programs will save significant time and effort by discovering those candidates who may withdraw or be rejected as potential LDs early in the process. The thesis of this chapter is that a robust psychosocial evaluation, one that includes assessment by the independent living donor advocate (ILDA), can frequently uncover issues that result in the LD candidate's withdrawal or elimination from the program. LD programs benefit when unacceptable LDs are identified early in the selection process, before they have undergone extensive testing or met with multiple health care providers. An initial evaluation process that includes participation by both the ILDA and the donor advocate team (DAT) is described. Using this dual approach—participation by an ILDA as well as DAT—has significant benefits compared to other modes of evaluation. The training that ILDAs should receive so they are able to complete a careful and thorough assessment of the potential LD is also discussed.

M. A. Clay (✉)
University of Massachusettes Memorial Medical Center, Office of Ethics (S3-205),
55 Lake Avenue North, Worcester, MA 01565, USA
e-mail: Marjorie.Clay@umassmemorial.org

Ethics and the Evaluation of Potential LDS

The ever-growing disparity between demand and the availability of transplantable organs as well as resulting suggestions for increasing donation, have stimulated much discussion in the transplant community [7–9]. In particular, the expansion of the LD pool to include donation between nonrelated and incompatible LDs and the emergence of commercial web sites designed to match LDs and recipients have once again raised ethical questions about the motivation and voluntariness of the LD's decision [10–12]. An example of this discussion is Biller-Andorno's recent paper, "Voluntariness in living-related organ donation" [13]. Biller-Andorno describes conditions that must be met in order for living organ donation to be considered a morally justifiable option for patients needing solid organ transplantation. After discussing the potential challenges involved in securing valid informed consent from LDs, Biller-Andorno proposes that "procedural safeguards" be used to protect the voluntariness of living donation decisions and suggests that "a clinical ethicist or an ethics committee might be helpful in integrating voluntariness-enhancing procedural steps into the algorithms that each institution usually develops for itself." Many published guidelines and consensus statements have offered similar suggestions, including the Centers for Medicare and Medicaid, whose requirements were designed to assure LD safety [14–21]. These guidelines and recommendations provide a reasonably consistent framework of principles for the evaluation of LDs. They generally suggest that transplant centers identify either an ILDA or an DAT to address ethical concerns and to ensure protection of the rights of the LD.

The evaluation of LDs at UMass-Memorial Medical Center (UMMMC) incorporates both components: an assessment by an ILDA as well as discussion by the DAT. The medical center ethicist functions as an ILDA and chairs the DAT, which consists of the LD coordinator, the LD clinical social worker, a hepatologist, a nephrologist, and the LD surgeon. With the exception of the LD surgeon who needs to know the health status of the recipient, the DAT is generally not involved in the evaluation or care of the recipient.

Evaluation proceeds in two stages for potential kidney LDs and in three stages for potential liver LDs. This discussion focuses primarily on phase I of both evaluations: The initial screening that is completed before LDs proceed to more extensive testing. In phase I, the potential LD meets with members of the DAT. The LD coordinator provides organ-specific education, takes a complete medical history, describes the evaluation process, and obtains consent for the evaluation, using a consent form that meets the requirements for the informed consent of LDs as recommended in the bylaws of United Network of Organ Sharing (UNOS) [22]. The LD coordinator also provides an overview of the donation procedure, the estimated length of recovery, and potential limitations that the LD may experience postoperatively. The LD then undergoes a psychosocial evaluation with the transplant program's licensed clinical social worker (LCSW), who determines decision-making capacity, evaluates for potential coercion, and assesses the ability of the LD and family to manage the emotional, financial, and physical stressors of donation. Specifically, the licensed clinical social worker (LCSW) prepares the candidate for the emotional demands of donation while attempting to anticipate and address any negative psychosocial outcomes that might result postoperatively. The LCSW also explores the relationship between the LD and the candidate (e.g., the balance of power and control between them, what motivated the LD to come forward for evaluation, and any fears he/she may have about the procedure). Phase I testing concludes with the ILDA consultation (one ILDA interview is required for living kidney donation, while two ILDAs evaluate living liver donors). The ILDA meets with the LD to provide contact with someone independent of the transplant program should the LD have any concerns about the donation process itself and/or the actions of any health care provider who has evaluated the donor. The ILDA also assesses decision-making capacity, focusing on the nature and extent of the pressure the LD feels about his/her decision to donate and determining the extent to which the LD understands and appreciates the impact of donation on his/her life. The ILDA gives the LD a list of questions developed by the DAT that are designed to help the LD reflect on the significance of donation from a variety of perspectives (Appendix 12.1, "Questions to Ask Yourself as You Consider Living Donation"). The ILDA evaluates whether the potential LD is realistic in his/her assessment of the burdens and benefits of living donation and attempts to correct any misleading assumptions the LD may have about the recovery process. Each provider concludes his/her consultation with a "Provider Sign-Off" sheet that incorporates the important evaluative components that the team member discussed with the potential LD (Appendix 12.2, "Living Kidney Donor Evaluation Independent Donor Advocate Sign-Off"). The potential LD also signs the form to verify that each item was discussed and to acknowledge his/her understanding of the education provided.

At the conclusion of phase I of the evaluation, the DAT meets to determine if the potential LD meets criteria for proceeding with evaluation. Although they may overlap at times, the questions asked by each member of the DAT are focused on different components of an LD's fitness for donation, and different kinds of information are elicited. The team discusses the potential LD's suitability for living donation, sharing information gained from all three interviews. Any remediable concerns that emerge during the discussion are assigned to an DAT member for follow-up. For example, if a potential LD has not yet developed a reasonably detailed after-care plan, an DAT member will call at a later date to check on the LD's progress.

If the DAT determines that the LD (1) has no contraindications, (2) is not being unduly pressured to donate, (3) has not received or been promised any "valuable consideration" for donation, (4) is fully informed about the risks and benefits of donation and understands the information he/she has been given, (5) is aware that he/she may withdraw from donation at any point in the process, including the morning of surgery, and (6) all concerns have been addressed, the LD may proceed to the next phase of the evaluation process. A formal, written recommendation is submitted to the Multidisciplinary Selection Committee documenting the LD's status as a candidate for living donation, based on the results of the phase I assessment. (Appendix 12.3, "Donor Advocate Team Report").

Although somewhat labor-intensive, this combined ILDA–DAT approach has demonstrated several significant advantages over approaches that rely on a single ILDA or DAT to evaluate potential LDs. Included among those advantages are the following:

1. Discussing information gained from three separate perspectives allows the DAT to develop a multidimensional understanding of the potential LD. If discrepancies exist between information given by an LD to two or more ILDT members, the LD can be asked specifically about the topic that elicited those divergent responses. In addition, any concerns that emerge can be remediated by helping the LD develop a plan to address them (e.g., smoking cessation, losing weight, and arranging childcare). If concerns were identified during the evaluation, a member of the DAT is assigned to check in with the LD to help resolve the issue. If the LD is successful in addressing concerns raised by the DAT, a follow-up DAT meeting is held during which the LD receives approval to proceed to the next stage of the evaluation.
2. A single person acting alone cannot veto an LD's candidacy for donation during phase I of the evaluation. Using a team approach reduces the effect of subconscious biases or assumptions that may negatively affect a judgment about an LD's suitability for donation and augments the possibly limited information that would be obtained from a single interview. For example, if an DAT member is concerned that a LD's personality, lifestyle, or mental health issues may impede recovery, that concern is discussed at the DAT meeting, and accommodations or options can be explored.
3. Separating the ILDA role from the LCSW role and ensuring that the ILDA is not part of the transplant program allows the LCSW to focus more attention on the LD's emotional stability and to spend more time exploring the LD's support system and coping skills. Adding an ILDA who is not part of the transplant program to the team ensures that the LD has someone who can clearly distinguish what is in the LD's best interests from what might benefit the program. For example, independence from the program enables the ILDA to vote against accepting a specific LD without fear of real or perceived repercussions. Being independent also means that the LD can discuss with the ILDA any negative experiences he/she might have had with members of the transplant program (e.g., perceived pressure, downplaying of negative or equivocal results from medical tests, unexplained delays because the provider is behind schedule, lack of respect, or inappropriate comments).
4. The DAT approach gives LDs three separate opportunities to find someone with whom they can connect and to whom they might be more willing to disclose important concerns or doubts. The importance of developing trust and eliciting these issues early in the evaluation process cannot be overstated.
5. Repetition of information about living organ donation, multiple opportunities to ask LDs about their knowledge of risks and benefits, and different approaches to the LD's support system and living situation help insure that the information gathered by the DAT is both accurate and complete. Repetition also reinforces

the importance of certain themes: the ability to withdraw from the program at any point, a realistic assessment of what postoperative recovery entails, and a commitment to remain in contact with the program for the purpose of collecting postdonation data.
6. The DAT recommendation saves time and resources by identifying LDs who are clearly not suitable or who have not fully committed to donation. These potential LDs are evaluated and screened out before proceeding to more extensive tests and meetings with other providers (hepatologists, nephrologists, and LD surgeons) during phases II and III of the evaluation.

Assessing Capacity to Consent

The most important task in the ILDA interview is to assess the LD's capacity to make a valid, informed decision about living organ donation. In order to accomplish that task, the ILDA must assume and blend the roles of investigative reporter, teacher, and counselor. As a reporter, the ILDA seeks the LD's story: Who is this person? Can the LD explain why he or she wants to donate an organ for transplantation? How did he/she arrive at the decision to donate? Did the potential recipient ask the LD to be evaluated as a potential donor? Does the LD feel internal pressure to donate, and if so, how ambivalent is he/she about the decision? How have family members and friends reacted to the LD's plans? Will the LD have adequate postoperative care and support? These questions and many others like them are aimed at assessing the information the patient has, as well as determining how the LD is using the information to plan for surgery and recovery. Multiple approaches can assist the ILDA during the interview, such as the use of open-ended questions ("How did you decide you wanted to be evaluated as a potential LD?"), modified role-play ("Imagine that someone in your family asks you to explain what is involved in donating an organ to another person. What would you say to them?"), and direct questions ("What are you most concerned about?"). This part of the interview also gives the ILDA an opportunity to supplement the information that the LD has collected from other sources, since he/she may have an incomplete or inaccurate understanding of the risks of donation, the length of time necessary to ensure recovery, the importance of postoperative lifting restrictions, and other similar topics. In this role as teacher, the ILDA checks and corrects the LD's knowledge base by asking questions ("Can you tell me about the risks of organ donation?," and "What do you know about the long-term effects organ donation may have on your health?"), posing hypothetical situations ("What will your family do if you have a complication from surgery and have to be out of work for much longer than you anticipated?"), and playing "devil's advocate" ("How would you respond to someone who says that healthy people should not be allowed to put themselves at risk of harm by donating an organ to another person?"). At the same time, the ILDA will ask questions that encourage patients to reflect further on their decision to donate, their motives and expectations, and the impact of this decision on their lives. This part of the interview requires that the ILDA assume a counseling role: listening intently to both what the LD says and does not say and asking questions that encourage the patient to think more deeply and/or explain more fully his/her thoughts and feelings about the donation decision (e.g., "What does the act of donating your kidney/lobe of liver mean to you?" and "What difference do you think it will make in your life?")

For the last 25 years, in multiple books and papers, Paul Appelbaum and his colleagues have been developing a comprehensive theory of informed consent derived from case law and empirically tested in a variety of clinical settings and with different patient populations [23–27]. Two components of their approach to informed consent are particularly relevant to living organ donation: first, the characterization of consent as a process, rather than as an event; and second, the clarification of standards for assessing decision-making capacity. According to their analysis of consent, the traditional "event" model sees consent as a discrete act, taking place at a circumscribed period of time, usually ending with the patient's signature on a form. In contrast, the "process" model views consent as a dialogue or negotiation between physicians and patients over the goals of treatment and how the patient chooses to address those goals. Acknowledging that the event model may be a better "fit" with how hospital- and clinic-based medicine is organized, Appelbaum and colleagues argue that because it is not patient-centered, it does little to foster a good doctor–patient relationship and even less to ensure that patients understand the information they have received [23]. Thus, while it may satisfy the "letter of the law (the minimal legal requirement)," it violates the "spirit of the law": active patient participation in the decision-making process.

In contrast, the process model offers a view of the physician and the patient both engaged in a negotiation about the choice of treatment. Each is a member of the treating team, and each brings values and expectations to the encounter [23]. The physician shares specialized medical information about the nature, purpose, risks, and benefits of the treatment options; the patient has contextual and historical information that explains how he/she will evaluate the information presented. Together, through what Appelbaum and colleagues call "a process of mutual monitoring," they decide on the best treatment choice for this particular patient at this specific time, not a "one-size-fits-all" recommendation made in the absence of the patient's participation [23].

Although developed as a commentary about obtaining informed consent for treatment, the event-versus-process distinction also usefully applies to consent for living organ donation. In the case of organ donation, the medical team has important medical information to convey about the donation procedure, its risks and possible complications, length of hospital stay, length of recovery process, and similar issues, while the patient has information about his/her health history, personal values, attitudes about donation, responsibilities, and expectations. A donation decision requires that the medical facts and the LD's personal history and values be brought together so that the LD can understand what the medical information means in the context of his/her life. As the evaluation proceeds, the LD gathers more detailed knowledge about specific risks of donation, given his/her unique health history, and also has the opportunity to discuss donation with a number of providers, all of whom are knowledgeable about transplantation. At UMMMC, LDs are also strongly encouraged to speak with one or more previous LDs who donated through our program, so they can ask questions about pain control, recovery, and return to previous levels of energy and activity. All of these components are part of the informed consent process, and are given enough time so that the LD feels well prepared for donation. The fact that living donation requires that a healthy LD put himself/herself at risk for the good of another person intensifies the need for this deliberate process of shared decision-making and also raises the stakes if the process is rushed, truncated, or ignored.

Applebaum and colleagues have also developed an evidence-based approach to assessing decision-making capacity that is useful in assessing LD consent [27]. They began by reasoning that the best way to assess capacity is to mirror the decision of a judge, if this case were being adjudicated during a competency hearing. "The key question to be answered," Appelbaum wrote, "is, 'Does this patient have sufficient ability to make a meaningful decision, given the circumstances with which he or she is faced?' " Analyzing case law, they found that competency adjudications typically involve four functional standards. In order to be considered competent, patients must demonstrate all four of these abilities: (1) the ability to make and communicate a decision, (2) the ability to understand the information that has been given to them, (3) the ability to give cogent reasons for their decision, and (4) the ability to appreciate the impact the decision will have on their lives.

Some of the most difficult ethical questions in medicine involve "continuum concepts": a single idea or term that encompasses a range of possibilities, moving from one extreme to another (e.g., from problems with nausea to death). These concepts require first, that we be able to draw a line on the continuum that marks an important distinction ("this," but not "that"), and second, that we be able to explain why we placed the line at that point, rather than at any other location on the continuum. Different people can draw different lines on the same continuum, and at times, the debate about which point is the "correct" place to draw the line can become rather protracted.

In many ways, the concept of decision-making capacity encompasses a similar continuum of possibilities. Most people would probably agree about the extremes of the range: A floridly psychotic individual does not have capacity, and neither does someone in a persistent vegetative state (PVS); an awake, alert patient with no impairments of cognitive function (e.g., no trauma, no narcotic or psychotropic drugs on board, and no congenital defects), on the other hand, probably does meet the criteria for capacity. It is the gray zone between the extremes that requires careful consideration and judgment. For example, consider the disclosure requirement of consent: How much information is enough to ensure a well-informed decision? Where on the continuum, from "what the transplant surgeon knows" to what Ingelfinger [28] famously referred to as "informed (but uneducated) consent," is the line that identifies successful disclosure and comprehension? In other words, how much information does the LD need in order to be both informed *and* educated? Is the ability to paraphrase what the LD has heard an adequate test of comprehension?

Similar questions can be asked about voluntariness. On a continuum that extends from threats of physical or psychological harm at one end (coercion, being forced to do something against one's will) to no overt influence at all, at the other, where do we mark the boundaries of "persuasion," "manipulation," and "simple influence"? Are we more willing to accept internal pressure, perhaps because it is rooted in sincere regard for the intended recipient, than we are willing to accept external pressure, in the form of conscious or unconscious manipulation by the recipient and/or the LD's own family? What of the LD who discovers that he/she is the only match, or the only medically acceptable LD, within the family? Does the fact that everyone else has been ruled out exert undue pressure on this LD to follow through with donation?

The ILDA Interview: Sample Questions

As noted earlier, the medical literature documents the great variation that currently exists among transplant programs regarding the use of procedural safeguards for protecting LD safety and autonomy. It is very likely that even more variation exists in the content of the ILDA interview itself. The following questions are representative of areas that should be explored during the ILDA interview, with a brief discussion of the information about the LD that may be elicited by them.

- *"How did you find out the recipient needed a kidney (or liver) transplant? Were you asked?"* With this question, the ILDA can determine whether the LD is under pressure to donate, whether the recipient has offered the LD any compensation (money, trips, and major purchases) as an incentive, or whether the LD feels any tacit or explicit pressure to donate. For example, if the candidate has been repeatedly calling the potential LD to see if he/she "has called the transplant center yet," or has expressed no reservations or concerns about the risks of donation to the LD, it is likely that the potential LD feels that he/she is expected to donate, regardless of his/her own preferences and/or the risks to his/her health. One potential donor was contacted after years of no contact by the wife of a man who needed a kidney transplant. The wife offered to fly the donor cross-country to our center for evaluation. During the ILDA assessment, the donor was hugely ambivalent. On the one hand, she had serious reservations about donation and kept mentioning a variety of practical concerns (e.g., the effect of missing so much time from work, the lack of income during recovery, and limited support available). Yet, she felt totally unable to admit to her friend that she did not want to donate her kidney. Even during the ILDA interview, the LD was unable to settle on a decision about donation, talking herself into and out of the idea several times. When the ILDA reflected the donor's indecision back to her, explained the importance of voluntariness, and reassured her that the program would not disclose information from the evaluation to the potential recipient's wife, the LD was finally able to admit how much pressure she had felt to proceed with the donation. She subsequently withdrew from consideration.

- *"How did you make the decision to donate your kidney (or lobe of your liver)?"* The ILDA asks this question to understand how the potential LD arrived at the decision to donate: What was the process? What factors did the patient consider as he/she made the decision? Has he/she fully considered the impact of the decision on the family, present or future employment, and future health status? Is the decision the result of an orderly thought process, or is it the result of an impulsive, though perhaps misguided, desire to help a friend or a stranger? Consider a man who, in the middle of a conversation with a woman he did not know, after hearing of her son's need for a liver transplant, immediately responded, "I am going to donate part of my liver to your son." When he called our program and was told that he could not be a living liver donor because he did not have a relationship with the woman's son, he decided during that same telephone conversation that he wanted to be evaluated as a nondirected kidney donor instead. One might be inclined to reject this candidate on the grounds that such a spontaneous decision to donate an organ to a stranger does not satisfy the third and fourth standards for assessing capacity (i.e., the LD could not give reasons for his decision, nor did he seem to appreciate the impact this decision would have on his life). However, as the conversation with the ILDA continued, it became clear that this decision was similar to other decisions he had made throughout his life. In other words, his decision was "authentic," congruent with values he had held for many years. He was, as his history amply illustrated, an impulsive, generous, and altruistic person who explained his reasons for wanting to donate by saying simply, "This is who I am. This is the kind of life I want to live."
- *"How has your spouse (family, friends, etc.) reacted to your decision?"* Living organ donation is an emotionally and physically demanding challenge. Does the LD have support from his/her friends and family members? Is anyone among the LD's family/friends expressing misgivings about the decision? Is anyone strongly opposed? When the LD is recovering from the donation procedure, will anyone be criticizing the decision, or belittling the LD for having donated? Will the donation have a negative impact on the LD's current relationships? These questions address two potential barriers to living donation: first, the context within which the donation is occurring, and second, whether the LD has expectations that he/she has not yet expressed.
- *"Have you talked to your supervisor about your need to be absent from work for an extended length of time?"* These questions are part of the ILDA's assessment of the financial impact that living donation will have on the LD. It is also an opportunity to encourage the LD to think about details he/she may not have adequately explored. Will the LD receive income during the time he/she is recovering from surgery? Does living donation represent a financial hardship for the LD/family? Does the LD have contingency plans in place if absence from work turns out to be longer than expected?
- *"What is your plan for postoperative care?"* Some LDs have vague plans for their recovery at home, following surgery. The ILDA assesses whether these plans are realistic and specific, and encourages LDs to develop such a plan if they have not yet done so. For example, it is disconcerting to hear a potential LD

say, "I think my brother will help out," as opposed to an LD who talks about a rotation schedule already created by friends and family members to ensure that someone will be available when needed.
- *"What are you most concerned about?"* How the LD answers this question can be very revealing. By listening carefully to what the LD says, and addressing the issue directly, the ILDA can gain insight into issues that may become barriers to donation. For example, if the LD mentions topics such as employment, child care, and financial concerns, it may be that he/she is conflicted about the decision in a way that should be addressed and resolved before proceeding with the evaluation.
- *"'What if' the transplant fails?"* Although transplant centers do not anticipate bad outcomes, no one knows what may happen in the future. This question allows the ILDA to assess the potential LD's emotional resiliency and coping strategies. The ILDA can also encourage the LD and recipient to have a "heart-to-heart" conversation about the possibility of adverse events, so that each knows that the other is as prepared as possible if an unexpected outcome does occur.
- *"'What if' you have a serious complication?"* Once again, the point of this question is to discover what resources the LD has for dealing with a difficult donation process. The ILDA focuses on the impact that a prolonged recovery would have on the LD's living situation, job, family, and finances, and encourages the LD to discuss this possibility with his/her spouse, significant other, or other person(s) who will be affected by an adverse event. For example, what will be the financial impact of a delay in returning to work? How will child care be handled if the LD is the person primarily responsible for child care? Will small children understand why their mother/father/grandparent cannot do the things they normally do?

How potential LDs respond to these last two questions can help the ILDA gauge whether LDs are beginning to appreciate the seriousness of their decision and the potential impact the decisions will have on their lives (one of the four standards for assessing decision-making capacity discussed earlier). For example, if LDs respond by saying, "Oh, that will never happen," or "I do not want to think about anything negative," or "The hospital makes you say that, right?" (treating questions about risks as simply a pro forma exercise rather than real possibilities), the ILDA can use their response as an opportunity to reinforce the idea that living organ donation is a serious decision with the potential for having unexpected, adverse outcomes.

ILDA Training

At UMMMC, the training of new ILDAs begins with the ILDA Training Manual, a compilation of the job description, relevant hospital policies, basic information about medical ethics, Health Insurance Portability and Accountability Act of 1996 (HIPAA), and samples of all the forms and documentation used for the initial evaluation, including the information packet that potential LDs receive

(Appendix 12.4, "Contents of ILDA Training Manual"). The medical ethics section of the manual is focused on organ donation and includes a pre- and post-test with vignettes of challenging cases, with correct answers and discussion of the cases provided so that ILDAs can assess their knowledge base (Appendix 12.5, "Medical Ethics Pretest"). During the next stage of the training process, the prospective ILDA supplements his/her understanding of the donation process by observing any or all members of the team as they interact with the LD: the LD coordinator, who does the initial intake interview and reviews the consent for evaluation; the transplant surgeon, who explains the surgical procedure, its risks and possible complications, as well as the postoperative follow-up plan; the LCSW, who discusses the LD's coping skills and the nature of the relationship between the LD and the recipient; and the ILDA, who assesses the potential LD's decision-making capacity, how well the LD understands the information he/she has received, and whether the LD feels under any pressure to donate. The prospective ILDA then interviews a potential LD while being observed by a more experienced ILDA, who provides feedback. The ILDA begins evaluating LDs independently when he/she feels ready to do so.

What should an ILDA know about medical ethics? No doubt every medical ethicist who is asked this question will respond with a different list, but it would be surprising if the following topics were not included on most of them: (1) the twentieth-century emergence of the principle of autonomy and its requirement of informed consent, (2) the distinction between intrinsic and instrumental value and its connection to autonomy, (3) the correlative theory of rights and duties, and (4) principles of distributive justice. While it is beyond the scope of this chapter to offer a detailed discussion of each of these topics, a few points about their interrelationships are worth noting, because the role of the ILDA is primarily derived from them.

ILDAs are charged with promoting and protecting the LD's autonomy. What is striking about this mandate is that it would not even have made sense prior to the twentieth century. For Hippocrates and centuries of practitioners after him, decision-making in medicine was guided by two values: beneficence and nonmaleficence. The most succinct formulation of these values can be found in his *Epidemics*: "Declare the past, diagnose the present, foretell the future; practice these acts. As to disease, make a habit of two things—to help, or at least to do no harm" [29]. On this view, patients are seen as the passive beneficiaries of the physician's art and experience. In fact, the less they are told about their situation, the better, as Hippocrates advises in *On Decorum*:

> Perform [the duties of the physician] calmly and adroitly, concealing most things from the patient while you are attending him. Give necessary orders with cheerfulness and sincerity, turning his attention away from what is being done to him; sometimes reprove sharply and emphatically, and sometimes comfort with solicitude and attention, revealing nothing of the patient's future or present condition [30].

Physicians following Hippocrates' advice would find the concept of informed consent quite alien, as Katz observes in his book, *The Silent World of Doctor and Patient*. Katz argues that doctors believed that the practice of medicine required them to attend to their patients' needs on their own authority, without consulting their patients about the decisions that needed to be made. He adds, "The idea that patients may also be entitled to liberty, to sharing the burdens of decision with their doctors, was never part of the ethos of medicine [31]." To illustrate the accuracy of Katz's observation, consider this reaction to the emergence of autonomy, one of many similarly impassioned pleas for a return to tradition [32–36]:

> We will argue that the currently dominant school in medical ethics, that of a patient autonomy-rights model... has been used to subvert values intrinsic to medicine, that it has done so without adequately establishing the merits of its case, and that the unfortunate result has been the attempted replacement of the historic medical value system by an ill-fitting alternative. [32]

However, regardless of how "ill-fitting" it may seem to proponents of traditional medicine, it is unlikely that patient autonomy will disappear any time soon. Increased access to education, the empowerment of women as they assumed factory jobs vacated by men going off to war (e.g., World War II (WWII)'s "Rosie the Riveter" phenomenon), and increased attention to civil and human rights all produced patients who were much less willing to place their lives in the hands of their physicians, at least without knowing what the physician planned to do. However, beyond these practical and political arguments for recognizing autonomy, strong personal and philosophical reasons also support autonomy's privileged status.

In broad outline, the argument proceeds in four steps. First, we recognize that autonomy is a value that derives from the fact that people want to choose for themselves how they will live their lives. It is a major part of what distinguishes being an object from being a subject; it distinguishes between being something that is acted *upon* from being someone who *acts* [= a subject/person]. Second, we acknowledge that persons/subjects have intrinsic value: value that is, in the words of Immanuel Kant, "in and of and for itself." This value is not the result of what the subjects do, they just *are* valuable, as Kant explains:

> The good will is not good because of what it effects or accomplishes or because of its adequacy to achieve some proposed end; it is good only because of its willing, i.e., it is good of itself.... [I]f even the greatest effort should not avail it to achieve anything of its end, and if there remained only the good will (not as a mere wish but as the summoning of all the means in our power), it would sparkle like a jewel in its own right, as something that had its full worth in itself. [37]

Later in the *Groundwork for the Metaphysics of Morals* Kant writes, "[the good will] must not be the sole and complete good but the highest good and the condition of all others, even of the desire for happiness." In other words, intrinsic value is what makes ethics even possible, because without it, we would be caught in an endless regress of derivative values. If each value derives its goodness from some other value, which derives its value from yet a third value, and so on, the only way to stop this chain of inferences is to reach something whose goodness is not derivative, but "just is" good in its own right. For Kant, that end point is autonomy: choices made under the guidance of reason.

The third step of the argument is to appreciate the practical significance of the distinction between intrinsic and instrumental value. Unlike human beings, whose autonomy is intrinsically valuable, objects acquire value only when they are being used as a means to an end. According to Kant, our "personhood" depends upon autonomy, the ability to govern ourselves, to make choices according to our own values. The reason Kant admonishes us to never treat a person merely as a means to an end is because to do so is to strip personhood away from him/her, turning the person into an "object"—a thing—whose only value is a function of its use. That is why Kant uses the personhood formulation of the Categorical Imperative as a test for the moral permissibility of actions: anything that passes the test (i.e., does not treat a person merely as a means) is morally acceptable, and we *may* do it, but anything that fails the test is not acceptable, and we *must not* do it.

The last step in the argument is to recognize that in fact, we do use people constantly: Our lives consist of networks of relationships within which we both ask for and provide all kinds of assistance to each other. Consent is the only way we can legitimately use another human being as a means to an end; it is the reason why Kant added the word "merely" to his Categorical Imperative ("Act so that you treat humanity, whether in your own person or in that of another, always as an end and never merely as a means"). To ask for consent is to acknowledge that other people have the freedom to say "No," and to pursue their own agenda instead. It is their decision, not ours, that permits us to use them as a means to other ends.

Without consent, living organ donation would be vivisection, mutilation, or battery ("unconsented to touching") [38]. To ask someone if he/she will consent to the removal of a kidney/lobe of liver for the sake of another human being is to accept the possibility that they may refuse (and this is why medical ethicists prefer the term "informed choice," rather than "informed consent"). Consent is authorization; it transforms what would otherwise be considered robbery (taking something from another person without permission) into altruism (the autonomous decision of a fully informed person to make a priceless gift).

The correlativity theory of rights and duties maintains that for every right we have, someone else has a duty. Each right makes a claim of some sort, on a person or a group. That claim in turn generates a duty on these other parties, either to act or to refrain from acting (= forbearance) in a certain way. The duty may apply to a specific, namable person, in which case it is called an *in personam* duty, or it may apply more generally to a group of people, referred to as an *in rem* duty. For example, if I owe you US$ 100, then you have a right to receive US$ 100 from me, and I have a duty to pay you US$ 100. Your right, seen from my point of view, is a duty. My duty, from your point of view, is a right. The claim that you are making on me is that I actually *do* something: in this case, I must pay you US$ 100. Rights that generate a duty to do something are called positive rights. In contrast, a negative right creates a duty to *not do* something, which we call a forbearance [38].

Given the ethical primacy of autonomy, and the fact that in the U.S., at least, it is also considered a right, the ILDA has two extraordinary duties: (1) to protect and promote the LD's freedom to choose whether to donate an organ to another person and (2) to place the LD's safety and well-being above everything else: the improved health and longevity of the recipient, the success of the transplant program, and the reduction of the UNOS wait list. It is a positive duty: It requires that the ILDA *do* something. Specifically, the ILDA must assess the validity of all three components of informed consent: disclosure, capacity, and voluntariness.

Conclusion

In summary, the ILDA brings his/her intellect, resourcefulness, and diligence to bear on ensuring that living organ donation is—and remains—an ethical option for the many people whose lives and health depend on the altruistic acts of others. With its focus on informed consent—reviewing the candidate's understanding of information disclosed as well as assessing the voluntariness of the decision—the ILDA interview should be the ethical bedrock of LD programs. A well-prepared ILDA can also serve an important gatekeeper role, by identifying problems that may prevent a candidate from proceeding to donation. In this chapter, we have characterized: (1) a successful two-pronged approach to the psychosocial evaluation, (2), the medical ethics content that should be part of the ILDA's training, and (3) examples of how these resources work together to prepare the LD for donation. Especially in an era when the demand for transplantable organs far exceeds the availability of deceased donors, the most important thing we can do is to ensure that living donation continues to be an ethically appropriate option for those in need of organ transplantation.

Acknowledgments This chapter could not have been developed without the assistance of Paula Bigwood, UMMMC Living Donor Coordinator, and Dina Jamieson, UMMMC Living Donor Licensed Clinical Social Worker. Dr. Adel Bozorgzadeh, Chief, Transplantation Services, has promoted the role of the independent living donor advocate from the very first day he arrived at UMMMC.

Appendix 12.1

Questions to Ask Yourself as You Consider Living Donation

We have developed questions for you to ask yourself as you consider living donation. If you want to discuss any of these questions with your Independent Donor Advocates or other members of the Donor Advocate Team, please call:

- Living Donor Coordinator—<name><telephone number>
- Living Donor Clinical Social Worker—<name><telephone number>
- Chair, Independent Donor Advocate Team—<name><telephone number>

Motivation

- Have I been totally honest with myself about why I want to donate part of my body to the recipient?
- Am I expecting anything in return for my donation? (e.g., gratitude? publicity? other kinds of attention? a better relationship with the recipient?) How will I feel if what I want to happen, does not?

Potential Pain and Discomfort

- Do I feel adequately prepared to deal with the pain and discomfort associated with this surgery?
- Will I be able to communicate my needs—both physical and emotional—to hospital staff and/or my family?
- Can I manage the recovery period without running into problems (e.g., boredom, anxiety, and nervousness)?

Financial Concerns

- Am I prepared financially for being out of work for months to a year?
- At what point will I become anxious about my lack of income?
- Do I have an adequate backup plan in case I have to be out of work longer than I expected?

Postdonation Concerns

- Do I have expectations about what this experience will do for me? Are they realistic?
- Have I thought about how I will feel if the recipient fails "to take care" of the kidney (portion of liver) I donated?
- Have I thought about how I will feel if the recipient has serious complications or does not survive the transplantation?
- Is my family/personal/professional life relatively stable and secure?
- If not, are there things that I can do now to improve the situation?
- Is there anything I can do now that will improve my recovery (e.g., lose weight, exercise more, and stop smoking)?
- Has anyone among my close friends and family shown disapproval or criticized me for wanting to make this donation?
- Will I be able to handle these reactions when I am feeling weak and/or emotionally fragile?

Family Concerns

- Have I spoken to my family about how they will cope if I should have serious, unexpected complications?
- Do I have a plan in place for my children and/or other dependents if I should have an unexpected outcome?

- Does my Health Care Proxy Agent know my treatment preferences if my condition should deteriorate so that I need advanced medical technology to survive?
- Does my family know who my Health Care Proxy Agent is?
- Do they understand that I have chosen that person to make medical decisions for me if I should become unable to communicate with the medical team?

Instructions for the ILDA: How to Introduce These Questions

You can introduce these questions at any point in the interview, but be aware that many people will begin reading them as soon as they receive them. If that happens, explain that these questions are theirs to take home and to use as they continue to gather information and consider donation.

One opportunity to introduce this list into the discussion is after you have asked the donor if s/he has any questions. Often donors will indicate that they are pretty overwhelmed with all of the information they have received, and will probably have questions later, after they have had time to think about their decision. Remind them that: (1) they are welcome to call any member of the donor advocate team (DAT), (2) you definitely want to help them come to an informed decision, and (3) the DAT developed this list of questions based on our experience with many potential donors. Offer to speak with any family member who may be especially uneasy about the potential donation. The most important thing is to reassure them that you are available to them as they come to a decision, to help in any way possible.

Note In Massachusetts, the Health Care Proxy is the only legally valid form of advance directives. ILDAs from other states may inquire about the person's Living Will (or other form of advance directive accepted by in which they practice.

Appendix 12.2

Living Kidney Donor Evaluation Independent Donor Advocate Sign-Off [1]

UMASS MEMORIAL MEDICAL CENTER Transplant Services **LIVING KIDNEY DONOR EVALUATION INDEPENDENT DONOR ADVOCATE SIGN-OFF**	NAME: ADDRESS: BIRTHDATE: SEX: UNIT NUMBER: PRINT CLEARLY IN INK OR STAMP WITH PATIENT CARD

Informed Understanding	Advocate	Patient
All of my questions and concerns have been addressed and answered.		
My family and people important to me have been given an opportunity to ask questions and express concerns.		
I have been given contact information for my Independent Donor Advocate and know that I can contact my Independent Donor Advocate to have any new concerns and questions addressed.		
I have a thorough understanding of the nature of the donation procedure, its risks and benefits, including rare but significant risks (i.e., death).		
I have been given questions to consider throughout the evaluation process.		
I have been informed that if I decide not to proceed with donation, information about my decision will not be disclosed to the recipient without my consent.		
I have been informed that my medical information will not be revealed to the recipient without my authorization. I also know that if I have a medical condition that might harm the recipient, the transplant team will not allow the transplant to occur.		
I have been informed that I may "opt out" of donation at any point in the evaluation process.		
I have been informed that it is a federal crime, subject to a $50,000 fine or five (5) years in prison, to transfer human organs for 'valuable consideration.'		
Comments:		

The information above was presented to me in a clear and understandable manner. I understand that I may call the transplant office with any further questions or concerns. I have been informed that I am under no obligation to donate my kidney and that I may withdraw from the program at anytime.

_____   _____   _____   _____
Patient Signature   Printed Name   Date   Time

_____   _____   _____   _____
Patient Signature   Printed Name   Date   Time

Evaluator Input	Yes	No
Evidence of coercion either by family members or others.		
The potential donor has capacity to give informed consent.		
The potential donor has not been offered monetary consideration for the donation of his/her kidney		
Comments:		

---

[1] Reprinted with permission from UMASS Memorial Medical Center.

Appendix 12.3

Donor Advocate Team Report[2]

	NAME:
	ADDRESS:
UMASS MEMORIAL MEDICAL CENTER	BIRTHDATE: SEX:
Transplant Services	UNIT NUMBER:
DONOR ADVOCATE TEAM REPORT	
	PRINT CLEARLY IN INK OR STAMP WITH PATIENT CARD

Present:_____

☐ Kidney Donor   ☐ Liver Donor

Potential Donor Name: _____ Age: _____
Recipient Name: _____ Age: _____
Relationship to Recipient: _____
Medical/Surgical History:_____

1. Any concern about coercion or undue pressure to donate	**Yes***	**No**
2. History of previous abusive relationship	**Yes***	**No**
3. Relevant Psychiatric history	**Yes***	**No**
4. Patient understands potential financial implications of donations	**Yes**	**No***
5. Any concern about financial inducement to donate	**Yes***	**No**
6. Patient has capacity to make decision to donate	**Yes**	**No***
7. Patient has an adequate understanding of risks, benefits, of donation	**Yes**	**No***
8. Patient understands that decision to donate is voluntary	**Yes**	**No***
9. Patient understands he/she can opt out at any time	**Yes**	**No***
10. Patient career requires heavy lifting or physical exertion	**Yes***	**No**
11. Patient reports sufficient post operative support	**Yes**	**No***
12. Reported ETOH abuse or dependence	**Yes***	**No**
13. Reported substance abuse or dependence other than ETOH	**Yes***	**No**

If applicable, list concerns to be addressed_____
_____
_____

For any **starred answer**, or **concern identified**, document resolution of issue on the reverse of this form.

DAT member assigned to follow-up on above concerns: _____

Potential donor may **proceed** with the donation process   **Yes**   **No**

If '**No**,' explain reason for negative recommendation._____
_____

_____   _____   _____
(Print: Donor Advocate Team Chair)   (Signature)   (Date and time)

---

[2] Reprinted with permission from UMASS Memorial Medical Center.

Appendix 12.4

Contents of ILDA Training Manual

Welcome to the Living Donor program 4
"Who's Who" in Transplant Services 7
Responsibilities of Independent Living Donor Advocates
    Job Description: Independent Living Donor Advocate 9
    Independent Living Donor Advocate Policy 11

Basic Principles of Medical Ethics
    Pretest for Medical Ethics 15
    Central Medical Ethics principles 19
    Rights 26
    Medical Ethics and organ transplantation 31
        Informed consent and decision-making capacity 33
            Guideline for Informed Consent and Patient Education 35
            Living Kidney Donor Consent for Evaluation 39
            Living Liver Donor Consent for Evaluation 45
        Answers to Medical Ethics pretest 51

Confidentiality, HIPAA and Protected Health Information
    Pretest 57
    Confidentiality 59
    Protected health information 65
    Answers to pretest 73

Evaluation Process
    Evaluation process flow chart 75
    Encounter forms 77
    Content of the interview 80
    Questions for reflection 85
    Checklist – Kidney 87
    Checklist – Liver 88

Appendix 12.5

Medical Ethics Pretest

This pretest will not be "graded": it is provided as a tool for you to assess your comprehension and retention of the material in this training booklet. You will have an opportunity to complete a "post-test" after you have completed this section.

1. Give an example that illustrates the difference between an *intrinsic value* and an *instrumental value*. Why is this distinction important in assessing potential living donors?
2. In response to the shortage of dialysis machines in the 1960s, Congress decided to underwrite the costs of care for *all* patients with end-stage kidney disease. This decision is an example of:
   A. Micro-allocation
   B. Macro-allocation
   C. Formal principle of justice
   D. Material principle of justice
3. The requirement of obtaining informed consent for evaluation as a Living Donor is based primarily on which principle?
   A. Beneficence
   B. Justice
   C. Nonmaleficence
   D. Autonomy
   E. Preservation of Life
4. The potential donor's right to information about the risks and benefits of Living Donation creates a _____ duty for the provider. In other words, the provider is required to _____

   A. Positive
   B. Absolute
   C. Negative
   D. Conditional
5. That physicians can overrule the patient's desire to donate a kidney because of a higher risk of developing diabetes at some point in the future is an example of:
   A. Nonmaleficence
   B. Paternalism
   C. Negative duty
   D. Beneficence
6. The current model of organ donation in the U.S. is an example of:
   A. An "opt-in" system
   B. An "opt-out" system
   C. A system that privileges justice over autonomy (i.e., places a higher value on justice)
   D. A system that values the public's best interest over the individual's best interests.

7. In Massachusetts, the standard of disclosure used to measure the validity of informed consent is:
   A. The Professional Community standard
   B. The Subjective Person standard
   C. The Autonomy standard
   D. The Reasonable Person standard
8. True False Only the courts can determine whether a person is competent or incompetent.
9. As an ILDA, you will be assessing the potential donor's decision-making capacity. What will you be looking for?
10. Describe what kind of duty is associated with the right to life (i.e., is it positive or negative, in rem or in personam). How does that characterization affect organ transplantation?

Note The next set of questions are based on cases, or composites of cases we have evaluated in our program. They are designed to give you practice with "real" situations, and to compare your answers with the original evaluation in the case.

11. Your patient tells you that he is receiving financial support from his father, the potential recipient, during the period that he will be out of work for the donation procedure and recovery. As the patient's ILDA, are you concerned about this exchange of money? If so, what will you do to address your concern? If not, explain why you are not worried about the exchange of money between recipient and donor.
12. Your patient is a young woman who plans to donate part of her liver to her mother, who has previously had two liver transplants secondary to alcoholism. During your interview, you hear about your patient's childhood, during which, at a very young age, she had assumed the role of parent to her younger siblings. She said her mother was seldom at home and often drunk or asleep when she was in the house. It becomes clear that your patient was the "responsible adult" in the family, and that she often took care of her mother, as well as her siblings. She has three young children of her own (aged 5, 7 and 9). Her husband is not supportive of her decision, in part because his job requires travel, and he is concerned about childcare. He also knows how many times his wife has been disappointed by her mother's apparent failure to take responsibility for her own health. As the patient's ILDA, what will you do?
13. During your interview with a young woman, you begin to notice that she is rather vague about the relationship she has with her children. As you ask more questions, she states, "I do not want to go into that," and refuses to offer further information. Her work history is erratic, also: after a significant period of unemployment, she has just begun a new business with her boyfriend and they appear to have unrealistic expectations about quickly they will become self-supporting. The boyfriend acknowledges that sales have been "slow," but they both believe they are "entering the ground floor of a business that will soon take off." The patient wants to donate a kidney to her mother, who has been on dialysis for 5 years. As her ILDA, what will you do?

14. Your patient today is a very pleasant woman who comes forward as a potential living kidney donor for her friend. When you ask about how she came to her decision, she says, "I thought it would be nice." She is unable to list any potential risks of kidney donation. She has a son who is 8 years old, but she said that the son's father is very involved and would probably take care of him during her recovery period. When asked who would take care of her following her surgery, she mentioned a brother, but did not provide details (e.g., whether she would stay at his house, whether he would visit her at her house). As her ILDA, what will you do?
15. Your final patient for the day is a young Hispanic man who comes forward as a potential living liver donor for his brother. He is very committed to helping his brother, but is reluctant to talk about the risks of the procedure and what is involved in the procedure itself. During your interview, he tells you that his wife is absolutely opposed to the donation. They have four young children from 2 to 12 years old. As she is so opposed to donation, they have not talked about how she would cope if anything bad were to happen to him (e.g., a complication that would extend the time he is off work, or his death). He explained his reluctance to talk with her, as well as his reluctance to learn about the procedure, by saying, "The more you know, the more nervous you get." He describes his mother, who lives in Puerto Rico, as being "kind of scared, confused, nervous" about his decision. As his ILDA, what will you do?

Answers and Discussion

1. Something has *intrinsic value* if it is valued for its own sake, as an "end-in-itself," and not because of what it can do. On most ethical theories, human beings have intrinsic value.
   Something has *instrumental value* if it is valued because it can be used as a "means to an end." It has no independent value apart from its use. If my goal is to hang a picture on the wall, a hammer has instrumental value for me: It allows me to achieve the end I desire. According to deontological ethicists like Immanuel Kant, it is immoral to treat a human being merely as a means to an end (i.e., to treat them as if they only have instrumental value).
2. *B. Macro-allocation*
3. *D. Principle of Autonomy*
4. *A. Positive duty*
   The provider is required to give the potential donor information that will enable to the donor to make an informed decision about living organ donation. The provider must also assess whether the donor has the capacity to make an informed choice and must take appropriate steps to ensure that the potential donor understands the information given (by using language appropriate to the person's educational level, providing a language interpreter for potential donors with limited English proficiency, etc.). Because fulfilling this duty requires that these actions

be performed, it is a positive duty. [A negative duty would be that which required the provider to *not* perform a particular action.]
5. B. *Paternalism*

Note If you answered "A" or "D," you are partially correct: certainly, these Hippocratic values are in evidence. However, in this case, physicians are (1) ignoring the potential donor's autonomy and (2) justifying that position by appealing to what is in the patient's best interests. Those two conditions are the definition of "paternalism."
6. A. *An "opt-in" system*
7. D. *The Reasonable Person standard*
8. *True*

Only courts can adjudicate 'competency.' Medical providers use the concept of 'decision-making capacity' to refer to the abilities that must be demonstrated before the courts will deem a person to be competent. If medical providers believe that the patient lacks capacity, s/he may ask Legal Counsel to petition the courts for a competency hearing and possible appointment of a guardian.
9. The four functional abilities required for valid decision-making capacity are:
   1. Ability to express a choice,
   2. Ability to understand relevant information,
   3. Ability to appreciate the situation and its consequences and
   4. Ability to rationally manipulate information.
10. The right to life is a negative, in rem right. It is negative, because it imposes a duty to *not* interfere with the person's life—e.g., to *not* kill that person. [If it were positive, it would impose a duty to do everything necessary to ensure that the person lives]. It is in rem because it applies to "the whole world" [everyone who belongs to the "universe of discourse"—in this case, everyone who is bound by American law].
    The connection with transplantation can be seen by asking, "What if we did believe that the right to life was a positive, in rem right?" In that case, we would have an affirmative duty (a duty to do) whatever it takes to keep a person alive. Minimally, it means we would probably have an "opt-out" system of distribution to ease the increasing discrepancy between supply and demand for transplantable organs.
11. It is illegal to exchange organs for money in the U.S.: in essence, to set a price on the value of a transplantable kidney or lobe of a liver. In addition, if the donor accepts money in exchange for his/her organ, questions can be raised about whether the decision to donate is voluntary, or whether the presence of money might lead a donor to make a decision that is not in his/her best interests. However, families regularly help their adult children through financial difficulties. The judgment you must make is very subtle: is the potential donor receiving what he might receive anyway, absent the donation? Or, does the amount of money exceed what would ordinarily be given by a father to his son? We are looking for the fine line between "supporting" his son during the donation/recovery period, versus "paying" his son for the donated organ.

Outcome Donor received approval to move to Phase II of the evaluation.

12. The characteristics common to children who have been "parentified" have been well described in the literature. While our respect for patient autonomy means we will accept her decision, it is important for this patient to reflect on her motivation for donation. Is she continuing her pattern of "taking care of everyone," including the mother who did not take care of her?

    One approach is to ask her, "If a deceased donor liver became available, how would you feel?" When the patient in the case was asked this question, she experienced how overwhelming her feelings of relief were. She began to consider the possibility that she did feel trapped by her mother's need, and that she really did not want to make the sacrifice that this donation would represent in her life. She acknowledged that her children were too young to understand the recovery process (her possible fatigue and limitations) and would be devastated if anything bad were to happen to her. Finally, the lack of support from her husband is a significant red flag. Living liver donation is an intense experience with an extended recovery time. Donors need support, nurturing, and assistance, and it is an open question whether this patient has adequate support for donating part of her liver.

Outcome Donor received approval to move to Phase II of the evaluation but has suspended the evaluation process to reconsider her decision.

13. It is not promising when a relationship with a potential donor begins with deception and/or secrecy. In this case, the potential donor had lost her house, her job, her marriage, and custody of her children because of her drug addiction, a situation that became clear during the donor advocate team (DAT) meeting. In "real time," the ILDA might point out that the uncertainty in this donor's life—whether and when her children might return, how the new business will fare—are challenging enough without adding the prospects of living kidney donation.

Note The ILDA interviewing this potential donor did not have information about her past. However, when the DAT met to discuss potential donors, the Donor Coordinator had gathered this information during her screening discussion with the potential donor. Even without that information, the ILDA believed that the donor's current circumstances were tenuous enough, along with her refusal to talk about her children, to suggest a postponement of the donation decision. The fact that her mother has been on dialysis for 5 years raises the question, "Why now?"

Outcome Donor did not receive approval to proceed to Phase II of the evaluation.

14. At this point, the patient does not appear to be a serious candidate for kidney donation. Before she is approved as a potential donor, she needs to be able to demonstrate that she understands (1) the risks of living kidney donation, and that she has thought about (2) what this donation means as far as its effects on her life. In addition, she needs to develop an adequate plan for her postoperative care (e.g., where she will stay, who will take care of her, whether her son will be with his father). The ILDA wrote, "If she shows herself to be committed

to the possibility of kidney donation, I would approve her as a potential living donor, assuming that the above conditions have been satisfied."

Outcome The DAT documented the conditions that must be met before the patient can receive approval to proceed to Phase II of the evaluation process.

15. One of the most important roles an ILDA has is to make sure that the potential donor is adequately informed about living liver donation, and also that he/she has a support system that will help him/her through a physically and emotionally demanding medical procedure. This patient met neither of those conditions at the time of his evaluation. The ILDA for this patient wrote, "My impression is that in his desire to help his brother, the donor has not yet carefully considered the implications of his decision, nor has he had the kind of conversation with his wife that I believe is required. Especially since he is the father of four young children, more planning and more preparation needs to occur before he is ready for surgery. I would also recommend a meeting between the donor, his wife, the transplant surgeon and an ILDA, for the purposes of (1) determining how informed the wife is about living liver donation, and (2) assessing the strength of her opposition, as well as the reasons behind it. Approval to advance to Phase II will depend on the completion of these requirements."

Outcome The meeting between the surgeon, the ILDA, and the couple occurred with the help of a Spanish-language interpreter (the wife had limited English proficiency). The donor was given approval to proceed to Phase II of the evaluation, despite the fact that his wife never wavered in her opposition. However, during the 2-week reflection period following acceptance as a living liver donor, the donor decided to withdraw from the program.

References

1. Levinson W, Pizzo PA. Patient-physician communication: it's about time. JAMA. 2011; 305(17):1802–3.
2. Johnson LL, Johnson AL, Colquitt JA, Simmering MJ, Pittsley AW. Is it possible to make an accurate diagnosis based only on a medical history? A pilot study on women's knee joints. Arthroscopy. 1996;12(6):709–14.
3. Peterson MC, Holbrook JH, Hales D, Smith NL, Staker LV. Contributions of the history, physical examination, and laboratory investigation in making medical diagnoses. West J Med. 1992;156:163–5.
4. Renz JF, Mudge CL, Heyman MB, Tomlanovich S, Kingsford RP, Moore BJ, et al. Donor selection limits use of living-related liver transplantation. Hepatology. 1995;22:1122–6.
5. Sterneck MR, Fischer L, Nischwitz U, Burdellski M, Kjer S, Larta A, et al. Selection of the living liver donor. Transplantation. 1995;60:667–71.
6. Beavers KI, Fried MW, Zacks SL, Fair JH, Johnson MW, Gerber DA, et al. Evaluation of potential living donors for living donor liver transplantation [abstract]. Am J Transplant. 2001;1:318.
7. Burr AT, Shah SA. Disparities in organ allocation and access to liver transplantation in the USA. Expert Rev Gastroenterol Hepatol. 2010;4(2):133–40.

8. Hayashi PH, Axelrod DA, Galanko J, Salvalaggio PR, Schnitzler M. Regional differences in deceased LD liver transplantation and their implications for organ utilization and allocation. Clin Transplant. 2011;25(1):156–63.
9. Yeh H, Smoot E, Schoenfeld DA, Markmann JF. Geographic inequity in access to livers for transplantation. Transplantation. 2011;91(4):479–86.
10. Singer PA, Siegler M, Whitington PF, Lantos JD, Edmond JC, Thistlethwaite JR, et al. Ethics of liver transplantation with living donors [comments]. N Engl J Med. 1989;321:620–2.
11. Washburn K. Maximizing LD potential: evolving organ procurement organization metrics and optimizing organ distribution and allocation in the United States. Liver Transpl. 2012;18:S1–S4.
12. Diethelm AG. Ethical decisions in the history of organ transplantation. Ann Surg. 1990 May; 211:505–20.
13. Biller-Andorno N. Voluntariness in living-related organ donation. Transplantation. 2011;92:617–9.
14. Dew MA, Jacobs CL, Jowsey SG, Hanto R, Miller C, Delmonico FL. Guidelines for the psychosocial evaluation of living unrelated kidney LDs in the United States: meeting report. Am J of Transplant. 2007;7:1047–54.
15. Adams PL, Cohen DJ, Danovitch GM, Edington RM, Gaston RS, Jacobs CL, et al. The nondirected live kidney LD: ethical considerations and practice guidelines. Transplantation. 2002;74:582–90.
16. Rodrigue JR, Pavlakis M, Danovitch GM, Johnson SR, Karp SJ, Khwaja K, et al. Evaluating living kidney LDs: relationship types, psychosocial criteria, and consent processes at US transplant programs. Am J of. Transplant. 2007;7:2326–32.
17. Bia MJ, Ramos EL, Danovitch GM, Gaston RS, Harmon WE, Leichtman AB, et al. Evaluation of living renal LDs: the current practice of US transplant centers. Transplantation. 1995;60(4):322–7.
18. Sterner K, Zelikovsky N, Green C, Kaplan BS. Psychosocial evaluation of candidates for living related kidney donation. Pediatr Nephrol. 2006;21(Oct): 1357–63.
19. Steiner R, Matas AJ. First things first: laying the ethical and factual groundwork for living kidney LD selection standards. Am J Transplant. 2008;8:930–2.
20. Erim Y, Beckmann M, Valentin-Gamazo C, Malago M, Frilling A, Schlaak JF, et al. Selection of LDs for adult living LD liver donation: results of the assessment of the first 205 LD candidates. Psychosomatics. 2008;49:143–51.
21. Medicare program: Hospital Conditions of Participation: requirements for approval and re-approval of transplant centers to perform organ transplants; Final Rule. Federal Register. 2007;72(61):15199–80.
22. United Network of Organ Sharing. Proposal to establish requirements for the informed consent of living kidney LDs. [updated 2013; cited 2013 April 15]. Available from: http://optn.transplant.hrsa.gov/PublicComment/pubcommentPropSub_293.pdf–application/pdf.
23. Lidz CW, Appelbaum PS, Meisel A. Two models of implementing informed consent. Arch Intern Med. 1988;148(6):1385–89.
24. Grisso T, Appelbaum PS. Assessing competence to consent to treatment: a guide for physicians and other health professionals. New York:Oxford University Press; 1998.
25. Berg J, Appelbaum PS, Lidz CW, Parker LS. Informed consent: legal theory and clinical practice. 2nd ed. New York: Oxford University Press; 2001.
26. Appelbaum PS. Assessment of patients' competence to consent to treatment. N Engl J Med. 2007;357:1834–40.
27. Grisso T, Appelbaum PS. MacArthur Competence Assessment Tool for Treatment (MacCAT-T). Sarasota: Professional Resource Press; 1998.
28. Ingelfinger F. Informed (but uneducated) consent. N Engl J Med. 1972;287:465–6.
29. Hippocrates. Epidemics. Book I, Section iii, 7. Trans. Jones WHS, The Loeb Classical Library. In: Reiser SJ, DyckAJ, Curran, WJ. Ethics in medicine: historical perspectives and contemporary concerns. Cambridge: MIT Press; 1977;7.

30. Hippocrates. On decorum. 16. Trans Jones WHS, The Loeb Classical Library. In: Reiser SJ, DyckAJ, Curran, WJ. Ethics in medicine: historical perspectives and contemporary concerns. Cambridge: MIT Press; 1977;8.
31. Katz J. The silent world of doctor and patient. New York: Free Press, Macmillan, 1984; p. 2.
32. Clements CD, Sider RC. Medical ethics' assault upon medical values. JAMA. 1983;250(15):2011–5.
33. Sandman L, Munthe C. Shared decision making, paternalism and patient choice. Health Care Anal. 2010;18(1):60–84. (Epub 2009 Jan 30).
34. Murphy JF. Paternalism or partnership: clinical practice guidelines and patient preferences. Ir Med J. 2008;101(8):232.
35. Sutrop M. How to avoid a dichotomy between autonomy and beneficence: from liberalism to communitarianism and beyond. J Intern Med. 2011;269(4):375–9.
36 Buchanan DR. Autonomy, paternalism, and justice: ethical priorities in public health. Am J Public Health. 2008;98(1):15–21. (Epub 2007 Nov 29).
37. Kant I. Foundations of the metaphysics of morals. Trans. Beck LW. Indianapolis and New York: The Liberal Arts Press; 1959;12.
37. Richards EP. Intentional torts. Program in law, science, and public health. Available at: http://biotech.law.lsu.edu/books/lbb/x134.htm.
38. Feinberg J. Social philosophy. Englewood Cliffs: Prentice Hall; 1973.

Chapter 13
Components and Timing of the ILDA Evaluation

Kathleen Swartz

The independent living donor advocate (ILDA) is responsible for representing, protecting, and promoting the best interests of the living donor. Prospective donors have the right to be given the tools to advocate for their wishes as they relate to living donation and the multidisciplinary team has the obligation to provide them. It is the thorough and successful evaluation of the donor candidates that facilitates this process. Living donors must be motivated, free of coercion, and well educated about the risks related to donation. The ILDA evaluation is focused on ensuring that the living donor is making both an autonomous and knowledgeable decision and on identifying any areas that may need further exploration or education by other members of the multidisciplinary team [1, 2].

In order to effectively fulfill the role of protecting and promoting the best interests and well-being of living donors, the partnership between the ILDA and the prospective donor must begin early in the process. Once the prospective donor contacts the transplant center and expresses an interest in living donation, educational materials and a health questionnaire are provided along with an explanation of the evaluation process and informed consent. Once blood typing and human leukocyte antigen (HLA) and crossmatch testing are completed, the multidisciplinary team evaluation is scheduled. The ILDA is introduced as a member of the multidisciplinary team and meets early with the donor candidate to assess their understanding of the evaluation process and provide any additional information to promote a voluntary informed decision about proceeding with the evaluation for living donation. At a minimum, the ILDA meets again with the donor candidate once they have met with members of the team, including the surgeon and nephrologist/hepatologist, to determine their understanding of the medical, psychosocial, and financial risks associated with living donation and their decision as to whether they wish to proceed.

K. Swartz (✉)
Trauma Services, Beaumont Health System, 3601 W. 13 Mile Road,
Royal Oak, MI 48073, USA
e-mail: Kathleen.Swartz@beaumont.edu
8242 Woods End Ct., Washington, MI 48095, USA

These meetings provide the ILDA the opportunity to gain the necessary knowledge about the prospective donor's motivation and educational needs to effectively assess their willingness and competence to donate. By meeting with the donor during the presurgical, inpatient, and postsurgical visits, the ILDA is able to reinforce earlier teaching and identify any additional concerns or situations that may arise. Effective evaluation begins early and is an ongoing process.

Potential donors must be educated on not only the risks associated with the act of donation itself but also those that are inherent to the evaluation before consenting to proceed. They must understand these risks and be allowed to ask questions without fear of bias and also that they may learn of medical conditions and/or unexpected results of paternity. Prospective donors must be given the opportunity to make a voluntary decision that is free from coercion or undue influence from the candidate, candidate's family, or the medical team. The ILDA must specifically ask the donor if they are feeling any pressure to donate and, if so, from whom. Living donation must be autonomous and free of coercion. The living donor advocate must carefully assess for any underlying pressures that may be influencing the donor's decisions. Often times, these pressures are unrecognized by the prospective donor and the ILDA must help the donor identify and evaluate them. Reluctance to answer questions freely, ambivalence related to living donation, or conflict with the intended recipient can all be signs of coercion and require additional investigation [1, 3]. Documentation by the ILDA must be sure to address any signs of coercion or undue influence, or needs to indicate that the prospective donor is free of these pressures and may continue with the evaluation process. An acceptable candidate for living donation must be making an autonomous decision. A thorough evaluation by the ILDA identifies the motivating factors influencing the prospective donor, which is essential in assessing the willingness to donate. Living donation is to be free from monetary or valuable gain, and the donor candidate must indicate that there is no such compensation involved. Informed decision making involves understanding all the medical, psychosocial, and financial risks that are involved with the process. The living donor advocate must be sure that the prospective donor not only receives all of this information but also has the competence to understand and evaluate any potential impact. Candidates must be assured that the decision to donate is voluntary and that they may withdraw from the process at any time up until the individual goes under anesthesia. Only after all of these areas are addressed can the prospective donor be allowed to make an informed decision to proceed with living donor evaluation [3, 4].

There may be instances when the ILDA begins the evaluation of the prospective donor prior to the initial team evaluation. With altruistic or unrelated donors, it is particularly important to identify the motivating factors for seeking living organ donation early on as this could also save the costs of medical tests and the medical team's time if the donor is not deemed appropriate by the ILDA. During a conversation with the transplant team, a prospective donor may ask questions or make comments that provoke concern related to coercion or pressure to come forward for evaluation. In order to promote and protect the donor's well-being, if any of these or similar circumstances occur, the ILDA evaluation should be initiated as soon as possible [5].

To promote honest and complete disclosure of information, prospective donors need to be evaluated in private. Even spouses and family members who are not related to the intended transplant recipient can affect the conversation. Providing a safe environment to share information invites open discussion without the fear of consequences [4]. Confidentiality is addressed at this time with the understanding that information received from the donor will only be shared with the multidisciplinary team members as needed. Independence of the ILDA, or that the ILDA has no interaction with or knowledge of any circumstances surrounding the intended recipient, is clearly explained. In some instances, the living donor advocate may be completely separate from the transplant center staff. The transparency of this independence promotes the notion that the ILDA is charged with looking after the safety and welfare of the prospective living donor and ensuring that they receive the education and information needed to make an informed decision that is in their best interest, and may not necessarily be in the best interest of the intended transplant recipient.

Free-flowing, bidirectional conversation is essential for a thorough evaluation and allows the ILDA to more accurately identify the unique strengths and potential burdens of the prospective donor. By asking open-ended questions, the living donor advocate invites responses that provide knowledge about the prospective donor, the information that they already possess regarding living donation, and the education that they are in need of in order to make an informed decision [4]. Entering the evaluation with only the knowledge that a prospective donor has come forward and indicating this to the donor allows the ILDA to initiate this type of exchange, while at the same time emphasizing independence. Allowing the donors to provide demographics (age, marital status, significant other, and children) and the type of living donation involved (related, nonrelated, or altruistic) gives the living donor advocate the opportunity to begin by exploring the decision-making process to better understand the donor's motivation.

The ILDA can begin to gain insight into the motivating factors by asking the prospective donor questions about how and when they learned about the intended recipient's need for a transplant; why the candidate needs a transplant; what the donor has learned about living donation; and how they personally came to the decision to be evaluated for donation. In related living donation, the underlying motivation usually stems from a sense of family and feelings of love and protection, whereas, in non-related living donation, donors may be motivated by a need to contribute to society or a sense of altruism as well as out of love or compassion [2, 6]. It is the role of the ILDA to initiate discussion that assists the prospective donor in identifying those factors that are influencing their desire to donate. There may be times when the donor identifies relationships they have with the intended recipient that need further exploration, such as employer/employee, members of organizations or faith communities, or solicitation from the Internet or media [5]. These types of relationships raise concerns that the prospective donor may be feeling pressure to donate and will require extended assessment. The prospective donor may not have identified the potential pressures these may invoke prior to evaluation and, therefore, may gain further insight with discussion. It is the role of the ILDA to assist the donor in exploring this possibility and identifying any implications related to donation. If the ILDA is not completing a full psychosocial evaluation (e.g., personal and family medical and psychiatric history, education, occupation), it may be useful to obtain a complete understanding of the donor.

The multidisciplinary team evaluation of a living donor candidate should allow for ongoing education, including repetition and reinforcement of the medical, psychosocial, and financial risks. The ILDA must ensure that the prospective donor receives this education and understands the process and procedure, along with identifying the associated risks and benefits that may be specific to the individual [1]. Asking the donor to explain the donation process and procedure and whether others have been evaluated as potential donors will assist the ILDA in identifying any areas that may need further education. This may also lead to further discussion that can be of help in determining the prospective donor's level of motivation. Those donors who have done research prior to the evaluation and have come with a list of questions may be highly motivated to proceed or they may be concerned about the associated risks. Prospective donors as well as the recipients must have a clear understanding of the risks associated with the surgical procedure. Asking them to identify and discuss these risks allows the ILDA to assess their level of understanding, as well as provide reinforcement.

The living donor advocate must assess the prospective donor's understanding about the intended recipient's medical condition that necessitates the need for a transplant and the treatment options, other than living donation, that are available. The donor may feel that living donation is the only option for the candidate. If the prospective donor is aware of alternatives to donation, they may have questions as to the length and availability of treatment and expected outcomes for the recipient. In these cases, the ILDA would need to ensure that the prospective donor receives the education and information necessary to make an informed decision and understands that there are other options available to the candidate.

The ILDA must determine if there are anticipated implications for the donor if living donation does not proceed as planned. Prospective donors may be fearful that if they do not go through with living donation, the relationship that they have with the transplant candidate, either family or mutual friends, may be negatively impacted. The donor may need assistance from the ILDA in recognizing this fear and its impact on the decision to donate. The prospective donor must be provided with a confidential and safe environment to discuss the implications they perceive should they decline to donate. The donor must be assured that they are in control of their decision to move forward with donation. They must be informed and must feel comfortable in the knowledge that they may withdraw from living donation at any time during the process. They must be assured that the ILDA will work with the multidisciplinary team to facilitate this in such a way that it does not negatively impact these relationships. Some transplant centers offer the option of a "medical out" for donor candidates. At the request of the potential donor, the center will provide a letter indicating a reason that the candidate is not considered medically suitable to proceed with living donation. This request remains confidential between the team members and the donor candidate [1, 4].

Once the prospective donor's motivation and the reasoning behind the decision making to be evaluated for living donation are assessed, the ILDA should evaluate the living donor's support system as it relates to this decision. Although this is an autonomous decision, it is important for the prospective donor to have spousal support in their decision to move forward with living donation. Living donation carries with it an increased risk of morbidity and mortality, and candidates may need the support of family and friends. In addition, there may be stressors placed on the household related to potential child-care issues, time commitments, assistance with transportation to and from the hospital, and clinic visits. This should lead to discussion regarding the prospective donor's employer and if living donation will have any impact on current or future employment or finances. Questions related to an employer's reaction regarding the potential living donation, whether the donor is knowledgeable regarding time-off-work policies, and whether living donation will affect the donor's occupation or employment need to be asked by the living donor advocate. The ILDA must ensure that the prospective donor understands and fully evaluates the impact that the decision of living donation may have on the spouse and family as well as their occupational status. Donor candidates must be cognizant of the fact that living donor evaluation may uncover issues with their own health that they were previously unaware of. These may be as benign as an increased risk of diabetes or as life threatening as cancer. The ILDA prepares the potential donor for the discovery of this type of information, which can potentially impact current and future health and life insurances, in addition to daily living [7, 9].

Postoperative recovery and discharge planning need to be discussed in the initial evaluation. The prospective donor must evaluate the impact of the recovery time and needs on themselves and the household. Discussion surrounding plans for postsurgical assistance with daily activities and driving arrangements should be initiated by the ILDA to ensure that the donor has identified the need for support during this phase and where that support will come from. The ILDA also needs to facilitate conversation surrounding the possibility that, should the recovery take longer than anticipated, additional support and resources may be needed. During the evaluation, the ILDA raises these issues and others that surround living donation with the goal of providing the prospective donor with the tools necessary to gather and assess the information needed to make a decision that is right for them [1].

All surgeries carry inherent risks. As protector and promoter of the donor's best interests, the ILDA must make sure that the prospective donor receives education and understands all the risks associated with living donation. As already mentioned, living donation carries with it an increased risk of morbidity and mortality. The donor needs to understand that there is no medical benefit to them related to living donation, but that there are risks. The ILDA must ask the donor about their understanding of these risks and discuss them as they relate to the decision-making process regarding living donation. Asking questions regarding the prospective donor's past experience with any hospitalizations or surgeries can give the ILDA insight into concerns and fears that the donor may have.

It must be identified that the living donation evaluation process itself has inherent risks. The ILDA must make sure that the prospective donor is aware that if the medical evaluation uncovers health information that the donor was previously unaware of and this information is of the type that medical personnel are required to report to governmental health agencies, the transplant center must follow through with this process as defined. The donor also needs to consider that there may be psychological effects related to identifying one's risk of a future health problem. The prospective donor may be deemed a noncandidate by the multidisciplinary team. The ILDA must disclose this to the donor candidate and make sure that they understand this possibility and the emotional impact it may have on them before proceeding with the evaluation [8].

Financial risk is another important component of the ILDA evaluation. Living donors may incur personal costs related to donation and these need to be identified. There may be transportation, including flights, and lodging costs if the donor is traveling a moderate-to-long distance for the donation. If traveling a shorter distance, there are likely gas expenses to and from the hospital for tests, clinic visits, surgery, etc. During the evaluation, time may need to be taken off work for testing by the prospective donor. There may be child-care costs, meal costs, costs of medications after discharge, and other nonmedical expenses. Household income may also be affected by time off from work in the postsurgical recovery phase. In protecting and looking out for the best interests of the donor, the ILDA needs to discuss this with the prospective donor and make sure that they have an understanding of these risks. The ILDA must ask the prospective donor if there is the possibility of financial hardship related to these financial risks should they choose to proceed with donation. A thorough evaluation allows the ILDA to determine if there are indications of high risk to the donor. Prospective donors with limited incomes and multiple dependents experiencing financial instability have been identified as high-risk candidates. Candidates must also be made aware that they may be subject to increased premium rates, or even denial, in relation to health and/or life insurance following living donation or evaluation [3, 7].

In addition to understanding the medical and financial risks that may be associated with living donation, the ILDA must help the prospective donor identify the psychosocial risks. Asking open-ended questions about how they might feel if the kidney they donated was rejected by the recipient or if the recipient was noncompliant with the medical regimen after donation facilitates discussion that will allow the donor to comprehend them. Should donation occur and the organ then fails to work in the recipient or is rejected, the living donor may experience a feeling of failure, regret, and/or grief. The prospective donor also needs to understand the possibility that the recipient's actions post donation may not optimize the gift that the living donor has provided. Identifying these scenarios during the evaluation provides the donor with the opportunity to realize not only the potential positive effects of living donation but also the negative consequences that may occur. The donor candidate should be made aware that the recipient may not either care for the donor's organ as they wish and/or be as grateful as the donor may expect, particularly depending on the candidate–donor relationship prior to surgery. The knowledge and understanding of these risks is essential if the prospective donor is to make an informed decision related to living donation [6].

The prospective living donor must not only understand that these risks exist but also evaluate the potential impact they may have on each individual. It is important for the ILDA to advise the donor of the importance of evaluating the benefit of having life, disability, and health insurance policies in place prior to proceeding with the living donor evaluation and making certain that they receive the education necessary to do so. With the increased risk of mortality and morbidity and the potential that unknown health conditions and diseases may be identified during the evaluation process, the donor must be educated on how this may impact insurability, as some insurers may classify this as a preexisting condition. Complications such as hypertension, proteinuria, or impaired kidney function following living kidney donation have the potential to affect insurability [9]. Ensuring that the prospective donor understands these risks and potential implications is imperative for informed decision making.

The prospective donor must be advised during the evaluation about short- and long-term follow-up requirements and understand the importance of this data for themselves and the transplant community as a whole [1]. The ILDA should ask questions related to current health care practices and lifestyle to gain insight into past and present behaviors that may indicate a need for further education or provide satisfaction that the donor has a clear understanding. Quality of life after donation should remain unchanged or even improved as research indicates that when compared with other healthy, motivated individuals, living donors have a similar quality of life [10].

Due to the "altruistic" nature of living organ donation, the indication that one is seeking any type of personal or financial gain represents a true conflict of interest. The ILDA must be sure to inform the donor candidate during evaluation that it is an unlawful act to receive any material or monetary gain that directly results from donation. A clear understanding of the prospective donor's motivation should lend insight and allow the ILDA to identify if there are any suspicions of financial or monetary compensation or other types of material goods that are tangible (e.g., car) or intangible (e.g., travel) expected in exchange for living organ donation. Assessment and documentation in this area are essential, as any indication of such an exchange or expectation would deem the prospective donor an unsuitable candidate for living organ donation.

The role of the ILDA is to promote and protect the best interests and well-being of the living donor. By conducting a thorough evaluation, the living donor advocate ensures that the prospective donor receives the education and information necessary to make an informed decision that is right for them. The ILDA gains insight and knowledge about the donor necessary to render an opinion about donor candidacy through the use of bidirectional information and education. The ILDA evaluation ensures that the living donor is motivated, autonomous, and educated. Recommended components of the ILDA evaluation are presented in Table 13.1.

Table 13.1 Components of ILDA evaluation	Type of living donor/relationship to intended recipient (related, nonrelated, altruistic)
	Knowledge/understanding of living donation process
	Understanding of intended recipient's medical condition as it relates to need for transplant and treatment options available
	Signs of coercion or undue influence
	Right to change mind at any time up until anesthesia/anticipated implications if living donation does not proceed as planned
	Willingness and competence to donate
	Possible financial or monetary gain, tangible or intangible
	Understanding of medical, psychosocial, and financial risks
	Support system including family and friends reaction/feelings
	Occupational status and employer's reaction/feelings
	Any anticipated impact on lifestyle
	Understanding/importance of long-term follow-up

References

1. Rudow DL. The living donor advocate: a team approach to educate, evaluate, and manage donors across the continuum. Prog Transplant. 2009;19(1):64–70.
2. Rudow DL. Role of the independent donor advocacy team in ethical decision making. Prog Transplant. 2005;15(3):298–302.
3. Bramstedt KA. Living donor transplantation between twins: guidance for donor advocate teams. Clin Transplant. 2007;21:144–7.
4. Sites AK, Freeman JR, Harper MR, Waters DB, Pruett TL. A multidisciplinary program to educate and advocate for living donors. Prog Transplant. 2008;18(4):284–9.
5. Dew MA, Jacobs CL, Jowsey SG, Hanto R, Miller C, Delmonico FL. Guidelines for the psychosocial evaluation of living unrelated kidney donors in the United States. Am J Transplant. 2007;7:1047–54.
6. Bosek MSD, Sargeant IL. Living kidney donor advocacy program: a quality improvement project. JONAS Healthc Law Ethics Regul. 2012 Jan/Mar;14(1):19–26.
7. Bramstedt KA, Katznelson S. Being Sherlock Holmes: the internet as a tool for assessing live organ donors. Clin Transplant. 2009;23:157–61.
8. Rodrigue JR, Pavlakis M, Danovitch GM, Johnson SR, Karp SJ, Khwaja K, et al. Evaluating living kidney donors: relationship types, psychosocial criteria, and consent processes at US transplant programs. Am J Transplant. 2007;7:2326–32.
9. Yang RC, Young A, Nevis IFP, Lee D, Jain AK, Dominic A, et al. Life insurance for living kidney donors: a Canadian undercover investigation. Am J Transplant. 2009;9:1585–90.
10. Clemens K, Boudville N, Dew MA, Geddes C, Gill JS, Jassal V, et al. The long-term quality of life of living kidney donors: a mulitcenter cohort study. Am J Transplant. 2011;11:463–9.

Chapter 14
Contraindications to Living Donation from an ILDA Perspective

Rebecca Hays

The independent living donor advocate (ILDA) participates to help ensure that all living donors are fully informed, willing, and uncoerced volunteers, building from the important components of assessment and interaction as described by Sites et al.—independence, transparency, partnership, and advocacy [24]. The role of an independent advocate is essential because of the unique context of, and potential pressures associated with, living organ donation internal for the prospective donor himself/herself, from the prospective donor's loved ones, and from the medical team. As an independent clinician, unbiased by either connection to the intended recipient or having a stake in whether or not the surgery occurs, the ILDA is tasked with the overall review of potential living donors' understanding of process, risks, and rights. As such, the ILDA acts as a safeguard and assures and reinforces that elements of informed consent are met. Fundamentally, then, living donation is contraindicated from an ILDA perspective when the prospective donor does not meet the standards of informed consent [1, 21] (Table 14.1).

This chapter will provide an overview of ILDA-identified contraindications to living organ donation, utilizing key concepts of informed consent categorized broadly as lack of intentionality (or desire to proceed), lack of understanding of risks/benefits, and lack of voluntary status (presence of coercion) [8]. Although all health care workers participating in the evaluation process agree that living donors should be ready and informed volunteers, the assessment of elements of understanding and preparedness can be challenging in practice. This chapter will explore these factors, will offer practice strategies for assessment, and will describe unique aspects of the ILDA role in doing so. Using both literature and case examples to explore differences between areas of relative risk and outright contraindication, the chapter will offer guidance for clinical practice. Finally, it will describe strategies for communicating contraindication findings to the prospective donor and transplant team.

R. Hays (✉)
Transplant Clinic, University of Wisconsin Hospital and Clinics, 600 Highland Avenue, Madison, WI 53792, USA
e-mail: RHays@uwhealth.org

Table 14.1 Contraindications to living donation from an ILDA perspective

1. Prospective donor does not want to proceed
2. Prospective donor lacks adequate understanding of risks associated with donation or the donation process
3. Prospective donor is not a willing and an uncoerced volunteer
(a) There is evidence of secondary gain
(b) There is evidence of coercive pressure

Background on ILDA Role and Practice

Before outlining specifics of these ILDA-identified contraindications, let us start with a brief overview of the ILDA role and purpose and a clarification of what the ILDA is empowered (and, conversely, not empowered or perhaps even qualified) to do. The ILDA serves as an unbiased resource for the prospective donor to learn more about the process and options; explores the prospective donor's understanding of surgical, medical, psychosocial, and financial risks; affirms understanding of process as well as follow-up recommendations; and confirms desire to proceed or assists with walking away (with the protection of confidentiality for the reasons why she/he does not want to proceed with surgery). Ideally, the ILDA supports and advocates so that all living donors are competent, fully informed, willing, and uncoerced.

To be clear: first, the ILDA role does not interpret medical or psychosocial risk profiles to make candidacy determinations (though if she/he serves in a dual role at the transplant center, these separate recommendations may be appropriate and necessary in the other capacity). Second, the ILDA does not trump prospective living donor autonomy to declare what is in his/her "best" interest (as in theory it would be in every person's "best" interest to avoid unnecessary surgery). It is not the ILDA, but rather the treating clinician (i.e., living donor surgeon), who formally completes the informed consent prior to surgery.

Individual transplant centers across the United States have operationalized the ILDA role in vastly different ways [25]. Other chapters of this book will explore recommendations for ILDA training, practice, and role throughout the living donation process. Certainly, during the evaluation process, the ILDA can participate in many ways to assist prospective donors throughout the process: via assessment, evaluation, psychoeducation, collaboration with transplant team members, and advocacy, all as central elements of practice.

In the varied and various ways that the ILDA role has been implemented, the ILDA must partner with potential donors to promote rights and understanding as part of the prospective donor's decision-making process. In so doing, ILDA also identifies barriers to prospective donors' provision of informed consent [15, 30, 31]. For example, the prospective living donor may not be able to understand or accept risks associated with donation. Essential to the ILDA role, then, is to be empowered to stop the donation process if elements of informed consent have not been met.

Of course, living donor candidacy criteria are defined by individual transplant centers. Previous research has shown broad differences in donor candidacy requirements and processes in the United States [5, 20, 25]. Provided the donor evaluation process is consistent with the Center for Medicare and Medicaid Services (CMS) and the United Network for Organ Sharing (UNOS)/Organ Procurement and Transplantation Network (OPTN) guidelines (and there has been a move within regulatory agencies and transplant professional organizations to increase degree of standardization in this process), individual candidacy decisions and criteria are determined by the transplant facility. Regardless of how contraindications are specifically defined, ILDA review of prospective donor readiness and understanding—including identified contraindications—becomes part of donor candidacy discussion, and should be addressed within teams and at donor selection meetings.

Informed Consent

Informed consent for live kidney donation is a prerequisite—essential for living donor transplantation from ethical, legal, and regulatory perspectives. In general, informed consent occurs when a competent person makes an autonomous choice about whether to access medical treatment, armed with adequate information and understanding regarding risks, benefits, and expected outcomes [2]. The patient's intention to proceed, understanding of process and benefits, and free will to decide are fundamental. However, as Valapour noted, these factors may be present along a continuum of clarity/confusion [32]. Informed consent can also be described as a reciprocal process between clinician and patient of information disclosure, processing, and decision making. Much has been written describing the challenges associated with determining adequacy of informed consent for living organ donation, a procedure lacking medical benefits for the participant and therefore demanding a high standard of careful process and communication. Living donor transplant has the added challenge of being a shared transaction, in which the living donor's informed consent must also include understanding of the intended benefits, options, and expected outcomes for another (the recipient) [4].

In "Informed consent in living donation: a review of key empirical studies, ethical challenges and future research," Gordon summarizes goals of the process as follows:

> The principle of respect for persons requires that potential LDs be competent and informed, and comprehend the risks to themselves of undergoing the procedure, as well as the risks, benefits and alternatives available to the recipient. The consensus conference on Living Kidney Donor Follow-Up emphasized the critical need to inform donors about risks specific to themselves. Further, potential LDs must be willing to donate and be free from undue pressure to consent to the procedure. Moreover, respect for autonomy means that LDs have the right to determine how much risk they are willing to accept, and conversely, that LDs (and the recipients) have the right to refuse the donation. [9]

In practice, though, living donor informed consent processes have been shown to vary widely across transplant programs in the United States and worldwide, with wild discrepancies noted in standards, consistency, and practice [9, 16, 32, 33]. In separate pieces, both Gordon and Rodrigue et al. identified significant "variability and deficiencies" in the consent process across the spectrum of living donor care [9, 20]. While many of the studies reviewed care prior to implementation of newer living donor safeguards (including OPTN Living Donor Informed Consent Guidelines; provision of follow-up care for living donors for 2 years; and implementation of the ILDA itself), concerns raised about variability in the quality of informed consent process continue to be valid. Regulatory and professional organizations have called for strengthened processes, and for standardized elements of disclosure and education, including separating the consent process for living donor evaluation from consent to proceed with donation (Table 14.2) [9, 15, 16, 27, 30–33].

Table 14.2 Guidance sources

Guidance sources	These references can be found at the American Society for Transplantation website, in the Living Donor Community of Practice section
CMS	Conditions of participation and organ transplant interpretive guidelines 2008 (pp. 77–85)
UNOS	Policies 12.4 (independent donor advocate (IDA)) 12.4.1 (IDA role) 12.4.2 (IDA responsibilities) 12.4.3 (IDA protocols)
OPTN	Guidelines for living donor informed consent http://optn.transplant.hrsa.gov/ContentDocuments/Living_Donor_Kidney_Psychosocial_Eval_Checklist.doc http://optn.transplant.hrsa.gov/ContentDocuments/Living_Donor_Kidney_Medical_Eval_Checklist.doc http://optn.transplant.hrsa.gov/ContentDocuments/Living_Donor_Kidney_Informed_Consent_Checklist.doc

CMS Center for Medicare and Medicaid Services, *UNOS* United Network for Organ Sharing, *OPTN* Organ Procurement and Transplantation Network

Elements of Informed Consent

Willing Volunteer

On its face, lacking desire to proceed is a straightforward contraindication to living organ donation. The living donor must be a willing volunteer. Valapour framed this component of informed consent as "intentionality," and defined it as an "absolute condition, that is, an act that is either intentional or not" (Table 14.3) [32]. Of course, at any time during the living donor evaluation process, the potential living donor has the right to stop the process. The ILDA (or, one would hope, anyone on the transplant team) would identify this as a contraindication, and assist the potential donor with walking away, while de-

Table 14.3 Basic components of informed consent

1. Intentionality
2. Understanding
3. Noncontrol (language beautifully outlined by Valapour [32])

signing a strategy amenable to the potential donor that preserves relations with the intended recipient.

However, sustained ambivalence and experience of "pressure" (internal and external) around organ donation decision making is not uncommon [7, 14, 33]. Importantly, the literature suggests that donors who describe ambivalence at the time of donation are at higher risk for poor psychosocial outcome [7, 26]. Transplant programs have integrated various strategies to assist prospective donors struggling with ambivalence, including a "cooling off period" [20], a "scaling system" of desire and readiness, referral to psychosocial providers for counseling/support, and, most recently by Dew et al., interventions utilizing motivational interviewing approaches [7].

The ILDA is ideally positioned to check in with the potential donor about the status of "intentionality" and stage of decision making at several steps in the donor evaluation process. The ILDA may meet with the potential donor early on to learn about motivation and conduct review assessment after the potential donor completes medical testing. The ILDA may also serve as the prospective donor's "voice" at donor candidate selection meeting: to forward lingering questions to members of the transplant team for discussion and input and also to articulate the prospective donor's desire to proceed (or not).

The profoundly ambivalent potential donor, who has not decided to proceed but has also not decided to close out the donation process, also benefits from specific aspects of the ILDA role and advocacy. Ultimately, a decision to proceed (or "intentionality") is necessary to be a living donor candidate. Given that informed consent is an affirmative action, for the purposes of living donor candidacy, "not deciding" must be the same as "deciding not to" proceed. As such, the ILDA can advocate for "cooling off" periods, and ways to ensure that the potential donor has had reflection time.

The ILDA also helps the prospective donor identify ways to resolve ambivalence. In some cases, the ILDA assists the ambivalent donor in accessing additional information about medical and psychosocial candidacy to aid his/her decision making. The ILDA advocates for this feedback, with the caveat that candidacy decisions have not yet been made. From an ILDA perspective, living donation is contraindicated until the prospective donor decides he/she wants to proceed. Holding to this standard during donor-candidate selection meeting helps preserve the "medical out" option.

Suggestion of Coercion

Prospective living donors do not decide to proceed in a vacuum. By definition, living donation decision making occurs with the hope of helping another. It is a shared transaction. Not surprisingly, then, studies have shown that contemplation about living donation is affected by feelings of pressure and obligation, both internally felt and externally imposed. These feelings may be positively expressed through role identification and aspirational identity: "this is what families do for each other" or "this is what [my faith] leads me to do." They may be felt internally as a weight associated with knowledge about benefits of living donor transplant for the recipient; pain seeing a loved one suffer; or desire to "save" another loved one from pressures to donate (most commonly in my clinical practice young adult children) [28].

Although these emotions can be experienced as difficult to weigh and sort, it is rather elements of external, coercive pressure that threaten potential donors' autonomous decision making. In a survey of 262 living donors, Valapour et al. found that 40% described feeling some level of pressure around donation [33]. "Influences affecting the voluntary nature" of informed consent ran along a continuum, with the mildest being persuasion, midline being manipulation, and most severe being coercion. Not surprisingly, data showed that living donors experiencing the highest degree of (presumably, external) pressure around decision making also had the highest rate of "unsureness" about whether they would choose to donate again [3, 7, 33].

Although a psychosocial evaluation during workup will certainly explore the prospective living donor's motivations and risk of experiencing pressure to donate, the ILDA evaluation serves as a secondary check to ascertain whether a potential living donor is free to choose to donate (or not) without inducement or fear of reprisal. Interviews elicit distinctions between internalized pressure often associated with living donor decision making and external pressure affecting potential living donor autonomy and safety.

When coercive pressure has been disclosed, the ILDA (and other transplant team members) must provide the prospective living donor education about necessary elements of informed consent and discuss ways to stop the donor process. In these situations, careful strategy and rehearsal about next steps is often helpful (see Case Example 1). It is also conceivable for a potential living donor to disclose others' efforts to induce him/her to donate, and being able to make an autonomous decision to donate (or not) despite this pressure. In other words, it is the prospective donor's perception of this pressure, and its influence on decision making, that is important in determining whether autonomous decisions are possible. If autonomous decisions are not possible, here, too, the ILDA assists with various options for walking away, including use of a "medical out."

> **Case Example 1: Presence of Coercion**
>
> *Details have been changed to protect patient confidentiality. The ILDA is a member of the Patient Relations Department at the hospital; nurse by training.*
>
> A 23-year-old man presents for donor evaluation; his sister is on the transplant wait-list for a third transplant. All team members note anxiety and pressured responses. His mother (recipient's mother too) contacts the transplant center repeatedly to request updates on his workup; she is advised of Health Insurance Portability and Accountability Act (HIPPA) restrictions. He believes donation is the "right" thing to do, and resents that it is "expected." He does not want to donate, but is not sure if he could live with himself if he does not. During ILDA phone assessment, he describes being "blackballed" until he proceeds with donation. ILDA labels this behavior as coercive, explains this is unacceptable, and suggests that the patient meet with the donor team members to strategize next steps. Donor evaluation process is stopped and medical out is provided, with rehearsal by both donor social worker and transplant coordinator.

Direct Payment

As outlined in the UNOS Guidelines for Living Donor Care, donor consent must include disclosure that "it is a federal crime for any person to knowingly acquire, obtain, or otherwise transfer any human organ for valuable consideration (i.e., for anything of value such as cash, property, vacations) . . ." [15]. As part of review of informed consent, then, ILDA assesses whether prospective donors understand these provisions, and in turn whether they agree to abide by them. Secondary gain as a factor in living donor motivation or decision making is a contraindication to candidacy.

The National Organ Transplant Act of 1984 (amended in 1988 and 1990, and colloquially known as NOTA) outlawed the sale of human organs [18]. Since then, as the organ shortage has grown, organ trafficking and international "transplant tourism" have been major ethical concerns for the United States and worldwide transplant community [14, 17].

Concerns about unregulated organ sales and transplant tourism continue to mandate careful evaluation and assessment of prospective donor's expectations, especially as more potential donors present to transplant centers without an emotional connection to their recipients (and so, presumably, less likely to observe the kidney transplant recipient benefiting from living donor transplantation). The number of first-degree relatives as living donors continues to decline [5]. Although in 1989, only 8% of transplant programs would consider a nondirected donor, by 2007, 61% of responding programs evaluated nondirected donors [20]. Recommendations from a UNOS, AST (American Society of Transplantation), and ASTS

(American Society of Transplant Surgeons)-sponsored consensus conference on the care of the living unrelated kidney donor recommended that evaluation processes and structure be fundamentally the same, regardless of the relationship (or lack thereof) between donor and recipient [6]. In all cases, including those lacking prior relationship, shared understanding of expectations and degree of (or limits to) future relationship between donor and recipient (including lack of financial relationship) be agreed upon prior to proceeding. During prospective living donor evaluation, the psychosocial assessment explores risk factors for secondary gain as a driving force behind prospective donor motivation. These in turn are linked to problems of pressure and/or coercion. Members of the transplant team should provide psychoeducation about NOTA provisions, and seek prospective donor response to the same, clarifying guidelines and options for next steps, including ways to walk away from donation process. If psychosocial assessment identifies areas of risk, including concerns about prospective donor transparency, the donor social worker may conduct further assessment, seeking consistency in descriptions of motivation, sustained interest and coping with a prescribed "cooling off" period, or consistency between desire to donate and other behavior (such as volunteer work, etc.). Recommendations regarding risk factors will be contained within psychosocial assessment and reviewed during donor candidacy meeting.

It is the ILDA role, then, to review prospective donor understanding of the guidelines, agreement to abide by them, and confirm prospective donor's desire to proceed with donation given these parameters. If any of these conditions are not met, ILDA presents this finding at donor selection as a clear contraindication to donor candidacy. For example, in rare cases, a prospective donor may disclose offers of secondary gain as coercive pressure or that he/she was unaware of NOTA provisions prior to presenting for donor evaluation (see Case Examples 2 and 3). As an independent and transparent advocate for donor rights and understanding, ILDA is uniquely situated to help these prospective donors and the transplant team craft a graceful way out that minimizes risk of negative impact, given that coercive pressure may be in play.

However, ILDA can also assist the prospective donor—and the transplant team—in sorting through considerations about secondary gain that can be confusing in practice. To summarize a few historic examples, a previous controversy about whether paired kidney donation constituted secondary gain was clarified only with the passage of the Charlie W Norwood Living Organ Donation Act in 2007 (Public Law 110–144), finding paired kidney donation acceptable under NOTA [18]. Similarly, it has been generally agreed that donors can be reimbursed incidental costs of organ donation, including travel and lost wages. Therefore, while it is clearly illegal to profit from donating an organ, getting reimbursed for expenses is acceptable. It is common for ILDA to help prospective donors clarify understanding of these general guidelines.

However, in other cases, what constitutes "valuable consideration" can be confusing. ILDA discussion with prospective living donors can identify areas of question. When in doubt, ILDA can help prospective donors access clarification, including hospital ethics consult. Following are a few examples from my own practice, without clear answers: if a prospective living donor gets a long-term increase in health insurance premium costs, presumably related to the impact of living donation, can the recipient cover these new costs? If a living donor delays accepting a new job in order to donate, can he/she be reimbursed potential lost wages? (see Case Example 4). In each of these examples, the prospective donor declared himself/herself unable to proceed without the assistance and wanted to comply with the law.

Defining the role of the ILDA here helps determine practice and next steps. After all, few, if any, ILDAs are attorneys expert in NOTA law; although all ILDAs should be well-versed in general concepts of medical ethics, not all ILDAs will be seasoned members of a hospital ethics committee. Therefore, in assessing secondary gain as a contraindication to donation, it is *not* the ILDA role to interpret NOTA per se. Rather, ILDA reviews prospective donor understanding of provisions and consent to abide by them, and partners with the prospective donor (and the transplant team) to clarify areas in question.

Case Example 2: Secondary Gain

Details have been changed to protect patient confidentiality. In this case, donor social worker is also an ILDA.

A 31-year-old woman presents for donor evaluation, hoping to donate to a distant cousin. She learned of the recipient's health status via a social media posting, and has been emailing directly with the recipient since then. During psychosocial evaluation, the prospective donor states calmly that the recipient told her insurance would pay a $ 20,000 fee for donation. As a result, finances are not a worry for her during her time off work. Donor social worker/ILDA clarifies that in the United States, no insurance will pay cash for a kidney, and in fact, this is illegal. Informed consent documents are shared to shed further light on the regulations. The prospective donor is dismayed. She feels "duped" by the recipient, and wishes to withdraw from donation. She states that the payment is not what drew her to donate, but that the false offer of cash leaves a "bad taste," and she will not trust future communications with the intended recipient. However, she does not want to confront the recipient, as she is afraid of family "backlash" for withdrawing.

ILDA collaborates with her and with the rest of the transplant team to end the donor evaluation. The clinician helps the prospective donor rehearse what to say within her family (though this rehearsal might not have been conducted by the ILDA had the ILDA not been a clinical social worker). The prospective donor is found to be "not a candidate" at donor selection, a finding which is transmitted back to her and (at her request) to the intended recipient.

Case Example 3: Secondary Gain

Details have been changed to protect patient confidentiality. In this case, the ILDA is a nurse coordinator who works as part of an independent living donor team (ILDT).

A 46-year-old man presents for donor evaluation, with intended recipient his brother. Intended recipient also owns the duplex in which they both live. Prospective donor is guarded, speaking in monosyllables when possible, and although each member of the ILDT gets the "feeling" that he is unenthusiastic, no one is able to engage him around these questions. Finally, during a follow-up phone call to share findings of the donor evaluation, prospective donor discloses that he has been advised that donating a kidney is the way he can avoid being evicted. He reports he "does not really have a choice." ILDA/coordinator is able to review concepts of secondary gain with him, and encourages him to reconnect with donor social worker for further discussion and intervention. Donor social worker helps prospective donor define elements of coercion and distinguish these from desired family roles and connections. In turn, donor social worker and ILDA/coordinator work together with prospective donor to identify ways to walk away from donation process. Prospective donor is found to be "not a candidate" at donor selection.

Case Example 4: Secondary Gain

Details have been changed to protect patient confidentiality. In this case, the ILDA is a chaplain who meets with donors at the end of the donor evaluation process.

A 22-year-old man accompanies his father to his transplant evaluation, expresses an interest in living donation at that time, and is advised that once his father is declared a transplant candidate, he can be scheduled for donor workup. Intended recipient's case is complex, and it takes months to meet candidacy criteria. In the meantime, the prospective donor is charged with minor crimes and sentenced to several months of jail time. Upon his release, he completes in-person donor evaluation. Briefly, his donor workup is WNL (within normal limits); he meets medical and psychosocial criteria, although he is noted to have a moderately high psychosocial risk profile. In reviewing informed consent documents with the ILDA, prospective donor notes that he was advised at a court hearing that "if I donated a kidney, the judge would take this under advisement" regarding sentencing for other, still-pending charges. Although prospective donor advised ILDA that this was not a factor in donation decision making (and ILDA found this to be believable, given prospective donor's longstanding interest in donation and status as caregiver for intended recipient), both the prospective donor and ILDA wondered whether this statement constituted "valuable consideration" in the context of living donation. ILDA assisted prospective donor in seeking input from the rest of the transplant team and, ultimately, the hospital ethics committee. Ultimately, prospective donor proceeded to donation, but did so after completing legal obligations.

Understanding Risks

As is outlined in UNOS policies for living donor care, the ILDA reviews prospective living donor understanding of the donor evaluation process; the medical, surgical, and psychosocial risks of living donation; and the understanding of treatment options and outcomes for the recipient [4, 15, 19, 31]. This has been identified as a key element in the care of living donors, and is of particular interest given the literature suggesting that past living donors lacked knowledge and understanding prior to proceeding [9, 20, 33]. As such, from an ILDA perspective, living donation is contraindicated if the prospective living donor does not understand the risks associated with evaluation and donation.

If lack of understanding is identified as a barrier to candidacy, ILDA should share specific concerns with transplant team members, advocate for prospective donor to receive additional assessment, education, or intervention as indicated, and conduct follow-up assessment. In general, lack of understanding may be attributed to cognitive deficits that preclude provision of informed consent, inadequate integration or understanding of risks/benefits as described by transplant team members, or evidence of significantly unrealistic expectations associated with donation. If, after follow-up assessment, the prospective living donor still cannot reflect back understanding of risks, expected outcomes, or significant aspects of the process, then elements of informed consent have not been met, and ILDA should summarize these concerns at donor selection meeting and recommend against proceeding.

Certainly, in the role of an independent, unbiased partner through the process, the ILDA is uniquely situated to help prospective donors assemble, and assess, global understanding of risks as described throughout the donor evaluation process and by many team members. ILDA checks in with the prospective donor about takeaways from education provided variously, and at many time points, by nurse coordinator, physician, and social worker. ILDA assesses whether the prospective donor has processed, and retained, fundamental points acquired throughout, including understanding of medical, surgical, and psychosocial risks of proceeding; need for follow-up care; expected outcomes for donor and recipient; and treatment options for the recipient. Assessment at this stage further allows prospective donor to integrate both globally understood risks of living donation and risks/impact specific to the potential donor's health history and risk profile (see Case Examples 5 and 6).

Case Example 5: Patient Understanding

Details have been changed to protect patient confidentiality. In this case, the ILDA is a social worker. Donor psychosocial assessment was conducted by health psychology.

A 27-year-old single man hopes to donate a kidney to his mother, presents as strongly motivated to proceed, and says he would be willing to undergo "any" risk to help his mom. He lives with his parents and works part-time. Health psychologist identifies some cognitive impairment, learns he was in special education in school—diagnosis unknown to patient or family—and has never lived independently. Medically, his workup is WNL (within normal limits)—nephrologist and surgeon note patient participation in interview, whether his answers were short. ILDA notes that the patient is unable to read the consent forms and has some difficulty processing information provided.

At donor selection, ILDA voices concerns about patient understanding, at which time, team recommends additional evaluation. Neuropsychology finds prospective donor limited but competent, recommends oral teaching and repetition. Prospective donor, accompanied by his father (who was previously ruled out as a donor), eagerly participates in additional teaching sessions (with coordinator) by phone. Prospective donor phones in to ethics consult, voices his desire to donate and ably answers questions about risk. He proceeds to donate and reflects back positively on the experience.

Case Example 6: Patient Understanding

Details have been changed to protect patient confidentiality. In this case, the ILDA is also a social worker.

A 57-year-old woman presents as a potential nondirected donor. Medical and surgical evaluation identified many complex risk factors; psychosocial evaluation is WNL (within normal limits). Discussion at donor selection centered around prospective donor as high risk medically, but team determined she was a candidate if she understood her risk factors. In the interview with ILDA after medical workup was complete, prospective donor stated repeatedly that she would donate "if you can guarantee I'll be OK." She was not able to reflect back teaching provided by nephrologist, and instead stated, "I've heard donors do great afterwards." Despite repeated efforts at teaching and engaging by multiple team members, she was not able to reflect understanding of risks associated with donation, nor of her specific risk factors. ILDA documented her lack of understanding of risks, and of the informed consent process generally, as a contraindication to donation.

The ILDA participation at this stage is also an opportunity to help the prospective donor voice confusion and ask questions. ILDA can forward concerns to other team members for follow-up. In these cases, lack of understanding may not be a permanent contraindication to living donation, but may instead trigger additional (or adapted) teaching, or evaluation. ILDA forwards concerns about prospective donor's lack of understanding to other team members, who can then arrange additional consults—for example, neurology or psychiatry, and/or tailored teaching to accommodate learning barriers identified during psychosocial assessment (most commonly at our center literacy limits) [10]. ILDA can also assist prospective donor in asking specific questions of a transplant team member.

It is also not uncommon for prospective donors to voice that risks are of "no concern," and that they want to donate "no matter what." Many prospective donors share that the "worst news" would be a medical rule-out during evaluation. Simmons et al., in research dating back to the 1970s and 1980s, found that living donor (LD) decision making centers on moral, rather than deliberative, reasoning [23]. It is sometimes a clinical and practice challenge, in these cases, to help prospective donors slow down enough to process information about risk. As such, part of the informed consent process is to assess whether donors are able to process information and whether they have actually integrated it.

Structured interview with the ILDA helps potential donors focus and reflect understanding back. The ILDA can further promote engagement by encouraging the potential donor to invite a family member (often more concerned than the potential donor himself/herself) to participate in this learning and teaching, or the ILDA can otherwise strategize creatively. Formal evaluation, with the goal of reviewing what has been learned and what will be involved in consenting to donate, promotes potential donor participation. In this context, it is rare for a prospective donor to decline to participate.

That said, psychosocial status risk profile certainly affects patients' ability to integrate understanding of risks. Some people may lack the maturity to identify themselves as ever vulnerable to risk; others may demonstrate "magical thinking" about what living donation will do for the intended recipient. Each of these factors could be described as a relative contraindication or risk factor, warranting careful psychosocial assessment and review, and the ILDA role in this will vary according to the ILDA's professional background and structure of the role on the team.

Documentation of Findings and Next Steps

Guidelines for ILDA practice outline documentation requirements and have been specific about content areas [15, 29, 31]. If ILDA identifies a contraindication to living donor candidacy during assessment, this finding should be summarized and should appear in recommendations. Rationale and evidence should be available for review by transplant team members and by the prospective donor upon request. In turn, ILDA should participate in donor candidate selection meeting to discuss findings and assist in care planning.

References

1. Abecassis M, Adams M, Adams P, Arnold RM, Atkins CR, Barr ML, et al. Live Organ Donor Consensus Group. Consensus statement on the live organ donor. JAMA. 2000;284:2919–26.
2. Beauchamp Tl, Childress JF. Principles of biomedical ethics. 4th ed. New York: Oxford University Press; 1994.
3. Clemens K, Boudville N, Dew MA, Geddes C, Gill JS, Jassal V, et al. Donor Nephrectomy Outcomes Research (DONOR) Network. The longterm quality of life of living kidney donors: a multicenter cohort study. Am J Transplant. 2011;11(3):463–9.
4. Council of the Transplantation Society. A report of the Amsterdam forum on the care of the live kidney donor: data and medical guidelines. Transplantation. 2005;29(6 supplement):S53–66.
5. Davis CL, Cooper M. The state of US living kidney donors. Clin J Am Soc Nephrol. 2010 Oct;5(10):1873–80.
6. Dew MA, Jacobs CL, Jowsey SG, Hanto R, Miller C, Delmonico FL; UNOS; ASTS; AST. Guidelines for the psychosocial evaluation of living unrelated kidney donors in the US. Am J Transplant. 2007 May;7(5):1047–54.
7. Dew MA, Zuckoff A, DiMartini AF, Dabbs AJ, McNulty ML, Fox KR, et al. Prevention of poor psychosocial outcomes in living organ donors: from description to theory-driven intervention development and initial feasibility testing. Prog Transplant. 2012 Sep;22(3):280–92.
8. Faden RR, Beauchamp T. A history and theory of informed consent. New York: Oxford University Press; 1986.
9. Gordon EJ. Informed consent for living donation: a review of key empirical studies, ethical challenges and future research. Am J Transplant. 2012;12:2273–80.
10. Gordon EJ, Bergeron A, McNatt G, Friedewald J, Abecassis MM, Wolf MS. Are informed consent forms for organ transplantation and donation too difficult to read? Clin Transplant. 2012 Mar-Apr;26(2):275–83.
11. Ibrahim HN, Foley R, Tan L, Rogers T, Bailey RF, Guo H, et al. Long-term consequences of kidney donation. N Engl J Med. 2009 Jan 29;360(5):459–69.
12. Jowsey SG, Schneekloth TD. Psychosocial factors in living organ donation: clinical and ethical challenges. Transplant Rev. 2008;22(3):192–5.
13. Living Kidney Donor Follow-Up Conference Writing Group, Leichtman A, Abecassis M, Barr M, Charlton M, Cohen D, Confer D, et al. Living kidney donor follow-up: state-of-the-art and future directions, conference summary and recommendations. Am J Transplant. 2011 Dec;11(12):2561–8.
14. Matas AJ, Delmonico FL. Living donation: the global perspective. Adv Chronic Kid Dis. 2012 Jul;19(4):269–75.
15. OPTN Guidelines for Care of Living Donors. http://optn.transplant.hrsa.gov/ContentDocuments/Living_Donor_Kidney_Informed_Consent_Checklist.doc. Accessed Oct 1, 2013.
16. Parekh AM, Gordon EJ, Garg AX, Waterman AD, Kulkarni S, Parikh CR. Living kidney donor informed consent practices vary between US and non-US centers. Nephrol Dial Transplant. 2008 Oct;23(10):3316–24.
17. Participants in the International Summit on Transplant Tourism and Organ Trafficking Convened by the Transplantation Society and International Society of Nephrology in Istanbul, Turkey, April 30-May 2, 2008. The Declaration of Istanbul on organ trafficking and transplant tourism. Transplantation. 2008 Oct 27;86(8):1013–8.
18. Public Law 110-144-December 21, 2007 (Charlie Norwood Act, amendments to the National Organ Transplant Act of 1984). http://optn.transplant.hrsa.gov/policiesAndBylaws/nota.asp. Accessed online October 1, 2013.
19. Rodrigue JR, Schutzer ME, Paek M, Morrissey P. Altruistic kidney donation to a stranger: psychosocial and functional outcomes at 2 US transplant centers. Transplantation. 2001;91(7):772–8.

20. Rodrigue JR, Pavlakis M, Danovitch GM, Johnson SR, Karp SJ, Khwaja K, et al. Evaluating living kidney donors: relationship types, psychosocial criteria, and consent processes at US transplant programs. Am J Transplant. 2007 Oct;7(10):2326–32.
21. Rudow DL. The living donor advocate: a team approach to educate, evaluate, and manage donors across the continuum. Prog Transplant. 2009 Mar;19(1):64–70.
22. Segev DL, Muzaale AD, Caffo BS, Mehta SH, Singer AL, Taranto SE, et al. Perioperative mortality and long-term survival following live kidney donation. JAMA. 2010 Mar 10;303(10):959–66.
23. Simmons RG, Marine SK, Simmons RL. Gift of life: the effect of organ transplantation on individual, family and societal dynamics. New Brunswick: Transaction Publishers; 1987.
24. Sites AK, Freeman JR, Harper MR, Waters DB, Pruett TL. A multidisciplinary program to educate and advocate for living donors. Prog Transplant. 2008 Dec;18(4):284–9.
25. Steel J, Dunlavy A, Friday M, Kingsley K, Brower D, Unruh M, et al. A national survey of independent living donor advocates: the need for practice guidelines. Am J Transplant. 2012 Aug;12(8):2141–9.
26. Switzer GE, Dew MA, Simmons RG. Donor ambivalence and post-donation outcomes: implications for living donation. Transplant Proc. 1997;29(1–2):1476.
27. The Joint Commission. Advancing Effective Communication, Cultural Competence, and Patient- and Family-Centered care: A RoadMap for Hospitals. http://www.jointcommission.org/assets/1/6/ARoadmapforHospitalsfinalversion727.pdf. Accessed online October 1, 2013.
28. Tong A, Chapman JR, Wong G, Kanellis J, McCarthy G, Craig JC. The motivations and experiences of living kidney donors: a thematic synthesis. Am J Kidney Dis. 2012 Jul;60(1):15–26.
29. Organ Transplantation and Procurement Network, Policy 12, Living Donation. http://optn.transplant.hrsa.gov/PoliciesandBylaws2/policies/pdfs/policy_172.pdf. Accessed online September 26, 2013.
30. US Department of Health and Human Services. Advisory Committee on Transplantation. www.organdonor.gov/legislation/advisory.htm. Accessed Oct 1, 2013.
31. US Department of Health and Human Services, Centers for Medicare and Medicaid Services. Requirements for approval and re-approval of transplant centers to perform organ transplants; final rule. Fed Regist. 2007;72:15198–280.
32. Valapour M. The live organ donor's consent: is it informed and voluntary? Transplant Rev. 2008:22; 196–9.
33. Valapour M, Kahn JP, Bailey RF, Matas AJ. Assessing elements of informed consent among living donors. Clin Transplant. 2011;25:185–90.

Chapter 15
Management of Conflict Between the Independent Living Donor Advocate and the Transplant Team

Roxanne M. Taylor

The role of the independent living donor advocate (ILDA) was created with the express purpose of providing the potential living donor with a contact person, within the formal transplant structure, who was not interested in the outcome of the potential transplant recipient but interested in the donor and donor's needs. The suggestion of an ILDA was made at the Amsterdam Forum in 2004, although no specific guidelines were provided at that time [1]. Since that time, the United Network for Organ Sharing (UNOS) has defined the ILDA role as one of promoting the best interests of the donor, advocating for the rights of the donor, and assisting the donor in understanding the consent process, the evaluation process, the surgical procedure, medical risks, psychosocial risks, and the need for follow-up care [2]. Again, the exact process of the ILDA functions within the transplant team is not clearly defined.

The role of the ILDA is a unique and unusual one. It is the job of the ILDA to assure that the potential living donor is making a well-informed, autonomous decision. The ILDA is expected to act in an ethical manner in assisting the living donor to make this decision. The ethical principle of non-malfeasance would require that the ILDA (as well as the transplant team) would do no harm to the living donor, either physically or psychosocially. However, because the act of donation can save or significantly enhance the life of another, the beneficence (doing good) of the act is considered by most to be a justification for the donation [3]. One must consider that any donation surgery is putting a healthy individual at risk for surgery and possible long-term health issues of their own for the benefit of someone else. The justification for this must be weighed carefully [4]. There must be respect for the donor and the donor's decision whether to donate. The ILDA must be sure that the donor's rights and values are honored and are never considered above those of the recipient's [3].

The reality is that all health care professionals want to believe that they are being an advocate for their patient. No matter what our role may be in the patient-care team, health care professionals have all been taught that the patient's needs and

---

R. M. Taylor (✉)
Maine Medical Center, 19 West Street, Portland, ME, 04102, USA
e-mail: TAYLORM@mmc.org

J. Steel (ed.), *Living Donor Advocacy,* DOI 10.1007/978-1-4614-9143-9_15,
© Springer Science+Business Media New York 2014

rights come first. However, communication failures between the health care team and the patient have at times caused preventable harm to both patients and caregivers. Many communication failures are the result of a hierarchical health care system, and many patients are unable to express their true feelings and fears to their providers. Improving communication with and within the health care team improves the quality of care and patient safety [5].

Schwartz describes a patient advocate as one who assists the patient through a clinical process by providing clarification, education, and advice. This person can help a patient steer through a complex system because of the patient's lack of understanding or knowledge. The patient advocate should be a member of the care team and be a voice for patients when they are not present. The relationship between the patient and the health care team should be one of care. The concerns and the best interests of the patient are the core of all care decisions. Because of the very nature of the role, the advocate may be adversarial and can promote discord among the care team [6].

Prior to the formation of the ILDA role and the formation of transplant multidisciplinary teams, the physician had the ultimate responsibility of deciding whether a person could be a living donor. The transplant surgeon has a relationship with the donor that must be based in trust that the physician has the health and life of the donor as their sole concern. Delmonico and Surman state that the physician has the responsibility of assessing the donor suitability by assessing their motives for donating, providing the donor with a complete process of informed consent, as well as exercising medical judgment of the risks to the donor [7]. This still holds true, but the current practice is that the overall suitability of the living donor is determined by the transplant team and not by a single practitioner.

No matter the structure of the transplant team, it is still in the educational makeup and nature of physicians to act as their patients' advocate. It is within their ethical practice to care for their patients' individual issues and address the root causes of the problems [8]. Physicians should promote healthy lifestyle decisions with a shared process of well-informed patients by discussing all treatment options and acting in the patient's best interest. Nurses are in a unique position to act as patient advocates because of the amount of time they spend with the patients and their background in patient-centered interdisciplinary care [9].

Both physicians and nurses have been part of the donor's care team for years, but many times, they were also involved with the recipient's care as well. Although they may think they are always acting in the interest of the donor, it is hard not to consider the recipient's often failing health. It would be very easy, but not necessarily intentional, for any member of the transplant team to imply that the recipient's life or well-being could depend on them getting transplanted. In addition, the donor may feel pressured, explicitly or implicitly, by the physicians and nurses in the transplant team and be afraid of speaking up about an issue of concern. It is also possible that the donor may understand the criteria for acceptance as a living donor and could possibly withhold information from the transplant team, either about their health status or about their motivations to donate.

15 Management of Conflict Between the Independent Living Donor Advocate ...

The formation of the ILDA role has allowed the potential living donor a person with whom, it is hoped, they can communicate—someone who, although a part of the transplant team, is never directly involved with the care of the recipient. In order to reduce the chance of error when dealing with living donors, the transplant team must build a culture of safety and quality and be designed so that system processes ensure that all information is communicated clearly and is understood by the donor throughout the donation process [5].

Disagreement among transplant team members can occur when weighing the medical and psychosocial factors that arise as part of the evaluation process. When an ethical dilemma occurs, there may be varying opinions about the course of action to be taken, and these may involve conflicting personal values, morals, beliefs, and medical judgments. If a disagreement does occur, there needs to be an exploration of all relevant information followed by an open discussion in which all team members can be heard and all acceptable options reviewed [10]. The question is always what is the best decision for the living donor.

In a national survey of ILDAs, the majority had reached a consensus in all cases with their transplant team, with some having to collect more information from the potential living donor or to discuss the case with an outside body to reach a final decision. Most ILDAs were part of the multidisciplinary selection committee, but some did not attend or only occasionally attended such meetings. Some were not even aware that this should be part of their role. There was some agreement on the duties of the ILDA role. The education of the ILDAs varied greatly, and the career backgrounds ran from medical professionals to members of hospital ethics committees to the clergy [11]. With little consistency in defining an ILDA, there is little doubt as to why there is confusion and sometimes conflict between the ILDA and the other members of the transplant team.

Possible Conflict Scenarios

A medical and surgical risk for the living donor varies from person to person and depends on their age and previous medical history. Surgical risks exist with any type of surgery and, although the mortality rate is low (0.03 %), deaths have occurred second to pulmonary emboli, infection, and bleeding. Post donation, future medical risks for living donors can be directly related to lifestyle health decisions, such as smoking and obesity, loss of the single remaining kidney from trauma or cancer, hypertension, and diabetes. Women may be at a higher risk of developing diabetes if they experienced gestational diabetes during pregnancy. Donors may have family histories of genetically transmitted kidney diseases that need to be fully explored to determine any degree of future problems [12]. The younger the donor, the more difficult it becomes to be able to fully predict the future health and risk for the donor. Certain minority groups may be at a higher risk for developing hypertension and diabetes [13]. It is the surgeon's and nephrologist's responsibility to assess the potential medical risk for each donor.

The decision could be made by the transplant physicians that a donor should not donate because the future risk to their health is deemed too great. This may be a straightforward decision for the physicians involved but may not be easy for the ILDA. There are many reasons why a donor may feel it is worth the risk to donate, and the ILDA must explore these reasons with the donor. The donor may be a parent, and their child's health will be much more important to them than their own. The recipient may be gravely ill, and the donor may feel it worth the risk of the surgery to save the life of another. In one study, it was determined that as many as 74% of donors were willing to accept a risk of death greater than the current 1 in 3,000; in fact, 29% were willing to take an almost 1/2 risk of their own lives in order to save someone else [14]. There should be written policies and practices that outline the short- and long-term risks for living donors that would allow the transplant team reasons to decline a donor if the medically acceptable criteria are not met and also allow the donors to make a free and informed decision to donate if they are medically suitable [13]. Using the same scenario, the ILDA may have an ethical dilemma in accepting donors that are medically marginal, fearing that the donor is putting himself at greater long-term risk. The donor may be willing to take a higher health risk that the ILDA does not feel is reasonable.

The formal psychosocial evaluation of the potential living donor is completed by a social worker, psychologist, or psychiatrist who is associated with the transplant team. The ILDA becomes part of that evaluation process by the very nature of the relationship of the ILDA and the donor; however, whether the ILDA performs the psychosocial evaluation varies from center to center. The ILDA may be privy to information that is shared by the donor that is not given to the other transplant team members. It is the psychosocial aspect of the donor's evaluation that is most likely to cause the greatest concern to ILDA and will also most likely be the greatest source of conflict within the transplant team.

Depression exists outside of the realm of donation and impacts 6.6% of all Americans within a given 12-month observation window [15]. It has been noted that depression is a risk of donation and affects anywhere from 5 to 23% of living donors within 4 years after donation. The frequency of depression in donors varied and was dependent on many different factors; it was prevalent in women than men, in whites as compared with non-whites, in donors who experienced complications, and in unrelated donors whose recipients suffered graft loss or death [16].

The difficulty of working with living donors is that they are human beings and come to the transplant programs to be evaluated as such. The relationship they have with the recipient varies from biological sibling, parent, child, spouse, close friend, to total strangers. In the study done by Fisher and colleagues, it was found that 71% of living donors believed they had a close relationship with their recipients, 28% thought their relationship was close to somewhat distant, and 11% felt that there was some tension or conflict within the relationship but chose to donate anyway. Some degree of family conflict was reported in 25% of the cases reviewed [17].

One question that is repeatedly asked of potential living donors is why they wish to donate. The motivations of living donors can be complex and varied but the main motivating factors appear to be altruistic, a desire to help another person have a better life. Most donors witness the stress, anxiety, and decreasing health of subjecting someone they care about to the rigors of long-term dialysis [18]. In one study of living liver donors, the donors were found to have high levels of altruistic, caring behaviors. In the group of donors used for the study, 70 % had recently donated blood as compared with 4 % of the general population of the United States and 62 % had already signed organ donor cards as compared with 37 % of adults in the United States [19].

How is the relationship between the donor and the potential recipient explored, and if the conflict is identified, how is this handled? Is there support of the living donor from their family in their decision to donate, and is there physical support available during their recovery immediately post donation? The ILDA should determine the support system available to the donor. One cannot assume that there is adequate support simply because the donor is married. Support from a partner can depend on their behavior, beliefs, values, and their attitude toward the donation [18].

In a study reviewing the motivations of living liver donors, DiMartini and colleagues found that the most concerning potential living donor was one who was ambivalent toward the donation. They worried more about the surgical event, the pain involved, the recovery period, and their short- and long-term health. Unlike most living donors, they had trouble seeing the positive emotional benefits of donating and focused on the negative physical effects of the donation. They were more likely to express negative feelings about the donation and had more issues post surgery. Their recommendation was that the ambivalent donor should be screened very carefully, further education should be offered, and counseling and extra time to think about their decision to donate was suggested [19]. In Rodrigue's measurement of living donor expectations, it is noted that donors who have high expectations of changes within their interpersonal relations, expectations of health consequences, and other life changes were at higher psychosocial risk and may suffer a harder "psychological fall" post donation [20].

Assessing the potential living donor's state of mind, exploring the relationship they have with the recipient, and determining their motivation are all within the role of the ILDA. This can be difficult when there are so few guidelines available. As per the Organ Procurement and Transplantation Network (OPTN) (UNOS) policy for evaluating living donors, the ILDA is to assist the living donor in understanding information about the psychosocial risks of donation, which can, but are not limited to, include the following:

- Assess for psychosocial issues that might complicate the living donor's recovery and identify potential risks of poor psychosocial outcomes.
- Determine that the potential donor understands the short- and long-term medical and psychosocial risks associated with living donation.
- Assess whether the decision to donate is free of inducement, coercion, and any other undue pressure by exploring the reason(s) for volunteering to donate and the nature of the relationship (if any) to the transplant candidate.
- Review the occupation, employment status, health insurance status, living arrangements, and the social support of the potential donor and determine if the potential donor understands the potential financial implications of living donation [2].

A literature review of 35 studies of psychosocial issues in living donors found no consensus in regard to the structure and method of psychosocial evaluations of potential living donors, although this is clearly a regulatory requirement [18]. The ILDA must be knowledgeable about the risks and benefits associated with all phases of the donation process [2], but there is no consistency in who performs this duty, what their professional or educational background is, nor is there a standardized assessment tool for them to accomplish this task.

The ILDA must explore all these potential psychosocial aspects as part of the donor's evaluation and make a recommendation to the transplant team of their suitability for donation. Living donors who have an unstable mental illness would not be a suitable candidate for donation, however if the donor is currently stable with medication treatment, seeing a counselor or psychiatrist should be considered for a second opinion. The ILDA could certainly have a differing opinion of the suitability of a donor with a history of depression than the rest of the transplant team. On the one hand, the ILDA may feel that a history of depression is too great for a living donor and may fear that the depression could worsen post donation. The ILDA may also feel that the risk of depression may worsen if the donor is not allowed to donate and the recipient's health declines. Lack of social support, family relationships, and conflicts with the potential recipient are all areas of concern that the ILDA may feel strongly about and cause them to hesitate in their decision to recommend a donor for donation to the transplant team.

As a part of assessing the potential living donor's understanding of the medical and psychosocial risks, the ILDA should evaluate the donor's ability to give informed consent for the donation. Most people do not have the medical knowledge or background to truly comprehend the full risks of any surgery, never mind one with the long-term implications of living donor nephrectomy. The general public must therefore put their trust into the competency and integrity of their health care providers. Informed consent is based in the ethical care of the patient and their right of autonomous decision making. Informed decision making requires that the patient receive knowledge of the intervention, the ability to process the information, and freedom to make a personal decision [21]. In addition, the informed consent and written educational materials must be in the language appropriate for the reading level of the donor so they have a full understanding of the risks involved and are prepared for the donation process [5].

It is the right of every living donor to be fully informed of all aspects and risks of living donation. As per OPTN Policy 12.2 and 12.2.1, the potential living donor must not only give consent to the donor nephrectomy but also give consent to be evaluated [2]. These policies were created to protect the rights of the living donor, and it is the clinical judgment of the ILDA to assess the potential donor's understanding of the procedure and the long-term health implications, and determine if there is any possible constraining or impelling influences on the donor's decision-making ability. The potential living donor is not only in a position to better the life and health of another but also in a vulnerable position as the decision to even allow them to donate is in the hands of the medical transplant team. This vulnerability can be compounded by poverty, a general lack of education, or a history of mental illness [21].

Clearly, it is possible that the ILDA may decide that a living donor either has not been completely well informed about living donation or lacks the capacity to make a well-informed decision about living donation. A donor may fully fulfill the medical evaluation criteria for donation but not meet the qualifications in an ILDA's judgment. This is a situation that may be resolvable with further donor education or may be an ongoing point of disagreement within the transplant team.

Not only the informed consent of the donor must be taken into consideration but also that which may cause conflict within the transplant team. It is possible that certain living donor behaviors or history may cause concern for the recipient and may place the living donor in a high-risk category. The living donor has the right to his or her privacy and the knowledge of high-risk behaviors may have the potential for adverse effects in personal relationships, employment status, and insurance coverage. The recipient also has the right to know if they are at risk for contracting HIV, hepatitis B or C, or any other infectious diseases. The disclosure of such behaviors can change the relationship with the recipient and cause the recipient not to accept the organ for transplant. Potential living donors must fully understand the implications of disclosing such personal information, and the ILDA must remain vigilant of the pressure not to reveal such information to the transplant team [22].

Conclusion

On the basis of an informal poll of other transplant programs as to their policy regarding disagreements between the ILDA and the rest of the transplant team, most programs had policies in place that gave the ILDA an option of seeking other counsel if an issue with a potential living donor did arise. The most common avenue was a second opinion from the hospital's ethics department, patient relations, physician-in-chief, or some other hospital administration department. Most noted that they had never had to do this. Issues were discussed at the donor selection committee and a mutually agreed upon conclusion was reached. Frequently, problems could be resolved by addressing more education with the donor or referring the donor for another opinion, such as a psychiatrist. Most programs also stated that the ILDA had the power to veto a donation, although again, they never had to wield this power in the face of team opposition.

The idea of having some type of grievance policy is also being addressed by UNOS. In the current proposal for policy changes, the proposed policy governing the ILDA must include a way to deal with any grievance the ILDA may have with regard to disagreements with the transplant team. The proposed policy states that the transplant program will provide for the ILDA to file a grievance when necessary to protect the rights or best interests of the living donor and to address any grievance raised by the ILDA concerning the rights and best interests of the donor [23].

The role of the ILDA has become more complex since its inception many years ago. Although the exact function and duties have been slow to be defined, this appears to be changing with each new UNOS policy and bylaw update. As the demands of the job become clearer, the professional background of the ILDA will need to become better defined as well. Currently, the role can be filled by almost anyone.

There are many reasons why the ILDA may have reservations about the suitability of a potential donor while the remainder of the team finds that donor acceptable, and there may be reasons why the transplant team may have issues with the suitability of the donor when the ILDA may not. We have the unique privilege of working with people who are literally willing to give of themselves and put their lives and health in the hands of the transplant team. This situation puts the responsibility of the donors' care in our hands, as we continue to improve access to transplantation for the recipients and we increase our knowledge of the risks and benefits of living donation [13].

The key to dealing with conflicts between the ILDA and the transplant team is that the ILDA must be a part of the team, with equal voting power in determining the suitability of all potential living donors. The members of a well-functioning team need to understand the role and responsibilities of each team member and respect each team member's judgment. An effective team discusses, evaluates, and seeks to make improvements in their process and thereby increases patient safety. The members of the team must feel free to speak up for living donors and themselves, and there must be true collaboration and respect [5].

References

1. The Ethics Committee of the Transplantation Society. The consensus statement of the Amsterdam Forum on the care of the live kidney donor. Transplantation. 2004 Aug;78:491–2.
2. OPTN Policies and By-laws. 14 May 2013. http://optn.transplant.hrsa.gov/PoliciesandBylaws2/policies/pdfs/policy_172.pdf. Accessed February 1, 2013.
3. Bosek M, Sargeant I. Living kidney donor advocacy program. JONAS Healthc Law Ethics Regul. 2012 Jan-Mar;14:19–26.
4. Cronin A. Allowing autonomous agents freedom. J Med Ethics. 2008;34:129–32.
5. Denham C, Dingman J, Foley M, Ford D, Martins B, O'Regan P, et al. Are you listening…. Are you really listening? J Patient Saf. 2008 September;4:148–61.
6. Schwartz L. Is there an advocate in the house? The role of the health care professionals in patient advocacy. J Med Ethics. 2002;28:37–40.
7. Delmonico F, Surman O. Is this live-organ donor your patient? Transplantation. 2003 Oct;76:1257–60.
8. Earnest M, Wong S, Federico S. Perspective: physician advocacy: what is it and how do we do it? Acad Med. 2010 Jan;85:63–7.
9. Breier-Mackie S. Who is the clinical ethicist? Gastroenterol Nurs. 2006 Feb;29:70–2.
10. Phillips S. Ethical decision-making when caring for the noncompliant patient. J Infus Nurs. 2006 Sep/Oct;29:266–71.
11. Steel J, Dunlavy A, Friday M, Kingsley K, Brower D, Unruh M. A national survey of independent living donor advocates: the need for practice guidelines. Am J Transplant. 2012;12:2141–9.

12. Davis C. Evaluation of the living kidney donor: current perspectives. Am J Kidney Dis. 2004 Mar;43:508–30.
13. Levey A, Danovitch G, Hou S. Living donor kidney transplantation in the United States—looking back, looking forward. Am J Kidney Dis. 2011;58(3):343–8.
14. Maple N, Hadjianastassiou V, Jones R, Mamode N. Understanding the risks in living donor nephrectomy. J Med Ethics. 2010;36:142–7.
15. Kessler R, Berglund P, Demler O, Jin R, Koretz D, Merikangas KR, et al. The epidemiology of major depressive disorder: results from the National Co-morbidity Survey Replication (NCS-R). JAMA. 2003;289(23):3095.
16. Lentine K, Schnitzler M, Xiao H, Axelrod D, Davis C, McCabe M, et al. Depression diagnoses after living kidney donation: Linking U.S. Registry data and administrative claims. Transplantation. 2012 Jul;94:77–83.
17. Fisher P, Kropp D, Fleming E. Impact on living donors: quality of life, self-image and family dynamics. Nephrol Nurs J. 2005 Sep/Oct;32:489–500.
18. Sajjad I, Baines L, Salifu M, Jindal R. The dynamics of recipient-donor relationships in living kidney transplantation. Am J Kidney Dis 2007 Nov;50:834–54.
19. DiMartini A, Cruz R, Dew M, Fitzgerald M, Chiappetta L, Myaskovsky L, et al. Motives and decision making of potential living liver donors: comparisons between gender, relationships and ambivalence. Am J Transplant. 2012;12:136–51.
20. Rodrique J, Guenther R, Kaplan B, Mandelbrot D, Pavlakis M, Howard R. Measuring the expectations of kidney donors: initial psychometric properties of the Living Donation Expectancies Questionnaire. Transplantation. 2008;85:1230–4.
21. Grace P, McLaughlin M. When consent isn't informed enough. Am J Nurs. 2005;105:79–84.
22. Gordon EJ, Beauvais N, Theodoropoulos N, Hanneman J, McNatt G, Penrod D, et al. The challenge of informed consent for increased risk living donation and transplantation. Am J Transplant. 2011;11:2569–74.
23. Proposed UNOS Policy and By-Law Changes. http://optn.transplant.hrsa.gov/PublicComment/pubcommentPropSub_320.pdf. Accessed May 17, 2013.

Chapter 16
Story Behind the Story

Barbara L. Rutt

"Who wants to hear a story?" This line spoken by Wilhelm Grimm in the movie *The Wonderful World of the Brothers Grimm* has captured my mind ever since I first heard it. I have always loved stories, and the stories behind the story fascinate me the most. These stories fascinate me because they are about real people telling, reminiscing, and sharing the why of who they are; as the listener, the stories make the connections I think I need as the one making the living donor advocate (LDA) assessment. Enough about me, let us proceed to what is needed for storytelling and how storytelling helps the LDA and the donor in establishing a relationship of trust and how the sacred story of the donor's life shapes his/her understanding, motivation, and decision making.

Stories draw us in, as we tell of things that happen in our lives and help us to make meaning of these episodes in our lives. These stories are rich resources that give insight into how we make decisions. In telling our life stories we become vulnerable. We may reexperience the feelings as we relive the experience through our remembering. We may also open our minds and hearts to reframe or understand more deeply, our beliefs, convictions, and responses to life.

We tend to have an idea of how we want our lives to flow, our life plan. When we tell the stories of our past and our plans, we become known to ourselves. Donors are, in essence, sharing a life plan that has taken a new turn by the decision to donate. In their stories there may be other factors, decisions they have made or life circumstances that are brought to mind that open their eyes to how their stories shape or reshape their lives. When donors tell their story, it is work—soul work. This decision for donation may change the life plan once again, depending on the outcomes of the process and surgery, thereby possibly changing the rest of the donor's story.

Storytelling may happen in groups, such as around the kitchen table or among a group of friends. The telling of one's story also happens one on one, when you share a piece of yourself with someone special or tell something about yourself to your child, physician, employer, etc. Storytelling may be informal or formal. The type of

---

B. L. Rutt (✉)
Lehigh Valley Network, Cedar Crest and I-78, Allentown, PA, 18105–1556, USA
e-mail: Barbara.Rutt@lvhn.org

story and the way it is shared depends on the purpose and the environment. The fact that it happens and that the memories are shared are what is important.

The purpose of the LDA interview has several facets: to be sure the donor is making an informed decision, to understand the motivation for the donation, to recognize the type of support system that may or may not be available, and to discover any aspects of coercion. Storytelling is the work of the soul; therefore, safety is required for the donor to be able to reflect and tell the sacred story of possible lost memories and experiences that may come forth and give meaning to their decision. In order for the donor to be able to share the story of his/her life, a safe environment is created by the LDA by explaining the interview process and encouraging the donor to ask questions of the LDA throughout the interview.

The tool used at Lehigh Valley Health Network begins with some basic information gathering, sharing, and an invitation for the donor to feel free to call anytime throughout his/her testing and discernment course. The LDAs tell the donors that we are available to support the donors and discuss questions they may have, all the way through surgery. Throughout the interview, the LDAs remind the donor to approach them when the donor has questions, concerns, or feels in need of support.

Once a safe environment is established, the donor begins to relax and the progression of integrating lives begins. In hearing the donor's story, the LDAs are adding a story to their own and weaving it into their understanding. As LDAs, we must be sure to ask for clarifications while hearing out the story, for we bring our own life experience, complete with its culture, motifs, codes, and imageries. Hence, we need to listen to the story as a stranger. We listen to the language, as a disinterested party, as someone who is hearing it for the first time without any judgment or bias.

Think back to a time when you heard a story for the first time. Where did it transport you? What were the facial expressions of the teller? What about the body language? Was the storyteller stiff, or was he animated? We need to ask ourselves, "How did all these pieces help our understanding of the story?" So it is as we listen to the donor's story and ask the questions needed to help them tell their story.

The stories of our lives are sacred to us as individuals. The stories tell of our love, our heartaches, the good and bad of our growth and development, and what makes meaning to us.

These stories tell of the relationships we have with ourselves, our family, friends, and enemies. Sometimes, family members and friends who voice their negative opinions for the decision to donate may be viewed as enemies.

As our donors come to us with their stories, they may transport us into their family situations; their tears can sometimes move us to tears, and their laughter can make us giggle. Do not misunderstand: We are not supposed to integrate ourselves into their story and have their emotions become ours. We are to listen to them with emotional understanding and empathy.

As they tell some of their stories, their body language reveals more about them than their words. We see the love, the fear, the compassion, and the energy they have for life in their facial expressions, tears, and body movements.

The first 5–7 years of an individual's life are considered the formative period of development. During this period, the framework for our decision-making as well as our worldview, our emotions, coping skills, and belief systems is formed. However, as discovered in the first altruistic story the LD could only vaguely share her life story prior to the age 19. After the age of 19 she was very detailed in her conversation. There are exceptions, and we must be vigilant with these exceptions, to gain a deeper understanding of our living donors and not set them up for misunderstanding because of our preconceived ideas of the natural framing of life.

The tool used by the LDAs at Lehigh Valley Health Network helps us to begin our conversations and encourages the donor to share the stories regarding different types of relationships. An example of the tool used is given here, along with some explanations. Each section addresses the principles that the LDA has to assess: motivation, finances, support, coercion, appropriate decision-making capability, and appropriate knowledge base.

Lehigh Valley Hospital

Potential Living Organ Donor Interview

Name: Date:

Phone #: *used as an identifier*

DOB: *used as an identifier*

Religion: *assists with answers to section II*

Local community of faith: *assists with section II*

Recipient Name: Relationship to Donor:

Living Donor Advocate:

Have you read the information booklet on living kidney donations?

P23 The page number is a reference to the page that specifically addresses the LDA. Many times the donors will say they have read the book and subsequently have no idea why they are being interviewed by the LDA. This helps the LDA know to ask other questions regarding the donor's knowledge of the material.

Do you understand what you have read?

I. Relationship with Self :

In this section, information is obtained regarding the donor's emotional and psychological aspects of living donation, issues of pressure to donate, medical conditions the donor may have had in the past, as well as the donor's understanding of the living donation process. Other areas for consideration are the donor's understanding of how the surgery and post-operative process may interfere with the lifestyle of the donor or future plans both physically and financially.

    A. Donor is able to identify and discuss major life events:

These events can be from childhood through adulthood. The event and description of the event assists in understanding who this person is and how the donor responds to memories of his/her life. Sometimes the donor has a difficult time thinking of an event, or deciding which one to choose, or will only name the event and must be prompted to share more information so the LDA can have an understanding of who this person is.

        1. Family of origin.

Describes the family make-up: birth mother/father; step parents; extended; single. Relationships between these individuals are also discussed.

        What lessons have your mother and father taught you?

Describes relationship to parents and values.

        2. Sibling relationships, then and now:

Frequently relationships as children change as we mature.

        3. Education experience:

Describes the formal education, does not negate life experiences and donor's education through their own readings. They may only have an eighth-grade education, with a college-level understanding through the reading they have done.

        4. Work history

Describes stability, growth, development.

    B. What kinds of things do you enjoy doing for fun? Relaxation?

    C. Have you ever experienced a serious illness? If yes, describe.

    D. Have you ever experienced surgery that required general anesthesia?

E. What would you say is your motivation for this organ donation? *Motivation is sometimes a difficult question for donors to answer other than "I want to help." A follow-up question of "Why?" brings about some discussion and adds the motivation to the story.*

F. How is the candidate helping you with the out of pocket expenses? Are you aware that you cannot receive payment of money or other compensation for being an organ donor?

G. Have you considered the effects of donation upon the following areas of your life: housing, childcare, transportation, follow-up visits, support, extended time off from work, or family planning?

H. On a scale to 1-10, what would describe your level of peace now?
Most donors are about a 7 or an 8 for the level of peace. Once in a while a 10 will jump out. Discussion on the level of peace extends the story and deepens the LDA's as well as the donor's understanding of the reasons for donation. This also adds understanding to the motivation of the donor.

(not at peace)   *(very much at peace)*

1   2   3   4   5   6   7   8   9   10

II. Relationship with a Higher Power:

Discussing the Higher Power contributes to the LDA's understanding of the donor's spiritual self. In addition, a deeper understanding of motivation and support systems is clarified. If the individual did not have a religion on the initial intake question, the first four questions are still applicable. Depending on the answers and discussion, the last question may be asked.

Sometimes a person's beliefs/ denomination can influence their decision for or against donation. Sometimes this can be to the point of coercion by the belief system. Prayer and what individuals pray about is personal. However, what a person prays about in general and how they believe their prayers are answered assists the LDA in assessing the donor's spiritual distress level.

A. Do you consider yourself a spiritual person?

B. Do you believe in a Higher Power?

C. In what image would describe this Higher Power?

D. Do you have a personal relationship with this Higher Power?

E. Do you participate in a religious denomination?

F. What do you feel is the greatest teaching of your religious denomination?

G. Do you know what your religious tradition teaches about donating one's organs?

H. How do you think belonging to this religious tradition is influencing your decision to become an organ donor?

I. Do you pray? What kinds of things do you pray about? Do you believe prayers are answered?

III. Relationship with Community:

The relationships in this area assist the LDA in determining emotional/psychological aspects, internal/external pressure to donate, and the type of support, motivation, and financial aspects. The donor will need emotional support prior to and post-surgery. Many times donors do not realize they also need this type of support. The donors are in the mindset of "I am doing a good thing," which they are, so emotional support is not sought after.

A. Do you live alone or with others?

B. From whom do you find your greatest support?

C. Have you discussed this organ donation with anyone? If so, with whom?

D. How do members of your immediate family feel about this organ donation? Have others expressed concern for you?

E. How do you think others (i.e., neighbors, co-workers) feel about this organ donation?

F. Does your current employer know of your decision to be an organ donor? Are they supportive? Do they know of the extended leave?

G. With whom do you share your most intimate fears and concerns?

IV. Relationship with Significant Other(s):

The internal/external pressure to donate, the medical/psychological conditions, the living donor process and perhaps the freedom and confidentiality to decline, financial aspects, as well as other options for the recipient are all discussed in this area of the interview.

A. Describe the most significant relationship in your life.
B. Describe the nature of the current relationship with the transplant patient *(this is not always known)*.

   1. Are there any familial ties to this patient?
   2. How long have you known this patient?
   3. How did you meet?
   4. On a scale from 1-10, how important is this person to you?

      Usually the individual is a 9 or a 10 on the importance scale. Occasionally, I have found a donor to rate spouse a 10, children 9, parents or siblings 8, friends 7 and so forth.

(less important)   *(more important)*

1   2   3   4   5   6   7   8   9   10

C. History of the need for organ donation.

   1. Did this person approach you to be a donor, or did you approach them?
   2. Five years ago, would you have thought that you would be an organ donor?
   3. What are your fears concerning this transplant surgery?
   4. Have you considered the possibility that the organ you are donating may be rejected? How do you feel about that? *Although this question is sometimes difficult for people to answer, it brings about wonderful discussions and opens many doors of understanding. The question helps the LDA as well as the donor understand motivation.*
   5. Do you feel that in any way you are being coerced into being a donor? By the patient? By family? Religious community? By the medical team(s)?

   Usually the donor will tell me they are not being coerced. They have not thought about it and may not realize there are different ways of being coerced. They may not realize that they themselves are so bent on donating they are not seeing the whole picture and hence coercing themselves. Therefore, I ask the following questions:

On a scale from 1-10, how free do you feel you are to be an organ donor?

(not free)   *(totally free)*

1   2   3   4   5   6   7   8   9   10

On a scale from 1-10, how free are you to walk away from this decision?

(not free)   *(totally free)*

1   2   3   4   5   6   7   8   9   10

What would happen to the relationship with the candidate if you were not to donate?

Interviewee's remarks: *The donor is free to add comments of areas we did not cover.*

Areas to Further Explore: *The LDA makes an assessment.*

_____   _____

Living Donor Advocate   Date

Let us take a closer look at the last two questions in the example given. It is easy to say you are free to be an organ donor. On the other hand, many donors have said they cannot walk away. They have given their word, and they would not back out once they have given their word. Is this coercion or commitment?

There are times donors will hear of the need and, emotionally, offer on the spot, or even later, to donate without knowing what is involved. These donors may feel obligated to continue because of their commitment to the candidate and not want to back out once they learn of the process. Throughout the process, donors are given education and an opportunity for counseling and for opting out gracefully or medically.

As we discuss this issue, the stories tumble out about how the freedom to walk away would be there if it were not for the commitment to their word. If there is a part in the process that says the donor cannot go forward, they have the freedom to walk away and not feel they have not tried to help.

The names in the following stories have been changed to protect the identities and also give credence to the personalities.

Story 1: Nonrelated

This is the story of a 41-year-old man. Connor wanted to help his stepdaughter have a better chance at life by receiving a kidney. Connor had read the book and looked online for information regarding the living donor process. He felt he understood what was expected.

Connor worked at Ground Zero post 9/11 to help with the aftermath. He recalled that experience as being filled with fear; he said, "it was something you had to do to understand." A quiet strength exuded from him as he sat in my office that day, in August, and shared his story.

We talked about his family of origin; he is the only male child, with three sisters. He remains close to one of his sisters; the others have moved away. His mother and father taught him right from wrong and to be fair, and his father taught him a strong work ethic. Connor finished high school and had on-the-job training with an electric company, where he has been working for the past several years.

For fun, Connor mows the lawn and plays video games with his son. To relax, he enjoys that backyard with the freshly mown lawn. If it is raining, he uses the Internet to relax. He has never had a major illness, and the only surgeries requiring anesthesia, have been minor.

With his motivation to help his stepdaughter, his wife to help support him through recovery, and a stable home, Connor rates himself a 10 on the peace scale. Moving onto relationships with the Higher Power, Connor considers himself a very spiritual person, which also helps with being at peace.

Connor says, "You cannot describe this Higher Power. It's bigger than the pictures you see in church." Although Connor does not have faith community, he has a prayer life. He and God have ongoing conversations. These conversations are about everyday life, family, problems, and joys.

In addition to God in his life, Connor lives with his wife, stepdaughter, daughter, and son. Although he has all these people around him, his greatest support is himself. He had discussed organ donation with his wife. She was a bit concerned. He also talked about it with his boss, who was supportive knowing about the possibility of extended leave from his job. Connor has not shared this with anyone else and he does not express his fears regarding organ transplant or anything else to anyone other than himself. He is a very self-reliant individual.

His most significant relationships in his life are his relationships with his children. They bring him tremendous joy and pride. He has known his stepdaughter for 17 years and loves her very deeply. On the importance scale, Connor rates the stepdaughter a number 10.

When the need for a kidney for his stepdaughter arose, Connor stepped up and said, "I am going to do this, she needs a kidney. Five years ago, would Connor have donated? He said, "Depending on the recipient, if family, yes." Connor does not have any fears regarding the surgery; however, we had this little question about considering the possibility of rejection. Connor's face became very serious, he was quiet for a moment, then said, "What can you do?" I prompted with "How would you feel?" Again he was quiet, then softly and hesitantly he said, "I'd be disappointed."

Connor was open—he was free to walk away from his decision. His desire was for this stepdaughter to be healthy. He was very willing to give of himself for his stepdaughter. His comment was "I will do my part for her to have a healthy life. It will be up to her to do the right thing to live healthy." Connor does not want to give his kidney to someone who will blow the chance on drugs, drink, and poor living. He wants to give his stepdaughter a chance to make something of her life. If his stepdaughter were to take up alcohol and/or drugs, Connor reflected he would be disappointed.

Analysis

Connor is very willing to give of himself for his stepdaughter. His comment, "I will do my part for her to have a healthy life. It will be up to her to do the right thing to live healthy," shows this willingness to help his stepdaughter achieve a healthy life. In our conversation, Connor also said that he does not want to give his kidney to someone who will blow the chance on drugs, drinking, and poor living. Connor truly wants to give his stepdaughter a chance to make something of her life. Although Connor states he is free to walk away, he holds himself to the decision. He feels he must help his stepdaughter and therefore by holding himself to the decision he is not free to walk away. This is his decision, and he feels he must help his stepdaughter. He will be disappointed and discouraged if the stepdaughter chooses to blow the chance he is giving her, but it is a risk he feels he must take as a father. I approved of Connor to move forward in the process.

Story 2: Sisters

Donna is a 49-year-old woman who was excited that her life was finally getting back on track. She had read the patient information booklet on living donation 3 years ago when she had planned to give her sister, Marie, her kidney. However, Marie got too sick then and the transplant had to be put on hold.

One major defining event in Donna's life was the death of her mother from diabetes and stroke at the age of 59. She does not want to see her sister die young as well.

Getting married was a very "big thing" in Donna's life. Her heartache was that she could not have children of her own. However, to her joy, she was invited to the birth of all of her nieces and nephews. If she was not in the birthing room, she has been involved in their lives. In Donna's words, "I get to spoil them and send them home." Donna looks out for her nieces and nephews and has good relationships with them.

When she and her sister were growing up, their mother was always home and their father was constantly working. Their father was always a loner, and still is; however, if you asked him to do something he was right there. Their mother controlled the house. Their father taught them hard work and that if you take a job, you do it. Their mother did not like to work. She kept the house, though Donna learned the crafts and cooking from her grandmother. Donna was close to her grandmother.

Donna has an older brother who was always doing the "boy things" and two younger sisters with whom she did the "girl stuff." She considers herself the fix-it person as far as relationships go. Marie is the younger sister and had a room to herself. The two older sisters, Donna and Jean, used to say she was spoiled because she had her own room. They socialized with their friends together, without Marie. The siblings are still fairly close, especially the girls.

After high school, Donna worked factory jobs. When she began getting laid off frequently, she went to school, took a medical assistant course and has worked with a cardiology group for 16 years. With her husband now retired, travel is the fun thing in her life. Donna also likes to cook, and crochet or knit cozy items for fun; to relax, she goes to the gym or to the movies.

Donna does not recall having a serious illness and never had a problem with anesthesia during the surgeries for her cleft palate, deviated septum, and kidney stone. Therefore, she does not see a problem with surgery now.

Marie has been sick for a long time; Donna's motivation for donating her kidney is to help Marie get her life back on track, help get her healthy. "No payment is needed or wanted, just seeing my sister healthy" is all she wants. Donna's level of peace is between an 8 and a 9, only due to the fact that the last time they were this close, something went wrong. Donna cannot be at peace until the day of surgery.

On intake, Donna stated she was a member of a congregation. In the relationship with a Higher Power, Donna went further to talk about her relationship with God. She is a spiritual person, believing that God is always there to talk to, anytime and anywhere. Her personal beliefs supersede her religious denomination's 'greatest teaching'. The church Donna belongs to has not influenced her decision. Her conversations with God are in regard to her family's health and safety and about work and relationships. Donna believes her prayers are sometimes answered.

Donna gathers support from her husband, a girlfriend at work, and her personal trainer. In addition to these three individuals, Donna has discussed organ donation with family and a few other friends. At first, her husband was distressed; however, after her husband spoke with Dr. Moritz, he understands the process, is more open to the donating, and is becoming supportive. Others have expressed concern asking how long Donna would be laid up and asked if she would be okay. Donna's employer is also aware of the donation, is supportive and aware of the possibility of extended leave. All in all, Donna's family and friends support her in her decision to donate her kidney to Marie.

Donna considers family her most significant relationship. There is a 20-year age difference between Donna and her husband, Tom; he is 20 years her senior, and this sometimes presents a significant barrier in their relationship, especially since his retirement. Tom likes to travel, and Donna prefers to be with family. Marie, Jean, and Donna are very close. And as mentioned earlier, Donna has been present or close by for the birth of her sisters' children and is actively involved in their lives. Donna rates Marie a number 8–9 on the importance scale. When Marie had the need for a kidney, Donna just said "I will do it." Marie never asked. The only fear about the surgery is the recovery time. If the kidney is rejected, Donna will be disappointed, but with the knowledge that she did what she could.

Donna says she is free to go forward and free to walk away. In her words, "Would I walk away? No! Am I free to? Yes! No one but me is keeping me here!. I have made this decision."

Analysis

This is the second time through the process for Donna and Marie. Donna is determined to help Marie get her life back on track and see her through to health. Donna places family on a high level of importance. Donna's only fear is that something will happen to Marie before the surgery can take place. The last time they were ready to go for surgery, Marie became too sick. Donna is ready to move forward in the donation process.

Story 3: Donor Exchange

Eileen, a 40-something business woman, came to the office for an interview. She wanted to donate her kidney to her husband, Skip. We were to find out later that she was not a match for Skip; however, a year later, we would find a match for Skip from Sondra. Eileen's kidney would go to Sondra's mother.

Eileen's Story

As Eileen discussed the major events in her life, I noted the amount of loss she was describing. Her divorce came at the same time as her mother's illness and death from a brain tumor. Her mother died 1 year after her diagnosis and after she had spent 6 months in coma. Her husband decided to divorce her during this time, and Eileen had little family support. Five years later, Eileen's dad died from lung cancer. His death was more sudden, as he was diagnosed was in May and he died 2 months later, in July. Her sister died of colon cancer 5 years ago. Eileen me Skip during her mother's illness, and her separation and divorce. Skip was always kind, listened and was a source of strength and compassion. Overall he was a strong influence and support during her times of distress.

Eileen's family of origin consisted of her mother, father, a sister, and brother. Her parents taught her honesty and responsibility. With only a couple of years between them, Eileen and her siblings had a close relationship. The sisters remained close as adults, the sisters became closer.

After high school and college, Eileen has worked in the banking and mortgage business. For fun, she likes to sail, snow ski, and walk. To relax, just sitting in the sailboat with her husband, Skip, feeling the water beneath her, it totally unwinds every part of her body. Eileen and Skip love to sail together and spend much time on the water.

When asked what her motivation is for organ donation, Eileen responded, "Love for my husband." Then she said, "Selfishly, I don't want him on dialysis, it will change our lifestyle. This is an opportunity to make a difference." If Skip had to go on dialysis, Eileen was afraid they would not be able to go sailing the way they had come to enjoy it.

Family, kids, and in-laws would be coming to help take care of the two of them when the surgery was scheduled. Eileen can work from home, if necessary. Therefore, Eileen was a number 10 on the peace scale, being very much at peace with her decision.

As a spiritual person, Eileen describes her Higher Power as a cloud that holds her up. She believes that the result of a relationship with her Higher Power is being a better person. Eileen does not believe one needs a connection with a church, faith group, or worship community, but a relationship with the God one holds dear. Eileen has a very active prayer life talking with God about friends, her husband, problems she may have, and asking for strength. Eileen believes all her prayers are answered.

Eileen lives with her husband and their cat. Her greatest strength is from her husband, and she shares her fears with him. She discussed organ donation with her children, Skip's folks, and a friend. The children expressed support, yet were nervous. Eileen's son said his biggest fear was that the doctor will come out and say both of them died.

When Eileen told her employer, she found much support. The manager's sister had donated her kidney to her husband. She says it was nice to have this kind of an understanding support.

The relationship with her husband has been the most open and honest relationship Eileen has ever experienced. Skip is the most important person in her life. When Skip's need for a kidney arose, Eileen initiated the conversation with Skip for a kidney transplant.

Eileen fears the needles and the catheter, then the waking up from the anesthesia, saying she is a bit "weak-kneed," but once past those things, Eileen does not seem to fear the surgery. As for the possibility of Skip rejecting her kidney, Eileen would not be happy about it, but knows she is doing all she can do to help him be healthy.

Unfortunately, Eileen was not a match for Skip. However, she was willing to be a donor to someone else who was in the same situation.

A year later, I met with Eileen and Skip as we introduced them to the other family in the donor exchange. Eileen was so grateful that someone was a match for Skip and that she could help someone else who was in the same predicament, of family not matching. It was wonderful to sit with these families as they met with each other, but I am getting ahead of myself.

Analysis

Eileen has suffered much loss in her life. Skip brings her love, support, and joy. His kidney disease is yet another loss, one that she can possibly help fix. Even though she was not a match, if there was a donor who matched, she may be able to donate to someone else in return. Eileen has considered herself free to move forward in the process once a donor exchange is found.

Sondra's Story

Sondra is a 20-year-old young woman who approached kidney donation with a matter-of-fact attitude. She was going to do this for her mother, end of story. She was a bright and energetic, even passionate, girl who needed to prove her love for her mother, and no one was going to stop her.

Sondra works out doing body sculpting and is working toward a muscle modeling career. Her only question in regard to understanding the materials and any questions she might have was how the surgery might affect the possibility of her plans.

As we talked about major events in her life, the day we met marked a very significant point, as she had been offered two full-time positions. She was processing which one would give her better room for growth and stability. Sondra also looked back at her childhood and some significant memories growing up. Two family vacations stand out, one to Puerto Rico and one that took them through 20 states. She recalls that they were great family times with her parents and her brother.

Sondra's family of origin was her father, mother, an aunt, and an older brother. She learned a sense of self, independence, and being strong. She is very close to her brother now, although, during childhood, he would tease her quite a bit.

Sondra started college and then thought about dropping out. When she found out there was a 'no return' policy on the money she had invested, Sondra continued, but changed her major to phlebotomy; she is now a certified phlebotomist. She goes out dancing or to the movies with friends and relaxes by watching TV. Sondra does not remember having a serious illness or surgery.

We then talked about the motivation question. Sondra said her mother has been through a lot of health problems and has the will to live. Sondra wanted to help her as get as healthy a life as possible. As I listened to the answers, they seemed to be covering more territory than Sondra was willing to share. What was she not saying? Now was not the right time to ask for more.

Then we talked about the effects of donation from the different areas of Sondra's life. Her initial response was "I can take care of myself." Remember, Sondra was taught independence and self-reliance. I reframed a bit and had her look at herself as the patient. After that, she was able to share that her dad and best friend had planned to help her and there were also members of her church who were going to make food. On the peace scale, Sondra is an 8. She is just nervous about the day of surgery. "Will I wake up?"

Sondra considers herself somewhat spiritual. She believes there is a God, but has not yet figured out how to have a relationship. Or what a relationship with God should be like. She attends the Methodist church and is confident that the members will help her family. Everyone at the church is supportive of her decision to donate. Sondra also believes in prayer and that her prayers are answered. She mostly prays for others, or when she is upset.

"Dad" is Sondra's biggest support. They have been through a lot together. He supports her 100%. The donor's mother seemed to worry about everything, but "Dad" just says, "We'll see." Sondra's father, one friend, and one aunt are privy to Sondra's fears. She does not share fears with many people.

Aunt Nell always was frank with Sondra. She told Sondra the truth, always opened her eyes to what was happening, and was always there to support her. Sondra's mother needed a kidney, but Sondra was not a match; someone else was, and Sondra was a match for that person's husband. Aunt Nell thought this was a good reason for Sondra to donate her kidney. Her mother is a 10 on the importance scale.

We talked about the possibility of her mother rejecting the kidney that she receives. With this Sondra started to cry and said, "At least the other person might still have their loved one." Sondra continued to cry. It was at this point that Sondra and I were able to make some headway through the strong front she presented.

Throughout the interview Sondra wanted to do the right thing. We began to explore the meaning of the 'right thing' and what it meant for Sondra to be closer to her mother. When Sondra was 11, Aunt Nell told her the truth about her mother's condition. Sondra's mother was seriously ill and close to death and no one wanted to tell Sondra. She could not even go to the hospital to see her mother. They all wanted to protect her. Sondra knew something was terribly wrong with her mother, but no one would answer her questions. No one until Aunt Nell took her aside and told her everything. After that time, Sondra was afraid to be close to her mom for fear of the hurt she would suffer if her mom should die. She shared how much she wants to be close to her mother. Her father has been both a mother and a father, but now she really wants a "mom." Aunt Nell is there, but she is not "Mama."

Analysis

In her vibrant young mind, Sondra shared that by giving a kidney to someone else who has someone to give a kidney to her mother, it is as if she is regaining her mother. It will not bring back her mother's lost eyesight, muscle strength, and other things that have been lost, but it is helping her mother to regain some health. Sondra is a determined young woman. I do not want to stop her process of donation. However, in order for her to go further she must come to terms with her feelings. Sondra was counseled to reestablish her emotional attachment with her mother, healing the longing for a relationship with her mother. Donating a kidney would not heal this longing for a relationship. We discussed ways in which she could develop a closer relationship with her mother.

Caution was recommended in completing this process as the relationship with the mother needed to be on a more secure footing before moving forward. When a donor match is found I would revisit Sondra's emotional attachment to her mother.

Postscript

Several months later when I was asked to introduce the families to each other, it was a beautiful, vibrant Sondra who led her mother into the room. She shared how close they had become over the last few months. Their relationship was on target for the surgery. Sondra's father was also happy they had been building their relationship. The "We'll see" had changed to, "Look at this."

As the families came together and introductions were made, we found that Sondra was donating her kidney to Skip and Skip's wife was donating her kidney to Sondra's mother. Among other information shared, they lived nearby one another, they shopped at the same stores, and they used the same place to have their laboratory results drawn. It was an amazing meeting.

Post transplant, the families stayed in touch. About a year after transplant, Skip was diagnosed with lung cancer and died. Sondra stays in touch with Eileen. Sondra's mother, Maria, is doing well.

Story 4: Altruistic Donor

Abbie is a 29-year-old single woman who has decided to donate her kidney. There is no one particular to whom she wants to donate, thus, it is considered a nondirected donation; she just feels the 'call' to donate her kidney. Abbie decided to live for God and serve people at the age of 19, and this is the next thing for her to do on her list.

Let us rewind a bit in telling Abbie's story. When asked about major events in her life, Abbie spoke of becoming a new person in Christ. She had been searching for something since graduation from high school, but did not know just what it was. When she became a Christian at the age of 19, the old way of living, the life she lived before went away and she started living differently. She called it being reborn. Abbie started becoming observant of the needs of other people.

Thus, when asked about her family of origin, there was not much to say other than that she grew up with her mother, father, and brother. Her mother was a homemaker and father, a computer programmer until just a short time ago. She could not think of anything her parents taught her. Abbie was a good student, and she said that her father said this was because her mother always read to her brother, Mike, and her. Abbie could not think of anything more about her family other than that Mike and she were close.

Abbie started college but dropped out when she became a Christian so she could study the Bible more. This is the subject Abbie would talk about, the Bible, and how God wants her to live and take care of people.

A couple of years ago, Abbie was going to help a friend's father and donate to him, but they were not a match. That is when she got the idea to be an altruistic donor. She does not have plans to marry or have children; she is not the same blood type as Mike or her father, so why not give her kidney to someone who could use it.

Abbie understands the risks of surgery. She has no fears or questions. She was going to donate a couple of years ago, but was in an accident and had to wait to heal. Abbie has people ready and willing to help her post surgery.

When her dad asked her why she would give her kidney to a complete stranger, Abbie answered, "Why not, they have a need and I can fill it."

Abbie believes God is asking her to do this. If it is not the right thing to do, there will be something wrong with her kidney.

Analysis

My initial assessment was that more consideration was needed to explore Abbie's relationship to family, especially her mother. She did not seem to recall major events in her life, nor conceptualize teachings she received from her parents. It was as though the first 19 years of her life did not exist. It was suggested to revisit Abbie's case, which was completed by social work and psychiatry. Abby was able to donate.

Postscript

Recently, I spoke with Abbie. We had a long conversation, followed by several e-mails. She helped me understand her point of view of the first 19 years of her life. To her, they did not exist because she was reborn to a new life in Christ. Abbie takes this literally. She takes the homeless home with her, feeds and clothes the poor, and gives away money to the people on the street asking for help. I just bet that if Abbie had another kidney she would donate again. Abbie donates blood and is on the bone marrow registry. She takes the Biblical command to minister to those less fortunate very seriously. Perhaps I was focused on the first 5–7 years of formation and not on the life formation she was living at present.

Story 5: Altruistic/Turned Down and Reapplied

In June 2012, Janet came to my office for the first time. She wanted to donate her kidney to anyone who needed it. Janet believes in what she calls 'giving back'; therefore, she donates blood as often as she can and is on the bone marrow registry.

When asked to discuss a major event in her life, Janet spoke about always wanting to be a mother. She has birthed seven children; one, in 1997, was stillborn. This death was very traumatic to Janet. Feeling that life inside of you and knowing how vital you are to the survival of that life is a powerful emotion. Janet shared that if she was young enough, she would consider being a surrogate for someone who could not carry a baby.

Presently Janet is in her second marriage. Her husband, Dan, was a contractor until recently when he became ill and had to have his foot amputated. He lost his job, the house went into foreclosure, and they had to move. Since Janet always thought she would be a mother and homemaker, she did not plan on working outside the home. Today, she is working at Amazon and doing surprisingly well. They want her to travel as a representative. All these factors have been an added stress on the family.

Janet's first marriage ended in divorce. They had three children who are now adults and on their own. Her first husband died recently, and she felt that she needed to support her children through the sickness and death of their father.

The story of Janet's family of origin was heart wrenching. Her father left shortly after she was born. The younger siblings have different fathers. Janet's mother beat the children frequently and a children and youth service was called numerous times. She found herself living under a children and youth service often.

As for her parents teaching Janet anything, Janet shared that because of the lifestyle, she has learned how not to be a victim and to live to do what is right for herself.

Should Janet be accepted as a donor, she is working on a plan for someone to take care of her, her husband, Dan, and the two children, aged 10 and 11, who are still at home. She has not strategized further than that at this point. I encouraged Janet to think what would happen if she is out of work for an extended period of time, since she is now the breadwinner for her family.

Janet turns to her Catholic faith in times of crisis. She is a member of a parish, gains support from the parish members, and sees them as extended family. She sees God as a guiding and caring being to whom she goes whenever she has a problem. Janet prays for the health and happiness of her family and believes these prayers are answered.

Because Janet always wanted to be a mother, it is not surprising to find that she gains her greatest support from her children. They all know about her decision to donate, but only her daughter will talk with her about the donation. Even Janet's husband does not want to discuss the kidney donation with her. The family understands that Janet wants to donate her kidney, but they do not like the idea.

Coworkers and neighbors do not know about this decision at all. Janet does not think of it as something she wants to share at this time. Eventually she will share, just not right now.

When Janet has a fear about something, the ones she turns to are her husband, Dan, and her daughters, in their mid-twenties. She can talk things through with them and they understand how she thinks. As Janet talks her fears through, they usually diminish.

The most significant relationship in Janet's life is her husband, Dan. He brings her joy. They were never separated in 20 years until Janet was asked to go to Tennessee as a representative for her company. This did not sit well with Dan. Janet has been asked to go on two other trips, one to Japan. Dan did not want Janet to go on these trips. Janet shared that since the amputation and trauma of losing his job, Dan has become more controlling. Now this decision to donate is not "sitting well" with him. Janet indicated that once he understands things more, he will go along with her decisions. He just needs time and information to understand.

When asked about any fears for the surgery, Janet was only mildly concerned about the anesthesia. She specified she has a hard time waking up after she has had anesthesia during prior surgeries. Otherwise, Janet had no concerns.

Janet wanted to know if I would be visiting her when she came in. I said I would if she would like me to visit.

Analysis

In our conversation, Janet indicated her husband's lack of support for Janet's desire to donate her kidney. She shared his becoming more controlling since his amputation. She has had opportunities for growth in the company and has had to turn them down due to Dan's not "allowing" her to travel. This is a woman who is driven to accomplish and to do "good" things for others—not for the notoriety, but for her own self-worth. I would suggest further exploration of Janet's need to give of herself and drive for accomplishments. Until this is done, I cannot recommend Janet for donation.

Revisit: April 2013

Janet came to my office a week early, since Dan was a patient in the hospital; he had broken his foot. She wanted to know if I would see her early. Janet had been staying at the hospital with Dan and had taken a break to come down to my office. She had her slippers on and was wearing sweats. She seemed much more relaxed than on her last visit.

I started the session by setting the parameters that we would be working with in this session. We would be discussing the different sections as last time (relationship with self, Higher Power, community, and significant other), but I would be asking different questions. This time the questions would be what has changed over the last 10 months and how has it changed.

A year ago Dan was a relatively recent amputee; now he is in the hospital with a broken foot. How is that impacting your family? Janet shared how she and Dan are more open with one another now, and that is why she is here with him and supporting him, and her daughters are caring for the two youngest sons.

Are you still donating blood and on the bone marrow registry? Janet reiterated that she has been donating blood since she was 18 years old. In fact when her daughter Terri donated her kidney to her husband, Max, Janet saw the blood mobile out front and ran down to donate because it was convenient. She is being consistent with her lifestyle.

I asked for more information about Terri's donation. How did that impact the family? Janet was emphatic with her explanation. This was an amazing turn of events for the family and for Janet.

When Max's kidney disease got to the point where he needed a transplant, Terri said she would donate and she was the match. Terri and Max would talk about what they were going through and invite Janet and Dan to go with them to meet other recipients and donors. Dan learned more about the process and this helped.

Later, Terri and Max had the surgery. Janet and Dan visited with them. Dan saw the incision and saw how Terri was recuperating. One day Terri and Max were visiting Dan and Janet, Dan saw how healthy Max looked—his color was better and his eyes clear. Dan hugged him and told Terri how glad he was that Terri had donated her kidney.

Since then, he has met and talked with the doctor. He has a much better understanding of what to expect and what Janet would be going through. Ten months ago, Dan would not talk about the donation. Now Janet and Dan talk.

Terri supports her mother's decision. The others support her because it is her choice. They are still not happy about it, but it is her choice.

If something were to happen to you when you run out on your extended leave, how would you survive? You are the breadwinner, you still have two young sons, you have a husband who is an amputee and has a broken foot. What is your plan?

Janet continues to depend on the older children to care for the younger ones and Dan. Terri, having been through the surgery, will be there for support. Dan is soon going to be on disability, so there will be some money coming in if she must be out of work longer than anticipated.

Analysis

Dan has moved to a more positive point of view toward donation since his daughter and son-in-law went through the process. The newness of his amputation and job loss has dissipated, and he is able to talk things through again, according to Janet. Janet implicated they have reached another milestone with the open communication, and the donation would not be detrimental to the family at this juncture. Janet joyfully announced, "My doctor has spoken with Dan and I have confidence he has given him the information he needs." If there are further questions from the transplant team of this family's dynamics, I would suggest having Dan come in for a conversation. Enough progress has been made with Janet to continue testing. While testing is being done, I would like to continue to speak with her in regard to her planning. Perhaps we could assist with financial counseling for a just-in-case scenario. I would like for them to be prepared.

Conclusion

Stories draw us in and capture our hearts. For just a few moments in time, the LDA is privileged to share in the sacred story of the donor. In those precious moments, we are blessed with heartache, joy, tears, and laughter. Then, we are asked to make a decision as to whether this person is really making an informed decision, or they just want to do this to help someone.

It is important for the LDA to know the Donor understands the donation procedure and is informed of possible complications, etc. The LDA gleans this information in the interview discussion. The Donor's relational story tells the LDA more about the reasons and their emotional readiness for the donation. You, the reader of these stories, may come up with a different analysis as well, as you may be even more objective than me.

So, who wants to hear a story?

Suggested Readings

1. Boisen AT. The living human document. In: Dykstra RC, editor. Images of pastoral care: classic readings. St. Louis: Chalice Press; 2005.
2. Gaydos HL. Issues and innovations 2 nursing practice. Understanding personal narrative: An approach to practice. J Adv Nursing. 2005;49(3):254–9.
3. Gerkin CV. Reclaiming the living human document. In: Dykstra RC, editor. Images of pastoral care: Classic readings. St. Louis: Chalice Press; 2005.
4. Hoffman PJ. The most altruistic living organ donor: A best friend. JAOA. 2011 Jul;111(7):445–449.
5. Kornfeld MZ (for Blanton-Peale Institute). Cultivating wholeness: A guide to care and counseling in faith communities. New York: Continuum; 2001.
6. O'Connell Killen P, DeBeer J. The art of theological reflection. New York: Crossroad; 2006.
7. Saijad I, Baines LS, Salifu M, Jindal RM. The dynamics of recipient-donor relationships in living kidney transplantation. Am J Kidney Dis. 2007 Nov;50(5):834–54.
8. Tong A, Chapman JR, Wong G, Kanellis J, McCarthy G, Craig JC. The motivations and experiences of living kidney donors: A thematic synthesis. Am J Kidney Dis. 2012;60(1):15–26.
9. Waterman AD, Stanley SL, Covelli T, Hazel E, Hong BA, Brennan DC. Living donation decision making: Recipients' concerns and educational needs. Prog Transplant. 2006 Mar;16(1):17–23.

Chapter 17
Living Donor Experience

Donna M. Kinzler

I have worked as a registered nurse for the past 24 years and as an acute care nurse practitioner for the past 13 years. I have worked primarily in surgical oncology and have cared for patients who were preparing to undergo or had undergone big abdominal surgeries in the hope of curing their cancer. Since I was used to working with surgical patients, in my mind, I approached my kidney donor surgery as a health care provider and not as a patient. Although I was a living related kidney donor for my sister 2 years ago, my living donor experience started many years earlier than my actual donor evaluation or the day of surgery. This chapter is as much about my sister, MC, and her experiences as it is about me, as we went through the experiences leading up to transplantation, together.

My earliest recollection of MC's kidney disease is of when I was in the third grade and she was in the fourth grade, as she is 14 months older than me. I remember her being in the hospital. That is as much as I knew at that time. Her kidney disease remained indolent until she was about 25–26 years old. She would go for her kidney doctor appointments all by herself and come back and report that all was well. She kept her disease to herself and did not want anyone to accompany her to her appointments. I would ask her how her appointments were; one day, instead of her usual response, she told me that someday she may need to have a tube placed in her abdomen. Working in the medical profession, I knew that was not good. I remember asking her questions that she was not able to answer. It was 22 years before her transplant that I had initially thought that someday I may need to be her kidney donor. As the years of her living with her kidney disease progressed and her creatinine increased, her physician visits also increased from yearly, to every 6 months, and then to every 3 months.

I had just started my Doctor of Nursing Practice program and was in class when I received a page from a number that I did not recognize. It was MC's nephrologist's office calling me to say that MC passed out during her iron infusion. This was her

D. M. Kinzler (✉)
DMK Legal Nurse Consultants, LLC, Pittsburgh, PA, USA
e-mail: DMKLNC@comcast.net

P.O. Box 858, Carnegie, PA, 15106, USA

first appointment for an intravenous infusion of iron. I arrived at the clinic and was informed that she had fainted from having the intravenous catheter placed and not from a reaction to the iron infusion. From that day on, she did not have a choice: I appointed myself to be her caregiver and would accompany her to every medical appointment.

I remember the day that MC's nephrologist told her that it was time to start peritoneal dialysis. Attempts to obtain insurance approval for transplantation prior to her starting on peritoneal dialysis were unsuccessful. MC was not approved to undergo kidney transplantation at the hospital where she received her care for the past 20 years, which was also the same institution where I had worked for the past 22 years. Her insurance would cover kidney transplantation in a neighboring state. I immediately went online to find out about the kidney transplant team and look up their statistics related to outcomes and complications. We both worked, thus, frequent travel for surgery and follow up would not be easy. We decided that MC would start peritoneal dialysis. As a health care provider, I was becoming increasingly disappointed with the health care system.

MC underwent her peritoneal dialysis catheter placement in November 2009. We wanted to become more involved with our local chapter of the National Kidney Foundation and had previously signed up to participate in our first Kidney Walk, which was scheduled for 2 days after her procedure. MC was not up to walking, so team members walked in her honor. This was the first team walk for "MC's Team." MC's insurance would be changing at the end of the year, so she would finally be able to undergo transplant evaluation at the health care system where she had been receiving her care. Throughout the next few months, we learned the art of peritoneal dialysis. We became experts at troubleshooting the dialysis machine alarms. She was able to continue to live with her kidney disease without anyone other than our immediate family and friends knowing what she was going through.

MC was supposed to have her kidney transplant evaluation in February 2010. For 1 month, she underwent the required testing. I scheduled all of her tests and would accompany her to the exams. All of the test results were back, but then we waited and waited. The transplant center never received her paperwork. I remember having a great deal of frustration as a health care provider that the health care system does not make things easy for patients. I expected things to run smoothly, and they did not. The one thing I learned is that I had to be my sister's advocate to get her scheduled for her transplant evaluation.

MC was finally scheduled for her transplant evaluation 6 months after she started on peritoneal dialysis. I awaited this day for months. During this evaluation, she never brought up living organ donation. That was okay because as her family caregiver, I had planned ahead. We would start with my mother and me as potential donor candidates. My sister, mother, and I went for the evaluation. We sat through meetings with multiple members of the transplant team. My main focus was the surgical evaluation. The surgeon primarily focused on the immunosuppression regimen after the surgery instead of the surgical procedure itself. I brought up living donor evaluation for our mother and myself and was told that someone would talk to us at the end of the clinic evaluation. My mother and I had our blood drawn for testing at the end of a long day and we left the evaluation feeling that it was uneventful.

A few weeks went by when I finally heard that I was a potential match for my sister and that I would need to undergo additional testing. This testing took a few months to complete. In the meantime, we finally received a letter from the transplant institute 3 months after her initial evaluation stating that my sister was added to the active candidate waiting list for kidney transplant. Months continued to pass, and we were doing well with peritoneal dialysis. Finally, my much anticipated phone call came; I was scheduled for my donor evaluation on September 24, 2010.

As a nurse practitioner working in a surgical practice, I was well accustomed to the new patient consultation and preoperative visit. I did my homework and was aware of the surgical outcomes for living related kidney donors from this center. As a health care provider, my thought was that I wanted a surgeon with excellent technical skills. I received a copy of the living donor consent form and read through it. I was prepared for what I read. I was warned that I would see the surgeon with another patient in the same room to discuss the risks and benefits of the procedure. I thought that this violated my patient confidentiality. Also, I was not sure that I would get the individualized patient care that I provided to my patients. After the consultation, I went to get my required testing. I went to work after the testing was completed and started to dissect the events of the day. I called my mother to let her know about my experience. Later that evening, I called a family friend who was a living kidney donor 2 years prior to my evaluation. I asked him how his overall experience was. He focused on postoperative pain issues. I thought his outlook as a patient was much different than mine as a health care provider, because I was more interested in health outcomes. The next day, I could not wait to obtain my test results. I just happened to pass my surgeon in the hallway and asked him about the specifics of my scan findings.

I met with my living donor advocate on a separate day. I remember thinking ahead of time that the questions would be rigorous. I remember the initial conversation thinking that more difficult questions would be asked but the overall questions were easy to answer. I answered honestly that I was not being compensated to be my sister's kidney donor.

I heard from my transplant coordinator by way of email when I needed to undergo another test. Finally, I heard in late October that I was approved to be my sister's donor. I made a few calls to tell my family members that I was approved. My sister and I decided on a surgery date after the upcoming holidays. I requested that our case be the first case of the day. Working in a surgical practice, I know that delays can happen in the operating room to cause the subsequent scheduled cases to be delayed. I did not want this to occur. We had waited for too long for this day. During this time, I took a new position at a different hospital. I was too nervous about starting a new job to worry about our upcoming surgeries.

We reviewed the surgery date at my sister's next nephrology appointment. We had less than 2 months of peritoneal dialysis to get through. The months leading up to the day of surgery were focused on learning my new job responsibilities.

I discovered on my own that I was able to take up to 6 weeks of donor leave in my new position. I did not have to worry about finances because I would be paid for my time off. I never thought about having a living will completed. One week before the surgery, I corresponded with my lawyer by way of email to let him know what I wanted in my living will. The Friday before the surgery, I told the two physicians who I worked with as well as my immediate supervisor that I would see them in 6 weeks. They were the only three people at my workplace who knew I would be undergoing donor surgery. It was Sunday, the day before surgery, and my sister was admitted to the hospital at ten o'clock in the morning to start the intravenous infusion of the medication to suppress her immune system. I went to the hospital with her in the morning and stayed to hear the conversation that her surgeon had with her. I asked if we were going to be on the same floor after surgery. I was told that recipients and donors with the same last name are usually on different floors after surgery. I asked her surgeon if we could be on the same floor so that I had easier access to check on her after the procedure. After this conversation, I went home. I never had any intense talks with my sister about what we were about to undergo. I am not sure what else I did that evening but I remember that the day did go by very fast. I remember being able to fall asleep easily. This surprised me because I thought I would be nervous. I woke up early so I could be at the hospital at 5 o'clock in the morning. Again, I did not feel nervous. I stopped to see my sister on the inpatient unit for a few minutes before arriving at the surgery unit. I was soon escorted to the operating room holding area where my sister also arrived. We were told that the operating room staff of the donor and recipient work as a team and like to meet both the donor and the recipient before the surgery. My only fear going into surgery was that the surgical staff would get us mixed up since we have the same last name. I remember my sister's nurse anesthetist asking her if she had a stress test done. I told her nurse anesthetist that she had it done months ago and the results were normal and should be in the chart. I instructed him where to call for the results. I was then told that I would be taken back to the operating room. I remember being very nervous about the staff not having this test result. How could the operating room staff take me back to the operating room if they did not know if the recipient was cleared for surgery? I know what can go wrong in hospitals and did not want anything to happen to my sister or me. I remember talking to my nurse anesthetist as she escorted me back to the operating room. This is the last thing that I remember.

I do not remember much of the evening of surgery. I remember waking up early the next day. I felt okay. The first thing I did was to evaluate how much urine I had out through the night. My pain occurred only when I moved, so I frequently relied on pain medication. I asked my nurse about my sister's condition and she told me that she was doing well. The surgeon came in to see me early in the morning and reviewed my laboratory results with me. My laboratory values were good. I got dressed and then walked down the hall to see my sister. I asked her how she was doing but never asked about her laboratory results or vital signs. She had a look of shock on her face and asked if we should have done this.

Two days after surgery, I was ready for discharge. I was concerned about hospital-acquired infection, and I did not want this to happen. I was discharged and out of the hospital by noon. I did not see my surgeon the morning of discharge because he was in surgery, but he stopped in to see my sister later that day. My surgeon called me the next day to see how I was doing. I did get the personalized care that I try to provide to my patients.

My sister came home from the hospital a day later. We convalesced at the same location. She was active and would stay awake while I would be in my room sleeping. I was happy to stay back in my room and alternate between sleeping and watching television. As I slept in, she had to get up early in the morning to be at the hospital to get her immunosuppression level evaluated. Before too long, she was able to go to our local hospital to get her laboratory levels checked. I thought about how complex postoperative medical regimens can be and how my sister and I were able to manage our care with the assistance of a caregiver who is also a nurse.

Recovering from surgery, I was still not active in my role as my sister's health care provider. I went to my postoperative visit one week after the surgery. I remember having to wait for 2 hours to see the surgeon. I could not imagine having my patients wait that long to see me.

As the weeks went on and we recovered from surgery, our caregiver left and we were on our own to take care of ourselves. I was able to take on the easy tasks as my sister's health care provider by monitoring her complex medication regimen. I had to return to work 6 weeks after the surgery. I remember going back to work and trying to pick up from where I had left off with my patients. I could not imagine going back to work before 6 weeks of recovery. I was tired after working all day and would go home and take a nap every evening. As the weeks went by, I was back to the usual business. I fully recovered from the surgical procedure. I felt good. By looking at me, one would not be able to guess that I had undergone donor surgery. I do not feel the need to tell people who I interact with on a daily basis that I am a kidney donor. If the issue would come up, then I would bring it up. I have no profound words to describe our experience. I am back to monitoring MC's health as well as mine.

My overall hope is that we continue to do well and live our lives free of complications from our surgical procedures. I hope that my sister's new kidney lasts her a lifetime. We do not live our lives any differently except for the fact that now my sister has her normal life back. We continue to have an annual celebration on the anniversary of our surgery and do something special with family and friends. I am in my fifth year as the captain for "MC's Team" and our Kidney Walk team continues to grow every year (Fig. 17.1).

My initial goal was to get my sister through peritoneal dialysis. My mission was successful. My primary goal was to get her to and through transplantation. We exceeded that goal. She has also become an advocate for her own health.

Overall, this experience has affected how I practice as a nurse practitioner. I have become a better clinician. I think about how I expected perfection from our health care teams and want to provide that same level of care to my patients. I have become more compassionate with my patients and their family members. The hospital I worked at was known for oncology and transplantation. I worked in oncology, but my personal life leads me into the area of transplantation, where I have learned a

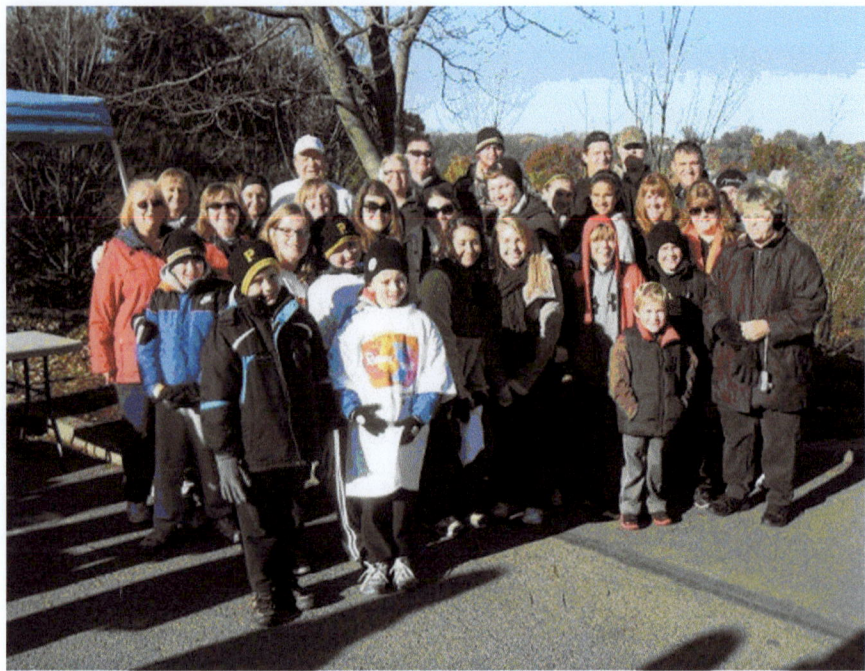

Fig. 17.1 "MC's Team" for the National Kidney Foundation Kidney Walk

lot along the way. Since undergoing my living related kidney donor surgery, I have worked with a patient who was going through her cancer treatment at the same time that her husband was going through a living related liver transplant from her son. I have also cared for patients with chronic kidney disease who are on hemodialysis and are subsequently being treated for their cancer. I became more connected to these patients and wanted to be sure that they were able to take care of themselves as well as their family members. I let these patients know that they need to advocate for themselves and their family members because the health care systems are so complex. I became disenchanted with the health care system from the day my sister had her peritoneal catheter placed and through our recipient and donor evaluation experiences. However, after surgery, I regained respect for the health care system. It got my sister and me through our surgical procedures without incident.

Part III
Living Donor Ethics

Chapter 18
Informed Consent for Living Organ Donation

Frank Chessa

Informed consent plays an indispensable role in health care, ensuring that the choices of patients and research subjects are respected. Informed consent is equally important for living donation, though it has distinctive features in this context. Unlike patients who give consent for treatment that benefits themselves, and unlike research subjects who may be motivated to advance medical knowledge, living donors are motivated by the desire to help another person, typically a family member. Understanding this difference in motivation is important to adapting the standard model of informed consent to living donation.

What is Informed Consent?

Informed consent is the primary mechanism to ensure that a person remains in control of what happens to his or her body. The basic idea is that a person's body is his/her own and he/she should be in control of what happens to it. A person who gives his/her informed consent to a medical treatment is in control because he/she understands the treatment being offered and freely accepts it. A person who gives informed consent to participate in a research trial is in control because he/she understands the purpose of the research and the risks and benefits of participating in it.

Courts and regulatory bodies have developed procedures for obtaining informed consent. Generally, these procedures aim to ensure that choices are made free of coercion, after rational deliberation, and with a good understanding of the consequences of the choice. As the chapter proceeds, I will elaborate on how the concepts of coercion, rational deliberation, and understanding relate to living donation. Now, however, I want to focus on a deeper aspect of choice. This is the idea that our choices are the most authentic when they are consistent with our core values.

F. Chessa (✉)
Department of Clinical Ethics, Maine Medical Center and Tufts University School of Medicine, 22 Bramhall Street, 04102, Portland, ME, USA
e-mail: chessf@mmc.org

If someone holds career advancement to be of the highest value in his/her life, yet consistently makes choices that inhibit career advancement, then there is a cause to worry that this incompatibility will lead to unhappiness and regret sometime down the road. Good decision-making means reflecting on one's core values and day-to-day choices so that they serve each other. Of course, each of us has multiple core values, and negotiating among them is not an easy task. Indeed, refining core values in response to new information and changing desires is a lifelong process. Nonetheless, it is important to be clear about the values that are the center of our lives and to reflect on how our current choices relate to the realization of these values. The process that supports a person providing informed consent—for living donation or anything else—should aim to help the person reflect on the relationship among their current choices, the consequences of these choices, and their core values.

What is Distinctive about Informed Consent for Living Donation?

Consent is an important concept in many aspects of our lives. One provides consent to medical treatment or to being a research subject in a clinical trial. One consents to an employment contract or a mortgage contract to purchase a house. Even in our personal lives, there are laws about consent to physical contact. In each of these cases, the processes that define *valid* consent vary. This is because what is at stake in each decision differs, as do the potential barriers to autonomous decision-making. Therefore, it makes sense to ask what is distinctive about the decision to become a living donor because the informed consent process for living donation should be responsive to the special features of the decision.

Informed consent for living organ donation has many features in common with informed consent for medical treatment, but it is also different. The primary purpose of accepting a medical treatment for oneself is to benefit oneself through the curing of a disease, healing of an injury, or the prevention of future health problems. In contrast, the primary purpose of donating an organ is to benefit another person. Donor nephrectomy carries surgical and long-term medical risks, yet there is no countervailing medical benefit for the donor (even though there are potential non-medical benefits such as a sense of achievement from helping another, enhanced self-esteem, closer emotional ties with family, etc.). For this reason, informed consent for living donation also has some important features in common with consenting to being a subject in a clinical research trial. Generally, one consents to being in a clinical trial in order to advance scientific knowledge, so that in the future others with the disease may benefit from improved treatments. The living donor also seeks to benefit another, but the beneficiary in living donation is generally an identifiable contemporary of the donor; indeed, in most cases it is someone to whom the donor shares a close emotional tie.

18 Informed Consent for Living Organ Donation

In living donation, the donor undergoes some harms and risks in order to benefit another person. This leads some commentators to suggest that proceeding with living donation requires strong ethical reasons that are independent of donor consent. Mark Aulisio et al. put it this way: "Harming an otherwise healthy person in order to benefit another person is *prima facie* wrong, and cannot be justified solely by the consent of the person harmed." [1]

This prohibition on harming a healthy person derives from the "first do no harm" principle in medical ethics. Overriding the prima facie wrong to proceed with living donation presumably requires that there be the potential for a great benefit and strong protections against harms to the donor. However, Aulisio is skeptical that the argument has been made: "Ethically [living donation] requires a high standard to proceed, which has yet to be developed." [1]

From the perspective of the donor, this approach may appear paternalistic. The idea is that living donation may be inappropriate even when it may benefit the recipient and the donor makes a fully informed, autonomous decision to donate—in essence, donation is wrong even if the donor wants to do it. Aulisio's argument goes too far. It is true that consent of the person harmed is not always sufficient to ethically allow harming the person. Nonetheless, there are many circumstances in which we allow the people to accept risks in order to benefit others, and in many of these cases a third party assists people in the activities that put them at risk. Aulisio's argument implies not that living donation is impermissible, but rather that the informed consent process should be exceptionally rigorous because the donor will not directly benefit but will assume some risks [2]. Others have pointed out that living donors do experience a strong psychological benefit from helping others, and thus it is a question of trading off risks and benefits, rather than merely accepting risks [3, 4].

In what ways should it be rigorous? This will depend on what the biggest barriers are to the living donor candidate making a knowledgeable, thoughtful, and voluntary choice. The especially close connection between donor and recipient provides the key, given that it gives rise to the greatest risks to informed and voluntary decisions. There are two ways in which the typically close family relationship between donor and recipient may inhibit free and informed consent. First, there is opportunity for family members (perhaps other than the recipient) to threaten material and emotional hardships on the donor. As an example, consider donation between two siblings, and the potential pressure that the parents could exert on the donor candidate, even as an adult. The implicit or explicit threats may be difficult for the potential donor to resist and difficult for the transplant program to discover. A second concern involves the close emotional connection the donor may feel with the recipient and other family members [5]. Family relationships can be complex and emotionally complicated, and it can take a good deal of introspection to detect one's "true" feelings toward one's family members. This raises the danger of the donor not being completely clear about his or her motivations for donation.

History of Informed Consent

The concern that family relationships form the primary barrier to free and informed consent for living donation stands in contrast to the context in which the rules for informed consent were developed. The primary threat to patient self-determination was not thought to be family members, but the medical profession itself. From its very early history, there has been a tension in the medical profession between telling patients the truth and withholding information in an effort to protect the patient and ensure his cooperation. For example, the advice of the Hippocratic Oath is to "speak to the patient carefully and adroitly, concealing most things." Thomas Percival, an English physician whose book *Medical Ethics* inspired the American Medical Association's (AMA) first code of ethics, wrote in 1803, "To a patient who makes inquiries which, if faithfully answered, might prove fatal to him, it would be a gross and unfeeling wrong to reveal the truth. His right to it is suspended, and even annihilated."

Communicating with patients has been closely tied to getting the patient to follow medical advice. So the early American physician (and signer of the Declaration of Independence) Benjamin Rush said, "Yield to patients in matters of little consequence, but maintain an inflexible authority in matters essential to life." Not everyone agreed with these paternalistic statements. Percival's critic, the Reverend Thomas Gisborne held that "the physician is invariably bound never to represent the uncertainty or danger as less than he actually believes it to be."

Given this history, it is not surprising that the medical profession has been skeptical about patient consent until relatively recently. However, the U.S.'s legal standards have long recognized the patient's right to consent to treatment. In 1914, the New York Court of Appeals ruled in favor of Mary Schloendorff, who consented to examination of a tumor under anesthesia, but not to its removal. Justice Benjamin Cardozo, ruling against the surgeon who removed the tumor, famously wrote, "Every human being of adult years and sound mind has a right to determine what shall be done with his own body; and a surgeon who performs an operation without his patient's consent commits an assault for which he is liable in damages (Schloendorff vs. Society of New York Hospitals 1914)."

This decision has provided the basis for informed consent in the legal cases since that time (though legal scholars debate whether consent should be grounded in rules against assault or in negligence). The term "informed consent" was used for the first time in *Salgo v. Board of Trustees*, Stanford University in 1957. This case turned on the question of which surgical risks should be disclosed to the patient. A central case that clarifies the level of detail a physician must provide about the risks of proposed interventions is *Canterbury v. Spence* 464 F.2d 772 (D.C. Cir. 1972). The decision criticized the view that "usual and customary practice" in the medical community should be used to set the standard for disclosure, instead of opting for a "reasonable person" standard. The reasonable person standard says that the risks of a treatment must be disclosed to a patient if a reasonable person would likely find these risks to be relevant to the decision about whether to undergo the treatment. Here is a central quote from the decision:

From these considerations we derive the breadth of the disclosure of risks legally to be required. The scope of the standard is not subjective as to either the physician or the patient; it remains objective with due regard for the patient's informational needs and with suitable leeway for the physician's situation. In broad outline, we agree that '[a] risk is thus material when a reasonable person, in what the physician knows or should know to be the patient's position, would be likely to attach significance to the risk or cluster of risks in deciding whether or not to forego the proposed therapy.' [6]

Canterbury carves out two exceptions to the risk disclosure requirement: (1) in emergencies and (2) when risk disclosure would harm the patient. Judge Robinson cautions about the overuse of the second exception—one should not withhold information about the risks of a procedure just because it might cause the patient some anxiety.

The current prominence of informed consent has more to do with its use in research, rather than medical treatment. This history can be traced to the trial of Nazi physicians at Nuremberg. A criticism of the physician-researchers—seemingly mild compared to the atrocities they committed—was that they did not give the subjects of their research the opportunity to choose voluntarily whether to be involved. The prosecutors at the trial claimed that voluntarily consent to participation in a research study was an international standard of medical research. Leo Alexander, MD, of Harvard University, authored an initial code for the conduct of research, which was adopted and expanded by the Nuremberg Court. The first principle of the Nuremberg Code laid out the basic of informed consent:

> The voluntary consent of the human subject is absolutely essential. This means that the person involved should have legal capacity to give consent; should be so situated as to be able to exercise free power of choice, without the intervention of any element of force, fraud, deceit, duress, over-reaching, or other ulterior form of constraint or coercion; and should have sufficient knowledge and comprehension of the elements of the subject matter involved as to enable him/her to make an understanding and enlightened decision.

This Nuremberg Code became the basis for the Declaration of Helsinki, the Belmont Report, and eventually the portion of the US Code of Federal Regulations that covers research ethics and set up the Institutional Review Board system of oversight.

It is worth noting that the standard of voluntary consent under conditions of full understanding was often violated in research performed before and even after World War II. The best-known example is the National Health Service study of syphilis in African-American men, which lasted for 5 decades from the 1920s to the 1970s. Poor, rural farmers from Tuskegee, Alabama were misled about the nature of the research study and were prohibited from receiving treatment for syphilis, all in the name of learning about the natural course of the disease. President Clinton offered a formal apology to the survivors of the research in 1997. Other examples in the U.S. of the violation of informed consent standards, include the Willowbrook Hepatitis research, radiation experiments on US servicemen, and widespread compulsory sterilization of women and men that occurred in many states between 1920 and 1970. One important lesson that should be drawn from these examples is that current regulations requiring informed consent—which have been criticized as bureaucratic and a barrier to provide beneficial services—are born from a less than honorable history in which basic human rights were violated by people in the health care professions in the U.S..

Elements of Informed Consent

It is useful to divide informed consent into five elements:
1. Decision-making capacity
2. Voluntariness
3. Disclosure
4. Understanding
5. Consent

Each element is necessary for informed consent, and if each element is satisfied, this is sufficient to show that informed consent has been obtained [7]. The elements are summarized below. The elements of informed consent can be a useful "checklist" to determine if informed consent has been obtained, though it should be remembered that informed consent is a process that happens over time and which may include multiple conversations and, potentially, the donor candidate forming different preferences at different times. Thus, a checklist approach should be integrated into the flow of the process.

Decision-Making Capacity

To be eligible to give informed consent, a person must have a decision-making capacity. Generally speaking, persons are assumed to have the mental capacity to consent to medical care or research unless they demonstrate characteristics that bring their capacity for decision-making into question. When it is unclear whether someone has the capacity to understand information and make a reasoned choice based on their values, a physician (typically a psychiatrist) can formally evaluate a person for decision-making capacity. A determination that a person lacks decision-making capacity is a clinical judgment, and thus is made by a health care provider such as a physician. (By way of contrast, a determination that a person is not *competent* is a legal determination made by a judge.) The most common criteria used to determine whether someone has capacity were set out by Applebaum and Grisso [8, 9]. As per the Applebaum–Grisso criteria, a person has a decision-making capacity if and only if they (1) can communicate a stable decision, (2) have the ability to understand information relevant to the decision, (3) can rationally manipulate this information, and (4) can appreciate that the information applies to oneself (e.g., does not have fixed delusions or magical thinking).

State laws vary on the specifics related to determinations of capacity and competency. For living donor informed consent, it is not necessary to have a court determine competency. Indeed, a formal medical evaluation for capacity should occur only if questions arise during the routine donor evaluation. (However, psychiatric expertise may be useful in the donor evaluation in other ways.)

Voluntariness

Consent is valid only if it is given voluntarily. A choice that is coerced through the threat of force or punishment is not voluntary. A physician who angrily threatens to abandon his/her patient unless the patient accepts the treatment recommended is acting coercively. Likewise, a grandparent is acting coercively if he/she threatens to disinherit a grandson unless he "steps up to the plate" to donate a kidney to an uncle. The grandparent may be within his/her rights to disinherit his grandson. Even so, the threat itself is coercive and it calls into question whether the grandson can give a valid informed consent. Sometimes, a promise of reward is thought to be coercive. For example, offering to pay US$ 50,000 to a mother whose children do not have enough to eat may be coercive if the mother cannot resist saying "yes" because of this reward. Concern about the coercive nature of payment is, in part, what is behind federal laws prohibiting compensation for organ donation.

Coercion by family members was one of the central reasons that the Center for Medicare and Medicaid Services (CMS) set up the rules for independent living donor advocates (ILDAs). Asking potential donors about why they are motivated to donate helps to rule out coercion: A person who speaks lovingly about wanting to help a friend or relative is probably not being pressured into the decision by a forceful relative.

Disclosure

A person makes an "informed" choice only if they have the information they need to make the choice. For treatment decisions, the information needed includes diagnosis, prognosis, the treatment options available (including the option of doing nothing), and the risks, benefits and burdens of each option. For research studies in which the subject does not expect to benefit, the information needed includes a description of the research and its potential to advance knowledge, what is expected of subjects who participate, and the risks of participating. Because living donors do not benefit medically from the removal of their kidneys, the information they require is similar to that of research subjects. They need information on the nature of donation and how it is expected to benefit the recipient, what is expected of them if they donate, and most importantly about the short- and long-term risks of donation.

A somewhat unique aspect of disclosure of information for living donation is that it might reasonably be argued that an informed decision requires having personal health information about the recipient. At a minimum, of course, the donor will now know that the recipient has (or is close to having) end stage renal disease (ESRD). However, a donor may want to know more. The donor may go through this thought process: *Donation is a sacrifice for me, but I am willing to do it if it will significantly benefit the recipient. I have been told in general terms that kidney transplant usually helps people with ESRD (by decreasing morbidity, mortality, and the discomfort and inconvenience associated with dialysis). But I want more detail, for example, what is the improvement in 10-year survival for people who have my recipient's health condition.* Typically, this sort of information would be provided directly by the recipient, but some recipients may not have a good understanding of this information and some recipients may be reluctant to talk about such personal issues with donor candidates. In the absence of the detailed information that they desire to make a decision, a donor candidate may simply decline to go forward. Alternatively, the recipient may allow her physician to disclose this information to the donor (sometimes in a meeting attended jointly by donor and recipient). Either approach is permissible. What is important to remember in this situation is (1) the recipients have the right to have their detailed personal health information kept private from the donor candidate if they so choose and (2) the donor candidates can decide that in the absence of detailed information they are not comfortable in going forward. I would caution ILDAs against making negative judgments about donors who want detailed information about benefits to the recipient as a precondition for donation. For some donor candidates, quantifying the likely significant benefit to the recipient is an important factor in making the donation decision.

Understanding

Presenting information to someone does little good unless the person understands the information. After all, the purpose of presenting information is so that patients and research subjects can make a reasoned choice about whether consenting to an activity is consistent with their core values. If understanding is not present, the consent is not valid. Persons in charge of obtaining informed consent must thus evaluate a person's understanding of the information presented. The "tell back" or "teach back" method is an effective and efficient way to evaluate understanding. One simply prompts the patient to explain the information they have heard. Within a few sentences, it is usually easy to evaluate a person's level of understanding of the material. If understanding is lacking, it is important to return to the disclosure process, varying one's approach and technique to successfully communicate the information to the patient.

Consent

All too often, "consenting" a patient means getting a signature on a piece of paper. A signature alone is not adequate to ensure that a person has given informed consent (although legally the signature may play this role). Giving consent means that a person has taken a mental action—they have made a choice to accept a treatment option, to become a research subject, or to donate a kidney. Making the choice—voluntarily, under conditions of full understanding, and for reasons that make sense internally to the person giving consent—should be an active and engaged process. Signing a form may be a necessary part of the process, but it should not be misunderstood to be the entire process.

CMS CoP Regarding Informed Consent for Living Organ Donation

The CMS has requirements for informed consent for living donation in their conditions of participation (CoP) tags X159–X168, with additional requirements for what the living donor advocate must discuss in tag X123 [10]. They allow transplant centers to determine whether the transplant team or the living donor advocate provides the required information and obtains informed consent. However, if the transplant team provides the information and obtains informed consent, it is the responsibility of the living donor advocate to confirm that the donor candidate has received the information, understands it, and has the opportunity to have follow-up questions addressed.

CMS requires that the information disclosed includes "all aspects of, and potential outcomes from, living donation." This broad requirement is further specified in the following list:

1. The fact that communication between the donor and the transplant center will remain confidential;
2. The evaluation process;
3. The surgical procedure, including postoperative treatment;
4. The availability of alternative treatments for the transplant recipient;
5. The potential medical or psychosocial risks to the donor;
6. The national and transplant center-specific outcomes for beneficiaries, and the national and center-specific outcomes for living donors, as data are available;
7. The possibility that future health problems related to the donation may not be covered by the donor's insurance and that the donor's ability to obtain health, disability, or life insurance may be affected;
8. The donor's right to opt out of donation at any time during the donation process; and
9. The fact that if a transplant is not provided in a Medicare-approved transplant center it could affect the transplant recipient's ability to have his or her immunosuppressive drugs paid for under Medicare Part B [10].

In addition, CMS requires the living donor advocate to discuss the following issues (which have been edited) with the donor:

1. Family or external pressures that impact the living donor's decision;
2. Donor's current medical history and his/her suitability as a donor;

3. Possible long-term clinical implications of the organ donation;
4. Living organ donation process;
5. Potential complications and general recovery from the surgery;
6. Financial aspects of living donation;
7. Options for the recipient other than an organ donation from a living donor; and
8. Required areas of informed consent for the living donor [10].

These two lists include much information that is important to the living donor's decision. However, they are quite extensive. The need to cover all of the topics, and the need to document that they have been covered, can lead the ILDA to spend a good deal of time "talking at" the patient or moving through the topics in a checklist fashion. Despite the natural inclination to complete the required elements, one should not forget that the most important aspect of the informed consent process is an open exploration of family relationships, motivations, expectations, hopes, and fears. In whatever manner the required information is communicated and documented, the informed consent process should not short-change real dialogue about the personal and emotional topics central to the donor's decision.

Several excellent models have been published that discuss informed consent in the context of the overall living donor evaluation [11-13]. These are essential resources in developing a specific script and evaluation tool for the quality of informed consent process in living donations.

Special Topics in Obtaining Informed Consent for Living Donation

I will end the chapter by discussing two ethical issues that may come to the foreground during the informed consent process for living donation. The issues are introduced by brief case descriptions.

Autonomy and the Voluntary Acceptance of Risk

Consider a woman who wants to donate a kidney to her 16-year-old son. All aspects of the donor evaluation are routine, except that the MRI shows a kidney stone of about 6 mm. This is just above the limit of what the transplant team typically allows, given that national guidelines suggest that there is a mildly increased risk for the donor in this circumstance. After a lively discussion of the evidence base, the transplant team rejects the woman's candidacy as a living donor. There are no other living donors for the recipient, and because of blood type and sensitivity, his wait for deceased donor kidney will be long. The donor candidate is unhappy with the decision, and she accurately argues that the evidence base is shaky and, indeed, even a pessimistic read of the data shows only a mildly elevated risk. Further, she says she should be free to decide to accept additional risk to greatly benefit her son saying, "it is *my* body and *my* life, after all." Members of the transplant team are sympathetic to the argument, especially because they judge the risk to be only mildly elevated over the baseline risk for other donors.

From the perspective of the living donor advocate, two questions seem fundamental: (1) Does the donor's informed and voluntary acceptance of additional risk tip the scales in favor of transplant in this case? (2) What does it mean to "advocate" for the donor in this case—does it mean supporting the donor's freedom to choose or seeking to override the donor's wishes for the donor's own good?

Fundamental to understanding the case is the basic distinction between the physician's right to offer only those treatments that promote the patient's best interest and the patient's right to refuse any treatments that are offered—in short, both parties to the transaction have veto power. Living donation requires a slight emendation of this distinction. While donor nephrectomy is never in the best medical interest of the donor, physicians have the right to offer donor nephrectomy at their discretion and only when the nephrectomy does not carry significant risk. In response to the first question, I would argue that the donor candidate's self-initiated and well-informed request to proceed with the transplant does provide an additional reason in favor of the transplant. The medical team, in this case, has the discretion to balance the slightly elevated risk against the donor candidate's strong desire to benefit her son. This is not to say, of course, that a donor candidate has a right to donate no matter the level of increased risk. However, it is to say that a strongly motivated donor may request that a transplant team waive some of their more conservative guidelines and ethically respond in the affirmative to this request.

The second question asks how a living donor advocate should respond to this situation. The advocates will likely find themselves caught in tension among several ethical principles. On one hand are the obligations to promote the patient's best interest and protect them from harm (often called the principles of beneficence and nonmaleficence). On the other hand is the obligation to promote the patient's right to self-determination (often called the principle of respect for patient autonomy). Some living donor advocates will have a preexisting predisposition to favor one set of principles over another. For example, those who think that an advocate's job is primarily to protect the donor from harm will not want to follow a patient's lead when they make suboptimal choices (this inclination is sometimes disparagingly called paternalism.) Other advocates may have a strong inclination to fight for the donor's right to choose, even if they personally do not agree with the choice. The point for all living donor advocates to remember is that both beneficence/nonmaleficence and respect for autonomy represent important ethical values. When they come into conflict, it may be necessary to grant temporary priority to one over the other, but this should be done only after all options for resolving the conflict, by honoring both principles, are exhausted. Even when one principle is deemed more important in a particular case, the importance of the "losing" principle cannot be forgotten.

Advocating for the hypothetical donor candidate, in this case, means making sure that the donor's arguments are fully heard by the donor review team and, if necessary, helping the donor request an appeal or file a complaint about the decision. However, it also means compassionately explaining the reasons for the decision to ensure that the donor candidate does fully appreciate the heightened risk. Perhaps it may be appropriate to recommend a "cooling off period" to give any immediate, highly emotional reactions of the donor time to subside. Waiting periods are often appropriate to make sure that the donor's decision is stable—meaning that it does not change due to arbitrary factors. This serves the purpose of informed consent.

Is Altruism the only Acceptable Motivation for Becoming a Living Donor?

Consider the following two cases:

1. A man is being evaluated to be a living donor for his ex-wife. The children from their marriage are still young. The man explains that he is motivated to donate for the good of his children—so that their mother can be involved in raising the children, and that she be as healthy as possible to participate in their lives. However, the man also explains that he has no desire to benefit his ex-wife. In fact, he blames her for breaking up the marriage and harbors very negative feelings toward her. Except for the children, he would be dead set against the donation.
2. A man is being evaluated to be a living donor for his ex-wife. The children from their marriage are still young. The man explains that he is motivated to donate for the good of his children—so that their mother can be involved in raising the children, and that she be as healthy as possible to participate in their lives. He also confides in you that he is still in love with his ex-wife. He muses, "Perhaps when she sees that sacrifice that I am making for her, she will take me back."

These cases illustrate atypical motivations for donation. In case 1, altruism is involved, but it is directed toward the children rather than toward the recipient. In case 2, altruism toward the recipient and toward the children may be involved, but there is also a strong element of self-interest—the donor is hoping to reconcile with his ex-wife. These cases raise two questions. Is the motivation of the donor relevant to the informed consent process? More importantly, do the motivations of the donor candidates in the two cases rule them out as potential donors?

The Applebaum and Grisso criteria for decision-making capacity do not include reference to acceptable or unacceptable motivations. Indeed, none of the criteria for informed consent—capacity, voluntariness, disclosure, understanding, consent—make a reference to acceptable or unacceptable motivations. On the standard criteria for informed consent, motivations are considered relevant to evaluating decision-making capacity only when they include unrealistic goals or are unlikely to be achieved given the choice that the person is making. It is the inconsistency between the goal of action and the likelihood that the goal will be achieved that signals that a person is acting irrationally. The content of the motivation, by itself, is neither rational nor irrational.

Nonetheless, there is a strong presumption in the literature on the evaluation of living donors that altruism is the only acceptable motivation. For example, the consensus statement on the live organ donor states that, "Transplant centers must ensure that the decision to donate is voluntary. Altruism has been the underpinning of live organ donations since its inception." [14]

The statement suggests that altruism is the only acceptable motivation for living donation, and even appears to conflate voluntariness and altruistic motivation. However, that all voluntary actions are motivated by altruism is clearly false. The more recent guidelines for psychosocial evaluation of living kidney donor candidates have a more open approach to donor motivation and informed consent. Dew et al. identify altruistic motivations as "lower risk/protective," and other motivations (such as recognition, or the desire to deepen a personal relationship) as higher risk [12]. Dew holds that certain nonaltruistic motives put donors at a higher risk of poor psychosocial outcomes, but does not suggest that nonaltruistic motivations rule someone out as being able to provide a valid informed consent [12]. Schroder and colleagues take a similar approach [15].

I would argue that it is possible to meet the criteria for informed consent for living donation even when the donor candidate's motivations are not purely altruistic. Further, in the evaluation of whether informed consent is achieved, one should look primarily at whether the donor's goals for donation are achievable and consistent with other goals and plans that the donor has.

This is not to say that all motivations are acceptable. There may be unacceptable motivations to donate—for example, the desire to be paid "under the table" and illegally by the recipient. Having this desire (and a plan to achieve it), does not mark a donor as irrational or unable to give a valid informed consent. However, it does mark the donor as an unacceptable candidate. Another way to say this is simply that there are criteria for an acceptable donor candidate in addition to the informed consent criteria. The informed consent criteria are not all inclusive.

It is beyond the scope of this chapter to delineate acceptable and unacceptable motivations. Because I believe that we are to some extent opaque to ourselves, I think that the concept of a completely pure, altruistic motivation is a fiction. Rather, I think that our actions are motivated by a bundle of reasons, and while there may be strongly altruistic strands in the bundle, it is acceptable to have a variety of other motivations as well. A full exploration of motivations with potential donors is always appropriate. During this exploration, a donor may even come to recognize that they have motivations of which they were previously unaware. Uncovering these motivations can be a real service to donors, and indeed some donors may reconsider donation after this process. This too serves the purpose of informed consent.

References

1. Aulisio MP, DeVita M, Luebke D. Taking values seriously: Ethical challenges in organ donation and transplantation for critical care professionals. Crit Care Med. 2007 Feb 1;35(2):S95–S101.
2. Aulisio MP. Response to spital. Crit Care Med. 2008;36(1):371–372.
3. Spital A. Letter: Ethical challenges to living organ donation. Crit Care Med. 2008;36(1):370–371.

4. Spital A. Donor benefit is the key to justified living organ donation. Camb Q Healthcare Ethics. 2004;13:105–109.
5. Sajjad I, Baines LS, Salifu M, Jindal RM. The dynamics of recipient-donor relationships in living kidney transplantation. Am J Kidney Dis. 2007;50:834–854.
6. Canterbury v. Spence 464 F.2d 772 (D.C. Cir. 1972).
7. Beauchamp TL, Childress JF. Principles of biomedical ethics. 6th Edition. New York: Oxford University Press; 2008.
8. Appelbaum PS, Grisso T. Assessing patients' capacities to consent to treatment. N Engl J Med. 1986;319(25):1635–1638.
9. Appelbaum PS, Grisso T. Assessing competence to consent to treatment. New York: Oxford University Press; 1998.
10. CMS CoP § 482.102, Patient and living donor rights. Downloaded October 3, 2012.
11. LaPointe Rudow D. The living donor advocate: A team approach to educate, evaluate, and manage donors across the continuum. Prog Transplant. 2009;19:64–70.
12. Dew MA, Jacobs CL, Jowsey SG, Hanto R, Miller C, Delmonico FL. Guidelines for the psychosocial evaluation of living unrelated kidney donors in the United States. Am J Transplant. 2007;7:1047–1057.
13. Sites AK, Freeman JR, Harper MR, Waters DB, Pruett TL. A multidisciplinary program to educate and advocate for living donors. Prog Transplant. 2008;18:284–289.
14. Abecassis M, Adams M, Adams P, Arnold RM, Atkins CR, Barr ML, Bennett WM, Bia M, Briscoe DM, Burdick J, et al. Consensus Statement on the Live Organ Donor. The Authors of the Live Organ Donor Consensus Group. JAMA. 2000 Dec 13;284(22):2919–2926.
15. Schroder NM, McDonald LA, Etringer G, Snyders M. Consideration of psychosocial factiors in the evaluation of living donors. Prog Transplant. 2008;18:41–49.

Chapter 19
Pressure and Coercion

Cindy Koslowski Brown

Living organ donation is a unique journey. Each experience is as distinctive as the individual who chooses to undertake it. For some, the journey may seem like a clear and paved road, without interruption or barrier, leading directly toward donation and the chance of extending the length or improving the quality of another person's life. For others, the path may be blocked, halting their progress and truncating their journey. And for yet others, the path toward donation may be ill-defined and wind in such a way as to make the journey unclear and the outcome uncertain.

In describing his/her personal journey, a potential organ donor might share that the initial decision to pursue donation was relatively simple because of his/her understanding that the risks to himself/herself were thought to be low and that the anticipated benefits for the intended recipient were thought to be great, as in the case of living kidney donation [1]. Some living donor candidates might share that they have had long-standing and emotionally close relationships with their intended recipients, and they wish to extend or improve the quality of that person's life. Yet other donor candidates identify their personal beliefs, their spirituality, or their family values as guiding forces in the decision to donate. Over the course of a discussion with the independent living donor team (ILDT), and particularly with the independent living donor advocate (ILDA), a donor candidate may discuss those situations and experiences in his life that serve as influences on his decision and motivation. Some of these influences may be clearly recognizable to the donor candidate and may be part of a solid foundation of appropriate decision making and motivation. Other influences may be more subtle and perhaps even imperceptible to the donor candidate [2]. And there may be yet other influences that exert such force that they are experienced by the donor candidate, or identified by the ILDA, as pressure.

Understanding what is influencing the individual donor candidate and how that donor candidate is impacted by those influences is a necessary component of a living donor's comprehensive evaluation. The ILDT and the ILDA must first appreciate

---

C. K. Brown (✉)
Department of Social Work, University of Michigan Hospital and Health Systems,
L1252 WH, 1500 East Medical Center Drive,
Ann Arbor, MI 48109-5268, USA
e-mail: ckoslows@med.umich.edu; ckoslows@umich.edu

that those influences on a living donor candidate can be direct or implicit. They can appropriately motivate, or they can cause pressure and result in emotional distress. The influences can sometimes be readily identified by the donor candidate, or they may instead be working outside the donor candidate's consciousness [2]. Understanding the complexity of how situations and experiences influence a donor candidate aids the ILDT and the ILDA in fully exploring the donor candidate's unique journey of living donation. It is through this careful and thorough exploration of what the influences mean for the individual donor candidate that the ILDT and the ILDA are then able to work toward the task of promoting the best interests of that donor candidate.

"The LDA must be knowledgeable of living organ donation, transplantation, medical ethics, and informed consent. The LDA is responsible for representing and advising the donor, protecting and promoting the best interests of the donor, and respecting the donor's decision and ensuring that it is informed and free from coercion." [3] Ensuring that a donor candidate's decision to donate "… is free from coercion" as defined by the Centers for Medicare and Medicaid Services (CMS) in its 2007 conditions of participation [3] is accomplished through the careful exploration of the influences impacting their decision to donate. Coercion is defined as "… the use of force or intimidation to obtain compliance" [4] and, most certainly, could be viewed as a form of untoward pressure. Although the definition does not specify, it is important to consider that the "use of force or intimidation" could be direct or implied. A potential donor could have been threatened quite directly by another in order to gain his compliance as might be the case when there is a significant power differential between donor candidate and intended recipient (e.g., employee to boss, child to parent, student to teacher, etc.). Consider, as an example, a young adult donor candidate who has been told by her parents that the financial support of her college education will continue provided she donates a kidney to her mother. The young woman may be considering donation not out of a desire to help her mother, but out of a desire to retain something that has been threatened—in this case, her continued college tuition; or consider an example in which a young man is told by his family that they expect that he will serve as a living donor to his sister and that they would be disappointed in him, if he were to refuse. The young man is left feeling that a decision not to donate would forever change the relationship between him and his family, so he may consider donating in an effort to retain his family's love and affection and not disappoint them.

These examples highlight very obvious instances of pressure and coercion, and in the absence of any other sincere motivation to donate or other relevant factors, the course of action for the ILDT is clear. Because these donor candidates may be considered to be pressured or coerced—being, in some way, threatened in order to gain their compliance to donate—they may not be considered appropriate candidates for living organ donation by some transplant teams, and their evaluation processes should be stopped in the interest of promoting the donor's best interests.

While clinicians should be attuned to the possibility of such flagrant examples of coercion, examples like these are unique in their clarity and simplicity. What is much more likely is that the situations and experiences influencing the donor candidate are more subtle, unspoken even. Consider a slightly different and more likely second scenario in which the same young woman considering donation to her mother is not financially dependent on her family. No such discussion or insinuation of financial support has occurred. The young woman has perhaps learned from her family, or from her mother's medical providers, about the benefits of living donor transplantation over deceased donor transplantation including the anticipated increase in graft function and graft survival [1]. This young woman may be further informed that her mother's renal function has declined to the degree that some type of renal replacement therapy is imminently needed, and if transplantation is not soon performed, she will be required to begin dialysis. Further, consider that serving as a living donor to her mother is highly regarded within her culture and that helping a member of the family is an expectation.

While the first example highlights an example of pressure or coercion, the second highlights more subtle influences at work. The many influences on the young woman in the second example appear strong and may exert such force on her motivation and decision making that they may be perceived as pressure. Janis and Mann discuss the difference between overt and subtle pressure of donors, noting that when the pressure is seen by someone as coming from an external source, he/she is less likely to determine that he/she must decide in favor of that particular choice. Conversely, if the pressure is more subtle or covert, "a person will attribute his choice of a course of action to himself, spontaneously develop fresh arguments in support of it, and act in a way that shows he is deeply committed to it." This is referred to as "bolstering." [5] Considering this, the course of action of not proceeding with donation in the first highly coercive example is likely clear to the donor team and more acceptable to the young woman herself. In the second example, however, fully appreciating the forces at play may be more challenging for both the ILDA and the young woman herself. If the ultimate course of action were to not proceed with donation because it was thought that those forces were creating undue pressure, then the decision may be more distressing to the young woman who has perhaps worked to "bolster" her decision to donate to her mother.

Appreciating that pressure exists in forms other than coercion from the recipient candidate is necessary for members of the team charged with the thorough evaluation of living donor candidates. While the ILDA is responsible for ensuring that the donor candidate is not being coerced, the ILDA must also appreciate the fact that the situations and experiences continually influencing the donor candidate cannot be avoided. It is through the careful exploration of these influences and how they impact the individual donor candidate that the ILDA determines whether or not they are experienced as pressure. The influences themselves will be perceived differently by each donor candidate, if he/she perceives them at all, and they may exist in the context of other very appropriate motivations to donate. Because proceeding with living donation is not without psychosocial risk like mood disturbance, relationship changes, financial strain, and suicides of donors after recipient graft loss [6], it is incumbent upon the ILDT to explore the myriad forces at play, both direct and subtle, and to understand the impact of these forces on the donor candidate's decision.

A number of situations and experiences that may influence a donor candidate will be discussed in the following section. The details have been changed to protect patient confidentiality. In some cases, the influences were ultimately thought to be a part of the donor candidate's appropriate motivation and careful consideration of donation. In others, the influences were experienced as pressure and caused distress for the donor candidate or were perceived that way by the ILDT and the ILDA. This list of situations and experiences is not intended to be exhaustive, and it primarily comes from this ILDA's clinical experience. The vignettes almost exclusively highlight living kidney donor candidates, but the issues discussed remain relevant to other living organ donor candidates as well. In addition, while the following situations have the potential to be of great influence and create pressure on the donor candidate, they do not suggest that a candidate in such a situation still could not be an overall appropriate donor candidate. Again, the exploration of the individual situation is warranted.

Case Example

Emily was a 36-year-old mother of one who presented for evaluation as a potential living kidney donor to her cousin. Over the course of the discussion with the ILDA, she shared that she had previously served as a bone marrow donor to her cousin and that his renal failure had developed following chemotherapy treatments for cancer. Emily talked about her willingness to donate bone marrow to him but acknowledged that living donor nephrectomy was "much more significant" and carried greater risks to her. Over the course of the meeting, she also explained that because of her prior act of bone marrow donation, her cousin and their extended family seemed to "expect" that she would now donate a kidney.

Emily went on to say that her cousin's medical team had additionally explained that she would be the ideal kidney donor to her cousin because her previous donation of bone marrow would have altered his immune system in such a way as to make it more tolerant of a kidney coming from her. The hope was that this could diminish his need for life-sustaining immunosuppressant medications or perhaps eliminate the need entirely. Emily shared that she felt great pressure from numerous sources. Emily discussed that while she cared very much for her cousin and that she wanted him to have an improved quality of life, she was greatly concerned about the impact of kidney donation on her life, her child's life, and her work. She talked about feeling "conflicted" because while she understood that her reservations about kidney donation were valid, she did not perceive that others in the family would find them as a justification for not proceeding with donation. Emily talked about feeling guilty about her reservations about kidney donation, particularly because she felt that she should "finish what she started." Emily noted that she had considered "just donating and getting it over with" but also feared "what she might be asked to give next."

This particular vignette highlights a number of influences that Emily perceived as pressure, and that impacted her consideration of donation. Her history as a previous bone marrow donor developed a foundation on which others viewed her as highly committed to helping improve her cousin's health. In Emily's view, the risks of bone marrow donation were quite acceptable in comparison to the expected benefit for her cousin, and she was quite agreeable to proceeding with this act. Emily perceived the risks of donor nephrectomy to be far greater, however, and for her, they did not sufficiently outweigh the potential benefits for her recipient. Her past act of bone marrow donation created for her family, and in some measure for herself, a sense that kidney donation would be the next logical step in the effort to help her cousin and that not proceeding would be viewed as selfish. Emily also felt that the information presented by her cousin's medical providers, likely intended as a means of helping her to make an informed decision about donation, was in actuality an additional source of pressure for her.

Fortunately, for Emily, she had a high level of insight into how these different forces were impacting her decision making, and she was willing to fully explore and discuss them over the course of several face-to-face meetings and phone discussions. Emily ultimately opted to withdraw from the donor evaluation process with the full support of the ILDA and the ILDT. Helping Emily to withdraw from the donor evaluation process in the least distressing manner possible while preserving her relationship with her family became the central focus, which was achieved ultimately.

Emily's case additionally highlights the incredible complexity of the influences that may be impacting a donor candidate, and while this chapter considers potential influences as distinct and separate issues, rarely are they identified or experienced as such.

Familial Influence

Fully understanding the role that a donor candidate's family and friends play in the donation process is a necessary component of the comprehensive donor evaluation. Understanding how a donor candidate's family and friends will be involved in his/her postoperative care is necessary to ensure that his/her needs will be sufficiently met [7]. A solid support network can also help a donor candidate weather many of the challenges they may face, both physical and emotional, as they proceed toward donation and recover afterward [8].

It is also essential to understand how those emotionally closest to the donor candidate feel about the decision to donate, and along those lines, what influence do they have on the donor's decision making and motivation. In some instances, the support network can itself be a source of pressure for the donor candidate.

Case Example

Danny was a 25-year-old man who presented for evaluation as a potential living kidney donor to his mother. He was the youngest of the four siblings in what was described as a close-knit family. When his mother shared at a family dinner that her diabetes had progressed to near end stage renal disease (ESRD) and that she was facing a need for renal replacement therapy, Danny and his siblings all asked about her treatment options. She discussed those options, including living donor kidney transplantation. Danny's oldest sister began discussion among the siblings about which of them would pursue donation to their mother. She talked about some of the medical issues that arose during her last pregnancy and her belief that this would preclude her from proceeding with donation. Danny's brother shared that he was being considered for a promotion within his company and that this would require more hours at work. He felt that his chance for the promotion would be significantly hindered if he were to take time off from his job to recuperate from surgery. Danny's other sister noted that as a new mom to twins, she did not feel that she could reasonably proceed given her new family responsibilities. Danny shared with the ILDA during his evaluation that his siblings all looked to him and suggested that since he had finished college, had been working for 2 years, and had no children or "other responsibilities," he could serve as a donor to their mother. Danny expressed to this ILDA that while he agreed that under the circumstances, he may indeed be the best candidate to donate, he was quite frustrated by his siblings' brief assessment and their ensuing expectation that he *would* donate. He noted that while he would have gladly offered to donate a kidney to his mother, with whom he had always been close, he felt that donation was expected of him by his siblings because they perceived that he had the fewest barriers to donating.

Danny's case highlights a situation in which the pressure he experienced was created by his perception that his siblings saw kidney donation to their mother as an expectation and that he seemed to be the most ideal candidate because of the life circumstances. Danny felt pressure from his family to proceed with donation, but let us consider situations in which the opposite is the case.

Reverse Influence

There are situations in which those who are emotionally closest to the donor candidate or who are themselves potentially impacted by the decision to donate may create a type of "reverse pressure" in which they actively discourage the donor candidate from proceeding with donation. It is not uncommon for those closest to a donor candidate to express some reservations about living donation, presumably out of concern for the risks to the donor candidate. It may be that those who are close to the donor candidate may ask helpful questions or suggest areas in which the donor candidate may need to gather further information to be well informed and make appropriate plans. There are times, however, when those closest to the donor candidate may have such significant concerns, for any number of real or contrived reasons, that they make clear that they are not in support of the decision. In these situations, the donor candidate is faced with the pressure of making his decision about the donation in the context of clear disagreement from those close to him. The donor candidate is then forced to consider the risk of not proceeding with the donation and potentially feeling guilt, anger, or other emotions versus the risk of a resulting discord in the relationship if he does donate.

Situational Influence

There are occasions in which the situation itself can create pressure for a donor candidate. Consider a situation in which a hereditary kidney disease has impacted all but one sibling in a family of four children who are all of adult age at this time. The healthy sibling presents as a donor candidate for his/her sister. He/she may share that they have been close throughout their lives and that he/she wishes to improve the quality of his/her sister's life by way of living donation. This healthy sibling may also talk with the ILDA and ILDT members about the experience of having watched his/her siblings endure the pain and other challenges of the disease over time. It may be that this experience has created a sense of guilt or perhaps obligation for the donor candidate and these feelings are part of his/her motivation and decision making.

An additional example of the significant influence that can be created because of the situation is also highlighted when there is a risk of imminent death of the recipient. Consider an example in which the family members of a woman noted to be in acute liver failure are offered the option of being evaluated as potential donors. The prospective donors are informed that the likelihood of spontaneous recovery by the woman has become quite unlikely and her chance of survival is low without liver transplantation. Although she is listed for deceased donor liver transplantation, the medical team explains that a compatible and satisfactory organ may not become available during the time that she remains an adequate candidate for the surgery. The family is informed that because of the dire circumstances, the transplant team is willing to consider living liver donation for the recipient.

The family, in this situation, is presented with what may be startling and frightening news of their loved one's prognosis, and in the context of trying to understand and reconcile this information, they are also being informed about an option that may save the life of the recipient. Facing what may be the imminent loss of a loved one can exert tremendous pressure. Though these evaluations may be some of the most complex in terms of the forces at play, they are also the ones in which time may prohibit the full exploration of the impact of these forces.

This example also highlights an additional force that factors into the consideration of living donor candidates. The mere existence of living donation as a treatment option for end-stage organ failure can itself create a sense of pressure. The knowledge that one could improve the length or quality of life of another human being by serving as an organ donor becomes a powerful influence [9]. The donor candidate may also be considering how he/she would feel if he/she opted not to proceed with donation and the outcome for the recipient were ultimately poor. To what degree this knowledge about the availability of living organ donation impacts the motivation and the decision making process may be discerned over the course of discussion between donor candidate and ILDA.

Spiritual and Cultural Influence

Exploration of a donor candidate's culture and spiritual beliefs may additionally uncover influences that might be experienced by the donor candidate as pressure; or, understanding the donor candidate's culture and spiritual beliefs may help the ILDT and ILDA more fully appreciate instances in which they perceive the donor candidate to be pressured. Living donation may be well supported, perhaps even highly encouraged, in a donor candidate's particular culture or within their spiritual views and practices, so understanding what these mean for that individual becomes the focus of the discussion.

Case Example

A 43-year-old Middle Eastern man presented for evaluation as a potential living kidney donor to his brother. From the beginning of the evaluation, he talked about donation as though it was an inevitable event and that he "had to" donate to his older brother. The ILDT understandably had some concerns about his perspective and felt that he might be feeling undue pressure. As the ILDA talked with the gentleman, he shared that within his culture of origin there is a great deal of emphasis placed on caring for and helping those within the family. He shared that it is expected that if one has the means to help a family member in need, that one would do so. Though he described the donation to his brother as an obligation as a member of the family, he also clearly articulated that he did not see this as a burden. Instead, he talked about feeling "honored" to donate to his brother. The donor candidate was ultimately approved by the ILDT to proceed, and after donating, he talked about his great joy in seeing his brother's health improve and much of his energy and vitality restored.

Influence Created by Providers or Process

As the receipt of a kidney from a healthy living kidney donor is widely accepted as the preferred treatment modality for someone suffering from ESRD [10], it should be expected that health care providers would work to promote living kidney donation as a treatment option. This emphasis on living organ donation is a necessary component in the education of a potential recipient and his support network as is the development of a structured evaluation process for both recipient and donor candidates. The manner in which information is presented or evaluations are conducted, however, may inadvertently create pressure for potential living donor candidates.

Case Example

Marisol is a 37-year-old woman who attended her father's kidney recipient evaluation and educational class. She and her two sisters, Rosa and Inez, sat with him throughout the meetings and interviews. They were informed together about the options of deceased and living kidney donor transplantation, the anticipated wait time for a kidney coming from a deceased donor, and the mortality statistics for recipients as they await a kidney from a deceased donor. Marisol and her sisters had always been emotionally close to their father, and they had generally been close to one another as well. Marisol understood the anticipated benefit that her father would derive by having a living donor transplant, and she was quietly considering the information that she had heard throughout the day. She was also considering that she and her husband had been trying to conceive for quite some time, and she was hopeful that she would become pregnant. She had been listening carefully to information presented about living donation, particularly information about the impact of donation on pregnancy. Marisol wanted to give continued thought to living donation and to talk with her husband and her physician before making an offer to donate.

Toward the end of the day, Marisol's sister inquired to the transplant team about how she could begin testing as she wanted to consider donation to her father. A team member provided Rosa with a laboratory requisition and explained that she could have her blood drawn for compatibility testing that afternoon. Rosa accepted the form, and Inez followed suit, also requesting the requisition. Marisol later shared with the ILDA that though she was considering offering to donate, she was not, at that moment, prepared to begin any testing. She stated, however, that because of the emphasis put on living donation throughout the day, and the manner in which the staff person provided the requisitions to immediately begin the testing process, she felt obligated to at least accept the requisition form and have her blood drawn out of concern for what her delay in doing so might mean to her father and her sisters.

Marisol later shared that she appreciated the information about living kidney donation that was presented throughout the day and that she felt it to be necessary, but she also felt that the process created a sense of pressure for her. She noted that because the team offered the opportunity to start testing on that first day with her father and sisters present, she felt that she had to undergo the blood testing. She explained that though she likely would have opted to initiate donor testing, she would have first given the decision additional consideration and preparation.

Marisol and her sisters all underwent testing to determine compatibility on the date of their father's recipient evaluation, and they individually received their results within a week. They discovered that of the three of them, Marisol was the only one who was compatible with their father.

Marisol's example highlights ways in which the process can inadvertently create pressure for potential donor candidates. Although not specifically for Marisol, her case alludes to an additional issue that should be considered within living donation programs, which is that not all people who undergo compatibility testing actually wish to be compatible with the intended recipient. Many well-meaning and concerned people opt to undergo blood tests to determine compatibility expecting that they will *not* be compatible. They may feel that by undergoing the tests they have demonstrated their concern and can then truthfully share their efforts with the intended recipient. Much to some of these people's surprise, however, they are indeed compatible, and before they have an opportunity to further consider the ramifications of this information, they are offered an appointment for their formal donor evaluation.

ILDTs might consider steps to be taken within their processes to minimize these occurrences. Before any testing begins, it may be helpful to include individual counseling sessions for any prospective donor about the possibility that he will be compatible and what the formal evaluation process entails. It may also be worthwhile for donor teams to consider asking that prospective donor candidates request laboratory tests or other initial testing on a day other than the recipient evaluation. Although the staff within living donor programs may be simultaneously working to streamline the evaluation process, the extra time and effort to counsel donor candidates and to minimize the pressure potentially created by the process are likely to be of great benefit in the long term.

Paired Exchange Influence

With the introduction of paired exchange programs in many transplant centers across the country comes the introduction of an additional source of potential pressure for some donor candidates. Paired donation programs may be attractive options to recipients who have a willing potential living donor who is not a "match" either by blood- or tissue-type incompatibilities. Some paired donation programs use sophisticated software programs that attempt to match an incompatible recipient and donor pair with another similar pair [11]. The transplants are then coordinated so that the living donors essentially "exchange" recipients.

Donor candidates considering living donation by way of such programs may experience an additional source of pressure to proceed, particularly once they are "matched" to an actual recipient or have been identified as a donor in a series of transplants. A donor candidate's knowledge that he has been identified as an essential part of a complicated process and that several very real human beings are impacted by his decision to donate can potentially create pressure for him. Understanding that if he exercised his right to withdraw from the donation process at that point, not only would his intended recipient lose an opportunity for transplantation but others would also not receive transplants, is necessary. Careful exploration with the donor candidate about the process as well as thorough discussion about his rights as a donor, including the continued voluntary nature of donation, is critical. The ILDA may also work to empower donor candidates to ask questions and express reservations that might arise regarding options for donation with which they might be presented.

It should be acknowledged that though the examples in the previous vignettes are intended to emphasize a primary influence for a donor candidate, most demonstrate a number of additional and no less significant influences at play—further highlighting the intricate and complex dynamics at work.

Assessment

Having an awareness of the many influences that may be at play is important for the ILDT and the ILDA. It is also paramount that the team working with living donors further appreciate that the mere presence of these influences does not mean that a donor candidate is suffering distress from the influence. Exploration with the individual is necessary to understand his unique perspective.

Though the evaluation process is formal, and the assessment should have structure, some of the most important information to be gleaned about the forces at work may come as a result of more open conversation with the donor candidate. When given an opportunity to speak freely about his particular journey, the donor candidate may offer some initial perspective on his feelings about donation that will then guide the remainder of the discussion. Early open-ended questions prompting the donor candidate to share information about how he came to consider donation may be quite fruitful. And while open questions may require more time on the part of the clinician, they often yield far more information than a questionnaire or a series of structured questions. This ILDA has additionally learned that offering a donor candidate opportunities to talk about himself/herself and his/her thinking about donation in a more open format early in the meeting helps to build a foundation for a solid therapeutic relationship. This approach can help the donor candidate to feel that he/she is a partner in a process, and empowering him/her to speak more freely may also reinforce the message that his/her perspective has great importance and value. Given that the role of the ILDA requires ongoing availability throughout the continuum of care [3], this initial investment of time can help forge a solid working relationship and a development of trust that may allow the ILDA to help the donor candidate explore his assumptions and beliefs.

As the discussion progresses, the ILDA may consider particular questions that may elicit evidence of undue pressure. The particular questions that follow have evolved from this ILDA's experience over time and are not meant to be an exhaustive list. This ILDA has also found that many of the following questions serve multiple purposes in terms of exploring and understanding a donor candidate's unique perspective.

Tell Me About Your Relationship with the Intended Recipient

Provided the donor candidate is considering direct donation to a known recipient or is considering donation on behalf of someone he knows by way of participation in a paired donation program, this request may be a helpful introduction to the discussion. Many donor candidates anticipate that they will be asked about this and are generally willing to provide a thoughtful response. The absence of a response or one that seems superficial might also indicate any number of potential areas of concern and, thus, requires further discussion. Follow-up questions about the duration of the relationship, how conflicts have been managed in the past, and whether or not the donor envisions any change in the relationship with the recipient following the donation, if he were to proceed, may be of clinical benefit. Conversely, the exploration of the anticipated impact on the relationship if the donor candidate were not to proceed may be telling. And though an initial response from the donor candidate might be that the "recipient would be fine with me not donating," this may not truly tell the whole story and may still warrant some continued discussion.

This ILDA has also found that a heartfelt discussion about the relationship between the donor candidate and the intended recipient can elicit emotional reactions from the donor candidate, sometimes to his own surprise. While donor candidates know within themselves the importance and the strength of their relationships with their intended recipients, finding the words to describe this to another person and hearing themselves say these words aloud can be quite powerful. One man in his early 50s who had worked his adult life in an auto assembly plant and had presented as quite stoic to other members of the ILDT began to cry as he described his relationship with his wife who was hoping to have her second renal transplant. In addition to being of clinical benefit, these are also moments in which this ILDA is reminded of the unique honor that it is to be witness to what donor candidates experience throughout this process.

How Did You Learn About the Recipient's Hope to Have a Transplant?

This question strives to uncover the context in which the donor candidate began to more formally consider donation. It may give some indication as to whether someone within the donor candidate's social network conveyed this information directly or if it may have been indirectly shared as might be the case for someone who learned during a church service along with other parishioners or someone else who noted a "status update" on someone's social networking site profile. Asking additional questions about what information was shared with the donor candidate might be productive in appreciating whether or not the donor candidate has a reasonably accurate perception of the situation and that they are not presenting as a donor candidate, based on misinformation.

Consider a case in which a young man was informed at a family reunion that he was "required" by the transplant center to be tested as a living kidney donor candidate to his aunt because renal transplantation was her "only" treatment option for impending renal failure. The young man contacted the transplant center to request evaluation, and when the details of how he presented for donation were revealed, he was informed that living donation is a voluntary procedure, that he could not be compelled to be evaluated as a donor candidate by anyone, and that despite his family's attestation to the contrary, his aunt could begin renal dialysis or wait for a deceased donor transplant as alternate treatments for her renal failure. He later learned from his family that his aunt did not wish to initiate dialysis and was eager to receive a preemptive transplant.

Does the Recipient Know that You Are Considering Donating? If So, How Did He Respond when He Learned?

Many donor candidates directly communicate with the intended recipient, or perhaps with someone close to the recipient, to share their decision to be evaluated; some opt not to do so until they have completed a portion of the evaluation process and have additional information. For those who have informed the intended recipient of their intent to be evaluated, understanding the intended recipient's reaction to this announcement may be clinically useful. Some donor candidates may share that the recipient appeared appreciative and that he perhaps expressed that there would be no negative repercussions if the offer to donate were rescinded. Some donors may talk about the intended recipient expressing relief or pleasure over the offer, and while some donor candidates may find this reaction to be quite expected and to have little influence on their continued consideration of donation, further discussion around whether or not the positive response creates any pressure to "see through" the offer to donate may be of benefit.

One woman shared that after offering to be evaluated as a potential donor to a long-time friend, her friend and his wife extended their effusive appreciation, even sending her flowers. The donor candidate shared that her friend and his wife began relaying her decision to consider donation to other people via their online social networking site, and while the donor candidate was pleased that her friend was so enthusiastic about transplantation, she admitted that his reaction created pressure for her. She stated that she felt committed to donating to her friend, but she recognized that any number of contraindications to donation could arise and preclude her from donating. She expressed concern about how "devastated" he would be if she were unable to donate. The donor candidate ultimately shared her feelings with her long-time friend and his wife, and they were able to navigate the situation in such a way that they all felt comfortable proceeding.

How Have You Been Treated Since Offering to Be Evaluated?

Understanding how people in the donor candidate's social network respond to the decision to consider donation or after the formal donor evaluation has begun can be of clinical benefit in discerning the presence of pressure. Do family members unexpectedly increase their contact with the donor candidate and seem more friendly or affectionate? Or, do they become surprisingly "hands off?" Are they behaving in an uncharacteristic manner toward the donor candidate? The presence of a significant change may be the clinically relevant issue.

One young woman shared that she had been estranged from members of her family for many years, and she had had contentious relationships with those with whom she maintained some contact. She stated that after offering to donate one of her kidneys to her grandmother, however, her family members became unexpectedly supportive of her and began including her in family activities. The young woman commented to this ILDA that their overtures seemed insincere, and she did not anticipate that they would continue to include her in family events or even maintain contact after donation. For many reasons this young woman opted not to proceed and asked to withdraw from the evaluation process during her meeting with the ILDA.

Under other circumstances, a young woman like this might have been very strongly influenced by the unexpected and desired affection being shown to her after offering to donate, and the hope that she might retain this affection might very well have prompted her to donate. If indeed the family had rescinded their affection post donation, it could be reasonably anticipated that the young donor might suffer emotional distress.

The influences at play for the donor candidate often come out over the course of a discussion and not necessarily in response to a particular question. However, it may still be of utility to directly inquire as to whether or not the donor candidate is feeling pressured by anyone or anything. Some donor candidates may answer in the affirmative from the outset, but most others may deny pressure and instead respond in such a way as to give the ILDA and the donor team some preliminary information about what forces are influencing him. Even a very resounding "no" response to the question can be quite telling. Though many donor candidates may be quick to state that they are making the decision to donate of their own free will and are not being "pushed" by anybody to donate, they may still be feeling the effects of the influences around them. As was previously discussed in this chapter, work by Janis and Mann suggests that it may be that subtle pressures are being experienced by the donor candidate. These subtle pressures may be leading the donor candidate to decide to donate and to develop a number of arguments in support of the decision to donate so as to "bolster" his decision [5].

Intervention

The role of the ILDA in the care of living donor candidates serves many purposes as have been defined by CMS. However, the mere presence of an ILDA as part of the care team for all living donors sends an important message that should not be underestimated. Understanding that there is an identified provider, whose only interest is the protection of their rights, reinforces for many donor candidates the importance of what they are considering and can offer significant support and comfort. One woman who presented as a donor candidate to her daughter commented, "Though I feel very comfortable with my decision to donate, I have to admit that it makes me feel even better to know that there is someone looking out for me and who would stand by me if I changed my mind."

Living organ donation is a voluntary procedure [12]. ILDTs discuss this repeatedly with donor candidates, and they can additionally reinforce this information by using language consistent with the message. Talking with donor candidates in hypothetical terms through the donation process and using language such as "If you proceed with donation…" rather than "When you donate…" reinforces that the donor candidate is not expected, by the ILDT, to donate and that they are not on an unstoppable trajectory toward donation. It serves as a reminder that there could be any number of barriers, both within and outside of their control, that may stop the donation process. The difference between "if" and "when" might seem to be a relatively subtle distinction overall, but the language ILDTs use sends very powerful messages.

The work done by the ILDA to build a therapeutic relationship and a foundation of trust can additionally help in the challenging situations in which the ultimate decision is to not proceed with donation. In situations in which the donor candidate makes the choice to not proceed, he may feel more empowered to express this to the ILDA and the ILDT, which can then allow for a more collaborative approach to withdrawing from the process.

In the event where the ultimate recommendation from the ILDA and the ILDT is to exclude a donor candidate from further consideration, out of concern for coercion or untoward pressure, and against the expressed wishes of the donor candidate, then that same therapeutic relationship may still offer some support. Overriding the decision of an otherwise autonomous adult and recommending against living donation may be one of the most challenging aspects of the ILDA's role, particularly when it may seem to some like a subjective assessment of risk. These are cases not to be taken lightly, and for the benefit of both the ILDA and the donor candidate, they require careful consideration and collaboration among the ILDT. The complexity of some situations may additionally benefit from the involvement of an ethics committee, if available, to help navigate the possible concerns. And while the potential risks to a donor candidate of proceeding with donation should be thoughtfully examined, so should the risks of being prohibited from proceeding. Meaning, the ILDA and the ILDT should alternatively consider the anticipated risks to the donor candidate, like emotional distress, if he is refused to make the donation by the ILDT.

In some situations, it may be appropriate to reconsider a donor candidate in the future. Perhaps the influence that was creating pressure was related to the timing or the situation as was the case for a young woman who presented as a donor candidate to her significant other within days of his diagnosis of acute renal failure. The ILDA and ILDT were concerned that the situation and the recipient's circumstances were creating significant pressure and impeding her ability to make a thoughtful decision about the short- and long-term consequences to herself. The ILDA recommended that she be excluded for the time being but noted that she could present for reevaluation after a specified time period, thus, giving her an opportunity to "cool off" and to allow the situation to stabilize so that she could more fully consider her decision. This young woman opted not to contact the living donor program again.

Conclusion

The journey of one who considers living organ donation is unique to the individual. While there may be situations and experiences in common, whether and how those situations and experiences are interpreted by the donor candidate requires careful exploration with the ILDA and the ILDT. Potential donor candidates may be impacted by situational, familial, spiritual, cultural, provider/process, and other influences. Influences impacting the donor candidate cannot be avoided. Such influences may be the basis of very appropriate motivation and decision making, while others may create distress or burden and be considered as "pressure." In some instances, a donor candidate may be coerced into considering donation as he/she may believe that something he/she values is being threatened, either directly or indirectly, and that donation is necessary in order to retain that valued item, tangible or otherwise.

Donor candidates may clearly perceive these influences and be able to articulate how they are impacted by them. Others may not be fully aware of the force that the influences exert, and it is through exploration between donor candidate and the ILDA that the impact is more fully understood and appreciation of the donor candidate's individual journey can be achieved.

References

1. Davis C, Delmonico F. Living-donor kidney transplantation: a review of the current practices for the live donor. J Am Soc Nephrol. 2005;16(7):2098–110.
2. Olbrisch M, Benedict S, Haller D, Levenson J. Psychosocial assessment of living organ donors: clinical and ethical considerations. Prog Transplant. 2001;11(1):40–9.
3. CMS COP 42 CFR Parts 405, 482, 488, and 498. Federal Register. 2007;72(61). http://www.cms.gov/Medicare/Provider-Enrollment-and-Certification/CertificationandComplianc/downloads/transplantfinal.pdf. Accessed March 9 2013.
4. Dictionary.com.http://dictionary.reference.com/browse/coercion?s=t&path=/.AccessedMarch 10 2013.
5. Janis I, Mann L. Decision making: a psychological analysis of conflict, choice, and commitment. New York:Free Press; 1977.
6. Schover L, Streem S, Boparai N, Duriak K, Novick A. The psychosocial impact of donating a kidney: long-term followup from a urology based center. J Urol. 1997;157(5):1596–601.
7. Schroder N, McDonald L, Etringer G, Snyders M. Consideration of psychosocial factors in the evaluation of living donors. Prog Transplant. 2008;18(1):41–9.
8. Dew M, Jacobs C, Jowsey S, Hanto R, Miller C, Delmonico F. Guidelines for the psychosocial evaluation of living unrelated kidney donors in the United States. Am J Transplant. 2007;7:1047–54.

9. Russell S, Jacob R. Living-related organ donation: the donor's dilemma. Patient Educ Couns. 1993;21:89–99.
10. Wolters H, Vowinkel T. Risks in life after living kidney donation. Nephrol Dial Transplant. 2012;0:1–3.
11. Paired Kidney Donation Program. http://www.uofmhealth.org/medical-services/living-and-paired-kidney-donation. Accessed March 9 2013.
12. Living Donation: Information You Need to Know. http://www.unos.org/docs/Living_Donation.pdf. Accessed March 10 2013.

Chapter 20
Financial Considerations

Jami Hanneman

It has been recognized that there is a potential for financial risks for the living donor. The goal of the independent living donor advocacy team (IDAT) is to ensure that the potential donor is aware of the financial risks. If risks are present, they should be reduced or eliminated so that the donor is not placed in a negative financial position. Financial considerations should be addressed with either the living donor social worker, financial specialist, or with the independent living donor advocate (ILDA). Patient-specific financial risks are typically assessed during the psychosocial and/ or ILDA assessment.

Kidney donors receive no medical benefit from their donation, though they assume all the risks of anesthesia and surgery. In certain familial situations, we cannot deny that there may be a tangible or emotional benefit to donation if the recipient is depended upon as the main financial contributor to the family. Circumstance such as paying for college tuition or a wedding may also put internal pressure on the family to pursue living donation.

A donor should not shy away from having a conversation with the recipient regarding any potential financial strains while the donor is recovering. After all, the donor volunteered a heartfelt gift and should not be left in a negative financial situation. Starting this conversation may be difficult as the topic is somewhat uncomfortable. The assigned ILDA or social worker should be consulted if any assistance with this is needed.

Out-of-Pocket Costs

Before starting the kidney donor evaluation, it should be explained as part of informed consent, what the donor is and is not financially responsible for. An estimate cost of any out-of-pocket expenses as well as any financial assistance

J. Hanneman (✉)
Kovler Organ Transplant center, Northwestern Memorial Hospital,
676 N. St. Clair St. Arkes Pavilion No. 1900, Chicago, IL 60611, USA
e-mail: jhannema@nmh.org

resources should be provided upfront. Certain testing such as age-appropriate cancer screening and follow-up on abnormal testing is the responsibility of the donor. If the person is without health insurance or subject to a high-deductible policy, these unexpected tests may be a financial burden.

Transplant center-specific costs should be considered. This could include parking and other driving expenses. Transplant center-specific billing policies that affect donor evaluation costs and postdonation follow-up need to be specified. This is especially true if the donor resides out of state and plans to do testing or follow-up at a lab or clinic closer to their home. Nonlocal donors will also need to figure in the cost associated with airfare, meals, and lodging.

Assessment of Donor Financial Risk

During the psychosocial assessment, the donor's financial situation needs to be evaluated. The clinician will use this information to determine the level of financial risk. The donor and/or the IDAT will need to decide if they are comfortable proceeding with this specific information. Employment status, debt, potential loss of income, Family and Medical Leave Act (FMLA) options, short-term disability benefits, and paid time off/sick leave should be evaluated.

Financial risk can fall onto a spectrum. There may be no financial risk if the donor receives 100% pay while on leave with the FMLA job security option. A moderate risk may occur if only 60% of wages are earned during recovery. The patient will need to decide if bills can be paid while receiving reduced wages. An example of high financial risk would be no FMLA or short-term disability options with no wage reimbursement. Based on how strenuous the job is, the patient may need at least 6 weeks off work. If the patient goes into debt during this time, there is an obvious financial contraindication. At that point, alternative options for the recipient should be exercised.

If the level of financial risk is unknown or difficult to assess, the donor should be encouraged to make a list of expenses to determine how much is owed while out on recovery. The donor may want to budget conservatively and may assume a return to work in a couple of weeks. However, not all donors are suitable to return to work this quickly and may require a longer recovery. Being optimistically cautious, preparing for the worst but expecting the best will reduce the risks of a future crisis.

The Uninsured Donor

Some transplant centers will not accept potential kidney donors who do not have health insurance. Others will, though specific informed consent must be obtained regarding the future health risk of the donor. The donor may wonder why health insurance is needed if their donor evaluation is covered under the recipient's insurance. Kidney donors need to plan for their future health, especially after the 2-year marker when transplant centers are no longer required to provide medical follow-up and the recipient's insurance is no longer financially responsible.

Case Study of an Uninsured Donor[1]

Ms. K is a young, healthy 31-year-old lady who flew in from Oklahoma to be evaluated as a kidney donor for her cousin. Ms. K is in between jobs and currently is without health insurance. She qualified for donor assistance to cover her meals, travel, and lodging. Her cousin has offered to cover her utility bills for 2 months. Ms. K has enough money saved to pay her rent for the next several months. The transplant center that evaluated Ms. K informed her of the risks involved in donating without health insurance. She made an educated and informed choice to proceed with donation.

One week after the donation, Ms. K met with the transplant surgeon who medically cleared her to fly back home to Oklahoma and finish out the rest of her recovery. Two weeks later Ms. K started to experience symptoms of a urinary tract infection. Based on her current symptoms and medical history, it was difficult to ascertain if her symptoms were directly related to her donation. The transplant center asked her to go to her local urgent care clinic as she was not established with a primary care physician. This communication with the donor and the transplant department was done via phone as the patient had already returned home.

As directed, Ms. K presented to urgent care, though was turned away due to the lack of health insurance and inability to pay. At that point, she was directed to the local emergency department. Ms. K expressed much hesitation to go to the emergency department because she was concerned about the billing. The transplant center did their best to medically manage the situation over the phone. However, managing medical care at a distance proved to be a challenge. We were dealing with out-of-state physicians as well as doctor's orders.

Two days later, Ms. K, who at this time had severe pain, went to the emergency department. Her physical symptoms worsened while she delayed treatment. She was diagnosed with a urinary tract infection and needed to undergo further medical testing to ensure her remaining kidney had not been compromised. She also continued to worry about payment for all the medical testing.

Eventually her condition was deemed to be donor-related and was covered by the recipient's health insurance. However, Ms. K's health was in jeopardy while guarantor information and diagnosis was being determined. If she had health insurance, she could have easily been treated immediately at urgent care.

---

[1] All identifying information has been changed to protect patient privacy.

Social Supports

The household annual income should be assessed during the psychosocial assessment. It may be that the donor is unemployed and the spouse is the main financial supporter. The spouse may be required to take an extended time off work to provide assistance and support during the donor's recovery. Financial risk within the family unit can occur, which will directly affect the donor.

Lost Wages

Lost wages are a concern for most potential kidney donors. There are no formal programs to reimburse for lost wages, though they may be legally reimbursed by the transplant recipient. In accordance with NOTA (National Organ Transplantation Act) (As amended by the Charlie W. Norwood Living Organ Donation Act -January 2008), Section 274e. "The term "valuable consideration" does not include lost wages incurred by the donor of a human organ in connection with the donation of the organ." [4] Any reimbursement for lost wages is an agreement through the recipient and the donor and typically does not involve the transplant center. Therefore, the transplant center cannot be held liable for any failure of the recipient to reimburse.

Potential living donors should be encouraged to take the Family and Medical Leave Act (FMLA) to protect their jobs while they are recovering from donation. Employee-specific benefits such as short-term disability and/or paid time off should be utilized for lost wages. Those with jobs that require strenuous activity and/or heavy lifting will need to take at least 6 weeks off work while under postoperative restriction. Before surgery, the patient should determine if any light-duty options are available, especially if recovery will not be paid in full.

Federal employees are eligible to receive 30 days paid leave for organ donation [7]. The majority of the states have also enacted organ donor leave laws that allow for time off.

Based off the state of residence there are tax deductions, leave of absence with pay, income tax credit and donated sick leave options [7]. A few states passed legislation allowing up to a $ 10,000 deduction on state income taxes for travel, lodging and lost wages associated with the donation [7].

Financial Assistance

Organizations such as American Cancer Society may be able to assist with free or low-cost cancer screenings and also provide funds for treatment. Centers for Disease Control National Breast and Cervical Cancer Early Detection Program

(NBCCEDP) provides access to breast and cervical cancer screening services to underserved women in all 50 states, the District of Columbia, five U.S. territories, and 11 tribes [1].

There are organizations that operate solely to minimize financial strain on the living donor. Due to limited funds, the potential donor does need to show financial hardship or need. The application for consideration must be submitted prior to the donation. A few of these organizations are: National Living Donor Assistance Center (NLDAC), Heal with Love, and American Transplant Foundation.

The NLDAC requires income verification of both the donor and recipient. Financial hardship needs to be proven and is assessed by 300% of the federal poverty guidelines. It is considered a payer of last resort, meaning that all other avenues of assistance, such as federal or state must not be available. If approved, a donor may receive up to $ 6,000 for transportation, meals, and lodging associated with their donation [10]. An accompanying person may also be included. Donor and recipient attestation forms need to be signed and placed in the patient's respective charts that document that no valuable consideration is involved.

Fundraising

Potential donors may choose to get involved in fundraising opportunities to assist in reducing the out-of-pocket costs related to organ donation. Organizations such as Help Hope Live [5] assist with various tasks related to fundraising, such as identifying potential networks within a patient community, creating flyers, and alerting the media to fundraising events. Any funds earned would be beneficial for the donor, so their expenses are paid while they are recovering and unable to work. It is recommended the donor keep a record of the monies given to them and how they are used for evaluation and pre- and post-surgical recovery.

Affordable Care Act

With the enactment of the 2014 Affordable Care Act, preexisting conditions associated with private health insurance are no longer of concern [8]. Preexisting conditions were previously of concern if a donor was looking to be covered under a private health insurance policy (nongroup coverage). The living donor would often be scrutinized by the insurance company for their donation, which was considered a preexisting condition and/or completely denied insurance.

Future individual life insurance policies may still be subject to higher premiums or denials based off a kidney donation.

Job Loss

Prevention against employment discrimination has not been implemented within the Affordable Care Act and may still pose a threat for a kidney donor. If a kidney donor suffers from job termination and is considered to be an "at will" employee, generally speaking, there is no recourse. Therefore, it is critical that the potential donor fully understand the financial consequences of their kidney donation.

Valuable Consideration

The National Organ Transplantation Act of 1984 (NOTA) prohibits buying and/or selling of human organs [11]. Specifically, "It shall be unlawful for any person to knowingly acquire, receive or otherwise transfer any human organ for valuable consideration for use in human transplantation [11]." It is a violation of federal law to offer or accept money or any item of value in exchange for a human organ to be used in transplantation. Criminal provisions include a $ 50,000 fine and/or 5 years imprisonment.

In 2007, Congress amended NOTA to include that paired kidney donation was not considered to be valuable consideration [11]. Lodging, transportation, meals, and lost wages are not considered to be valuable consideration. A living donor may be legally reimbursed for any reasonable costs associated with lodging, transportation, meals, and lost wages directly related to their donation.

It is the role of the transplant center to inform each potential living donor that selling an organ for transplantation is a felony. If it is found that a candidate is engaging in such activity, their candidacy should be terminated.

Valuable consideration laws are meant to protect the safety of the patient and the integrity of the transplant institution. The concern is to prevent a vulnerable person from making a rash decision out of desperation without considering long-term consequences. As shown in the China iPod scandal, exploitation of vulnerable people places lives at risk. A 17-year-old boy in China sold one of his kidneys so he could buy an iPhone and an iPod [2]. Out of a $ 35,000 payment for the kidney, the donor received just $ 3,500 [2]. Participants involved were held as criminally liable and stood trial. In this case, the patient was motivated by financial gain and seemed to have little concern about risks or future health. After the kidney was taken out, he suffered from renal failure [3].

Our primary concern is that if a potential kidney donor is being motivated by financial gain, they may not be forthcoming during the medical and/or psychosocial evaluation. Out of fear of being denied monetary compensation for their organs, a patient may conceal a preexisting condition wherein the procedure would render them at risk. Indeed, if the donation is not altruistic in nature, but rather done for monetary reasons, the donor may be too hesitant, ashamed, or uncomfortable to follow up. This presents a clear risk to the patient's health and future wellbeing. Failure to follow up with patients places the center at risk of noncompliance. This situation is unacceptable, and we must do our utmost to prevent it from happening.

Canadian Program

Canada has found a way to reduce the financial concern related to lose wages related to organ donor recovery. In 2006, Canada launched the Living Organ Donor Expense Reimbursement (LODER) program, which was designed to help alleviate non-medical expenses accrued by the living donor, especially lost wages [6]. For Canadian residents only, lost wages will be reimbursed after proof of income is verified. This program may drastically reduce the number of living donors who withdraw or are excluded due to high financial risk.

References

1. American Cancer Society. Stay healthy. c2013. www.cancer.org. Accessed: 16. Feb. 2013.
2. Fox News. Boy, 17, sells kidney to buy iPad 2 in China [Internet]. c2011. http://www.foxnews.com/tech/2011/06/02/boy-17-sells-kidney-to-buy-ipad-2-in-china/. Accessed: 15. Feb. 2013.
3. Gambino L. Chinese boy 'sells kidney to buy iPad'. The Telegraph. c2012. http://www.telegraph.co.uk/news/worldnews/asia/china/9191325/Chinese-boy-sells-kidney-to-buy-iPad.html. Accessed: 20. Feb. 2013.
4. Heal with love. http://www.healwithlovefoundation.org/. Accessed: 15. Feb. 2013.
5. Help hope live. http://www.helphopelive.org. Accessed: 15. Feb. 2013.
6. Klarenbach S, Vlaicu S, Garg A, Yang R, Clark K, Dempster T. A review of the economic implications of living organ donation: donor perspectives and policy considerations. 2006. http://www.organsandtissues.ca/s/wp-content/uploads/2011/11/Economic_Living_Organ_Donor_Klarenbach.pdf. Accessed: 16. Jan. 2006.
7. Legislation [Internet]. Transplant living. C2013. http://transplantliving.org/living-donation/financing-living-donation/legislation/. Accessed: 15. Feb. 2013.
8. American Medical News. Living organ donors shouldn't have to pay for their altruism. C2012. www.amednews.com. Accessed: 5. Feb. 2013.
9. National Breast and Cervical Cancer Early Detection Program (NBCCEDP). Centers for Disease Control and Prevention. http://www.cdc.gov/cancer/nbccedp/. Accessed: 15. Feb. 2013.
10. National Living Donor Assistance Center. c2007. http://www.livingdonorassistance.org/. Accessed: 12. Jan. 2013.
11. Prohibition of organ purchases. The National Organ Transplantation Act; 98-507 42 U.S.C. 274e. 1984. Title III § 301.

Chapter 21
Autonomy, Agency, and Responsibility: Ethical Concerns for Living Donor Advocates

Rosamond Rhodes

The Problem

The most basic commitments of medical ethics are that health professionals should act for the good of patients and society and in doing so, at least try to avoid harm. Living organ donation seems to run afoul of both the principles of beneficence and avoiding harm. The surgery does not provide a medical benefit to the organ donor, and in fact, it can potentially impose significant harms: risks, pain, disability, impaired function, and disfigurement.

From the recipient's perspective, living organ donation provides a tremendous life-saving benefit. From the living donor's perspective, organ donation may achieve an important good in that it promises to save a life. From the donor's perspective, the anticipated benefits provided by the transplant can be worth the risks and harms. From the perspective of a transplant program and the medical professionals who support its activities, with expertise and careful screening of recipients and donors, the risks and harms of living organ donation can be reasonable relative to the anticipated benefits.

Thus, for the donor as well as for transplant professionals, the critical ethical factor for living donor organ transplantation is that donation should be voluntary, and the donor should be acting autonomously. If a living organ donation was not voluntary, there would be no reason to view the action as good in the donor's eyes, and, in most cases, no reason to see the potential risks of pain, disability, impaired function, and disfigurement as anything other than ethically unacceptable harms. Thus, to more fully explain what is required for the ethical conduct of living donor organ transplantation, more has to be said about the concepts of voluntariness and autonomy.

R. Rhodes (✉)
Department of Medical Education, Icahn School of Medicine at Mount Sinai,
One Gustave Levy Place Box 1076, New York, NY 10029, USA
e-mail: Rosamond.rhodes@mssm.edu

Voluntariness and Autonomy

A living donor advocate (LDA) has serious responsibilities. On the one hand, the LDA has to ensure that donation decisions are voluntary and not coerced. On the other hand, the LDA has to help the would-be donor to explore and evaluate their decisions by probing their reasons so that their choices are actually autonomous and reflect their values and priorities. Both responsibilities require a clear understanding of the concepts of autonomy and voluntariness.

For ancient Greek and Roman moral philosophers, it was critical to understand the circumstances that must obtain for someone to be held responsible for what they did. Aristotle explained that people should only be praised or blamed for their voluntary actions. In his terms, an action is voluntary only when "the moving principle" originates from the agent. He explained that when some physical force caused an outcome, what occurred was not a voluntary action. For example, when a train lurches and you fall onto someone's foot and cause pain, what you did is not voluntary and you should not be blamed. He also explained that when nonculpable ignorance is involved, what occurs is not a voluntary action. For example, if there is no reasonable way for you to discern that the medicine you administer to a patient is contaminated, your administration of the contaminant is not voluntary. You should not be blamed for the illness that the patient suffers as a consequence.

Aristotle and the Stoics extended the concepts of voluntariness and responsibility to self-creation, in the sense that they believed individuals are responsible not only for their actions but for their characters and their motivatons as well. According to them, by acting as you do, you develop habits or inclinations to take pleasure in certain behaviors and to act in similar ways in the future. Similarly, you become pained by other behaviors and develop an aversion to them. In this way, you create your own disposition and develop your own tendencies to act as you then do. Because these results are consequences of your own previous voluntary actions, you are responsible for who you are. In this light, we can understand professional training as not just mastery of a body of knowledge, but also as the development of the habits and attitudes that we associate with professional responsibility.

For Aristotle, an act done in response to pressure is still a voluntary act [1]. Given the nature of the action and the nature of the pressure, what is done may be more or less excusable. Aristotle provides two telling examples. First, he describes a ship captain who finds himself in a storm. The captain must decide whether he should throw his goods overboard or not. If he does, he loses the goods and incurs a significant financial loss, but he also increases his chance of surviving the storm. If he does not, his chance of surviving the storm is diminished, but if he survives he still has his goods. Clearly, the captain does not choose to be in a storm, but given the circumstances and the pressures that they impose, the choice of what to do is his. Whichever course he chooses, his action will be voluntary and he should be held responsible. Aristotle's second example is a man threatened by a tyrant. The tyrant demands that the man do something shameful, and he threatens to harm his family if the man should refuse. Clearly, the threat is unwelcome pressure, but in

Aristotle's eyes, the man's response is voluntary. Imagine that the shameful act is writing an ode of praise to the tyrant, whereas the threat involves serious physical harm or death to a loved one. That shameful act could be more excusable than if the threatened harm is only tickling a loved one with a feather or less excusable if the shameful act is far more reprehensible.

The concept of voluntariness is now closely related to the concept of autonomy. Autonomy was originally a political concept rather than a concept used in discussions of individual action. In Classical Greek writing, "autonomy" was used to describe civic communities that were self-governing and independent of any other political authority. In the Renaissance and Early Modern Period, "autonomy" was still used as a political concept, but then it designated independence from a religious authority.

In the Modern Period philosophers such as Hobbes and Spinoza employed the concept in their writing, but without using the term. Autonomy, or self-governance, does not take hold as a moral concept by that name until Immanuel Kant (1724–1804) used it. For Kant, autonomy is the distinctive capacity of individual rational beings. It is the power of legislating for oneself, of giving oneself moral rules for governing one's own actions. Autonomy in this self-rule sense is the distinctive ability that gives beings their moral worth and makes their actions and choices worthy of respect.

Three senses of autonomy can be distinguished in Kant's use of the term. In its primary sense, autonomy is a self-regulating ideal. As an autonomous agent, I should always consider my actions in terms of rules that I would endorse for all similarly situated individuals, and I should conform my actions to the principles that I endorse. In its secondary sense, the concept defines how I ought to treat others. In dealing with other adults who are capable of autonomous action, I should respect their choices, presuming as far as possible that their choices are directed by autonomy and conform to the principles that the person has endorsed. The third sense of autonomy defines how one ought to treat those who are not now capable of autonomous action, but who may be in the future. Their autonomy should be promoted, and they should be guided to act autonomously.

In contemporary philosophical literature, numerous authors have tried to refine the concept of autonomy and clarify what it means to be a moral agent. In doing so they have put forward an array of different accounts, some very similar to others and some that present a somewhat distinctive view of what autonomy entails. The samples that I describe below illustrate the scope of these different positions on what autonomy entails.

Harry Frankfurt has famously put forward the view that an autonomous action conforms to a higher-order volition [2]. In other words, Frankfurt asks us to consider whether we would will ourselves to be guided by the desire that we are acting upon. For example, you may desire a slice of pizza, but would you will yourself to be moved by that desire? If yes, perhaps because it will satisfy your hunger, and you love pizza, and it is an affordable snack, having the slice is autonomous. If instead you would will to be free of the desire and able to resist the temptation, eating a slice is not autonomous. In Frankfurt's view, autonomy is about being the master of one's desires. Someone who is dragged about by desires is a slave to passions and not free.

Gerald Dworkin offers a similar account of autonomy that uses the concept of future-oriented consent [3,4]. In determining whether you or another is acting autonomously, Dworkin asks you to imagine whether the agent would be happy with the decision tomorrow. Using the pizza example again, if I would be upset when my jeans would not zip up tomorrow and tell myself that I should have resisted the pizza yesterday (all three slices of it), then my indulging in it yesterday was not autonomous. Using a medical example, imagine a Jehovah's Witness patient who refuses blood transfusions if needed during surgery. If that patient explains that he would believe a great harm had been done to him and would not want to live if he awoke to the news that his life had been saved with a blood transfusion, we should take his refusal to be autonomous and respect his choice.

Christine Korsgaard relies on a very Kantian notion of autonomy [5]. She explains autonomous action as acts that are considered and reflectively endorsed. For her, an impulsive or thoughtless choice is not autonomous. For Korsgaard, only an action that has been duly considered and evaluated, and found to be something that I would not consider wrong when done by another in similar circumstances would count as autonomous and worthy of respect from others.

Several authors have explained autonomous action in terms that suggest being true to myself or consistent with my values, goals, and commitments. Bernard Berofsky uses the terms self-authorization, self-realization, and self-expression to explain that I act autonomously when my action coheres with my view of who I am [6]. If I am astounded by something that I did and say to myself, "Eating that pizza was not like me at all. I'm a vegan and I regard my body as a temple," then eating the pizza was not autonomous. Similarly, J. David Velleman explains autonomous action as an expression of identity [7]. For him, an action is autonomous when I can identify myself with the action and when it fits with how I describe myself as self-narrator of my life. Marina A.I. Oshana offers a similar account [8]. For her, when there is an absence of alienation, the action was autonomous. When I appreciate that I did it, that it was not the fever or the alcohol that made me do it, it was my choice, then the action is mine. When instead I think, how could I have done that, it is not like me at all, then the action is not autonomous, it belongs to some alien other, and I am not responsible for the outcome.

Each of these views has something to it that rings true, but also some shortcomings. For example, Frankfurt's higher-order desire model and Dworkin's future-oriented consent model work well with the Jehovah's Witness whose priorities are clear and fixed. When an agent is more ambivalent and then makes a choice, it is not at all clear that the model is useful.

For example, if someone chooses to be a living liver donor and the transplant recipient develops primary nonfunction, would the donor be happy with yesterday's decision tomorrow? Or, if someone decided against being a living donor and their loved one died from liver failure, or received a successful transplant with a cadaveric organ, could we be confident that their decision conformed to their higher order volition? No answer is obvious. Thus, many of our actions and choices do not fit neatly into the Frankfurt and Dworkin schemes. If pressed, they might conclude that choices reflecting ambivalence are not autonomous. That stand would go too far in the direction of excluding adult actions from responsibility.

Korsgaard's view also seems too demanding. Although we may carefully deliberate about what to do when we face difficult dilemmas, most of what we do throughout the day is far more spontaneous. Most of the actions we perform are not carefully considered in terms of moral rules that we might endorse. Ultimately, this view appears to set too high a standard and exclude most of what we do from being worthy of the respect of others.

Berofsky, Velleman, and Oshana's views seem to have the opposite problem. Instead of limiting the actions that merit respect, they would excuse actions from responsibility whenever the agent subsequently denied identity with them. According to their positions, whatever I do when I am not feeling myself could not be counted as autonomous and could not be blamed. That seems far too cavalier.

Lessons from Being a Living Donor Advocate

As an LDA my task involved interviewing potential living liver donors to determine whether or not their decision to be a donor was informed and voluntary. In philosophic terms, I was trying to assess whether the donors' decisions were autonomous and genuine expressions of their agency. By the time they reached me, potential donors had typically spent weeks, months, or years contemplating their donation, speaking with doctors and family members, reading the literature, and surfing the Internet to explore the experiences of others. If any, these donors' choices bore the marks of careful deliberation and considered judgment. Their decisions to undertake the significant risks and harms involved in donating up to 70% of their livers were not rash, impulsive, or whimsical.

In my tenure as an LDA I drew on what I had learned from the philosophic literature on autonomy. For the most part, philosophers present their positions on autonomy and agency as vying theories or models of how to correctly conceptualize the decisions for which people can be held responsible. Donors' accounts of how they reach their decision to donate and the variety of conceptual terms that they employ in describing their thoughts and their motivation suggest that many of the standard views of autonomy and agency are all similarly flawed. To the extent that the individuals explaining their organ donation decisions have reliable insight into their own mental processes, the range of ways in which they characterize their decisions challenge all of the simplistic conceptions of autonomy. My experience of serving as an LDA and witnessing their testimony provided me with significant insights into the concept of autonomy. Some examples from the interviews that I conducted have been informative in that they illustrate the variety of ways that people experience and conceptualize their donation decisions.

Several of the potential donors who I interviewed made statements like this, "Of course I'm afraid and would prefer not to, but this is the right thing for me to do." Such declarations perfectly expressed Frankfurt's notion of autonomy. These potential donors were in control of their desires and their choices to become living donors conformed to their higher-order volitions. They willed that their actions be governed not by fear, but by their conceptions of their moral duty.

Similarly, a number of potential donors made statements such as, "I couldn't live with myself if I didn't try to save her." They perfectly illustrated Dworkin's future-oriented consent view of autonomy because their choices expressed their consistent priorities and the commitments that they expected themselves to value in the near and distant future.

Other potential donors explained their decisions in other ways. A few explained their decision by saying, "My family expects it of me." Such statements raise questions about pressure and coercion and the limits of autonomy. Is pressure from others (e.g., family members) inherently different from situational pressure (e.g., the ship caught in the storm, a dying loved one), or the internal pressure of personal hopes or expectations (e.g., for survival, recognition, maintaining relationships within the family), and if so, how do any of these forces undermine agency or diminish moral responsibility? When I probed these statements for signs of coercion, the donors' replies revealed that there was no outside pressure. In fact, the potential donors' decisions amounted to reflectively endorsed commitments to act in ways that their families would expect them to behave. In Korsgaard's terms, they chose to act in accordance with the rules that they and their families, and possibly society, embraces.

Many of the potential donors I interviewed articulated the same reason for donating verbatim. They said, "I want to be the kind of person who helps people." Such proclamations expressed Berofsky's view of autonomy as self-authorization, or self-realization, or self-expression. These donors viewed their actions in terms of the kind of self that they wanted to mold themselves into being.

One donor explained her choice to donate to a fellow parishioner who she did not know well by saying, "I am a Christian, like a good Samaritan I help my fellow man." Her pronouncement fit perfectly with Velleman's account of autonomous action as an expression of identity. This donor identified her choice as fitting with how she described herself and the story of her life as she tells it. Being a living donor is not alien to her, it is part of who she is in her own eyes.

Then there were the haunting assertions, "I have to. I couldn't do anything else. I have no choice." Again, the words themselves appear to express force, coercion, the opposite of autonomy. They do not fit with any of the accounts of autonomy that I have identified in the literature. These people, often parents contemplating donation to a child, seemed to be acting with freedom and authentically expressing their clear and definite priorities, yet their statements would tend to disqualify their actions as autonomous according to most models. To me, however, they expressed strong and unwavering commitment to a child as the parent's highest priority. These parents had no choice and could not do anything else because nothing else was as important to them as saving their child.

In the end, the lesson that I learned from talking to living donors was that autonomy does not fit one narrow definition. Taken together the different living donor responses suggest that the standard philosophical approach of trying to describe what is essential to agency or what an autonomous decision is, does not account for the range of human experience. Faced with the variety of ways that donors characterize their decisions, theorists would either be pressed to stretch the envelope and redescribe personal experience in terms compatible with their favored view or deny that many, many choices that others would count as paradigmatically authentic or autonomous have that status. In light of this experience, autonomy appears to be a nest of concepts with a family resemblance, and voluntary choices may reflect different senses of autonomy. Donors who are in control of their choices, actions, and wills are autonomous. Those donors' decisions are autonomous and worthy of respect. When medical standards for living donation are met, such donation decisions should be accepted.

In sum, autonomy is the *ability* to be a good ruler over oneself. For someone to be autonomous, she/he must have:

- The *ability* to adopt values, principles, and goals
- The *ability* to understand and appreciate the relevant facts of the situation
- The *ability* to reach a conclusion that makes sense
- The *ability* to abide by that conclusion

Someone who can do all of that is capable of acting voluntarily and can be held responsible for her/his actions.

The Responsibilities of a Living Donor Advocate

Understanding of the concept of autonomy and the elements that comprise voluntariness are critical tools for LDAs, but they are merely elements for enabling advocates to do their work. Assessing autonomy is, however, only one element of an LDA's work. The LDA's job is to help the donor. This involves two responsibilities related to autonomy. One is to assess the autonomy of the donor and the voluntariness of the donation decision. As I explained above, this assessment is necessary because unless the donation is voluntary, taking an organ from a living donor is unjustifiably causing harm.

The LDA's other responsibility is to help living donors to reach decisions that are consistent with their values, goals, and priorities, and to make choices that are authentic and that fit with the donors' own narratives. Both tasks require the advocate to enter the interview without a personal or institutional agenda, without preconceptions and assumptions, and with a nonjudgmental regard and a sincere commitment to helping the donor. Both tasks involve attentive listening and observation, as well as reflection on what is being said and not said. Two examples from my experience as an LDA will help to explain.

A Case of Assessing Voluntariness[1]

SC, a 41-year-old Asian woman from China, was being evaluated as a liver donor for her husband. His illness had disabled him so that he could no longer work and she had to leave her job to care for him. As part of her donor evaluation, SC had already met with the transplant team's medical doctors, surgeons, transplant coordinators, a psychiatrist, and a social worker. Each one had tried to explain the risks associated with living liver donation. In every conversation SC had signaled early in their explanation that the medical professional should stop explaining because she did not want to hear those things. These team members were concerned that SC's decision would not be voluntary unless she was fully informed as to the risks involved.

In my interview with her, SC described her husband as being a good man. She also volunteered that they have one son who is an outstanding student attending one of the city's elite high schools. She and her husband need money to cover his tuition costs at a good college. When I asked her to tell me about the risks associated with living liver donation, she became obviously upset and waved at me to stop my line of questioning. I did, but I asked her why she did not want to talk about what could happen. SC explained that if you talk about bad things, or even think about them, they would happen. Later in our conversation I asked her about others with whom she had discussed her decision. She mentioned that her husband wanted her to be a donor. She had also shared her decision with her own parents who did not want her to be a donor because they were worried about what might happen to her. She had not discussed the matter with her son, although he knew what was being contemplated.

At one point during the interview, SC asked me, "How often do the bad things happen?" I responded honestly, but I pointedly avoided naming the specific complications, and just spoke in terms of the very bad things, and the things that were bad, but not the worst. In the end, SC said that she had not yet decided what to do and that she was still thinking about donation.

By listening to what SC said, trying to understand her reasons, and discern what she was trying to convey, I concluded that SC was acting autonomously and that her decision would be voluntary. Even though she refused to articulate the specific risks involved in liver donation, what she had related convinced me that she was adequately informed to make the donation decision. She had told me about fearing that saying or thinking about the complications would cause them to happen, she had revealed her parents' anxiety, and she had asked about the frequency of complications. Taken together, this communication told me that SC knew what could happen. Whether her refusal to name or hear the possible consequences named was a matter of culture or personal belief did not matter. What did matter was that SC was aware of what could happen and that her choice to be a donor reflected her own values. SC's final statement that she was still deliberating

---

[1] Details have been changed to protect patient confidentiality.

about the donation decision also gave me confidence that her ultimate decision would be thoughtfully considered.

A Case of Helping a Donor Reach an Autonomous Decision[2]

MV, a 36-year-old man, was being evaluated as a liver donor for his father. He had been largely estranged from his father since age 8, when his father abandoned him and his mother to start another family. Later his father abandoned the second family to start a third family. The father, who recently developed liver failure, now has a 5-year-old child with his new partner. He had contacted MV requesting him to be a living liver donor so that he live and be a good father to his newest child. He made all of the arrangements for MV to come into the transplant center and be evaluated as a donor.

MV last saw his father when he visited MV's family about a year earlier. MV is married, and he has three young children. He explained his decision to donate saying, "I want to be a good person, the kind of person who helps people, and he's my father."

In my conversation with MV, he appeared to be well-informed about the risks involved in liver donation. He volunteered that he, his wife, and his mother have all been researching liver donation on the Internet. His wife and mother do not want him to donate, but they will support him in whatever decision he makes.

Although MV's words sounded as if they reflected an autonomous decision, listening to the simplicity of his statements and the absence of emotion in his description of his father's history and request suggested that further probing was in order. I asked MV whether, besides his father, there were others who he wanted to be good to and help. Then came his declarations of love for his wife and statements about how she was always there for him, in fact, waiting outside of my office. Then came the photos of his children and the expressions of pride in their accomplishments. Then came the photo of his eldest son on a dirt bike. And then MV said, "I spent more time with my son last weekend than my father spent with me in my entire life."

In the end, I told MV that in being a good person and helping others he needs to consider all of those who will be affected by his decision. In effect, I gave MV permission to change his mind about donation and licensed him to consider the consequences of his decision more broadly. That permission allowed him to more fully explore his options and to choose a course that was consistent with his priorities and image of himself. He left my office thanking me and saying that he had a lot to consider.

---

[2] Details have been changed to protect patient confidentiality.

Conclusion

Medical decisions can be much more serious than other decisions, they may need to be made very quickly, and their consequences can be enduring. Although in ordinary life we should generally presume that adults have autonomy and the capacity to decide for themselves, assessing patient decisional capacity is a medical responsibility whenever a lot is on the line. Typically, medical professionals assess the decisional capacity of patients who refuse critical medical interventions. In living donor transplantation, medical professionals also have to assess the autonomy of the living donor and the voluntariness of the donor's choice.

The assessment of living donors by LDAs is an ethically challenging activity. It requires a deep understanding of voluntariness and autonomy to sort out when a donation decision should be accepted. It involves an attitude of nonjudgmental regard and requires setting aside preconceptions, assumptions, and agendas so that the advocate can listen to what is being said and take in what the donor is trying to convey. Without that understanding and perspective, donations may be accepted as voluntary when they are not. This is a serious moral hazard for transplant programs that perform living donor transplantation. Great care must be taken to see that it does not occur.

References

1. Aristotle. The Nicomachean ethics. Translated by David Ross and edited by Lesley Brown. New York:Oxford University Press; 2009.
2. Frankfurt HG. Freedom of the will and the concept of a person. In: Christman J, editor. The inner citadel: essays on individual autonomy. New York: Oxford University Press; 1989. pp 63–76.
3. Dworkin G. The concept of autonomy. In: Christman J, editor. The inner citadel: essays on individual autonomy. New York: Oxford University Press; 1989. pp 54–62.
4. Dworkin G. The theory and practice of autonomy. New York:Cambridge University Press; 1988.
5. Korsgaard CM. Reflective endorsement. In: Korsgaard CM, editor. The sources of normativity. New York: Cambridge University Press; 1996. pp. 49–89.
6. Berofsky B. Identification, the self, and autonomy. In: Frankel PE, Miller FD Jr., Paul J editors. Autonomy. New York: Cambridge University Press; 2003. pp 199–220.
7. Velleman JD. The self as narrator. In: Christman K, Anderson J, editors. Autonomy and the challenges of liberalism: new essays. New York:Cambridge University Press; 2005. pp 56–76.
8. Oshana MAL. Autonomy and self-identity. In: Christman K, Anderson J, editors. Autonomy and the challenges of liberalism: new essays. New York:Cambridge University Press; 2005. pp 77–97.

Chapter 22
A Practical Guide: Role of the Independent Living Donor Advocate: Protect or Advocate or Is it Both?

Betsy B. Johnson

Thomas has a history of multiple health issues. When he was a young, he had leukemia and he received a bone marrow transplant from his sister, Susan. At the time, Thomas was 8 years old and his sister was 10.

Thomas is now 25 years old and married to Nancy. His sister, Susan, is 27 and married to Bill. Thomas has experienced a decline in kidney function and will need a transplant. His nephrologist wants him to have a transplant before he has to start dialysis, as this would be better for him. As Thomas received bone marrow from Susan, a donated kidney from Susan has a great chance for success.

Thomas has been seen by the transplant team; and he and his wife are excited that Thomas may be able to avoid dialysis by receiving a kidney from his sister. All that needs to happen next is that Susan contact the transplant center and get started with her workup.

After several weeks, Susan calls and asks about the living donor process. An appointment is set up with the independent living donor advocate (ILDA), and Susan brings her husband, Bill, with her to the initial meeting. Bill and Susan both inquire about all that is involved in donating a kidney. Bill states that although he and his wife are young, he is concerned about Susan's long-term health in case she donates her kidney. Bill also shares his concern that his wife could be seen as an organ farm for her brother. It seems to Bill that everyone is just assuming Susan should and will give a kidney to Thomas. Bill asks, "Does it stop with a kidney? What if Thomas needs a liver at some point? Susan didn't have a choice as a child to give her bone marrow, but she now has a choice about donating a kidney." Susan and Bill are both assured that if Susan does not want to go forward with donating a kidney to Thomas, her decision will be respected and supported.

A week later, the transplant social worker receives a call from Nancy, Thomas' wife. Nancy states she had a tense conversation with Bill, Susan's husband, and cannot believe that Bill is expressing concerns about Susan giving Thomas a kidney.

B. B. Johnson (✉)
Division of Transplantation, Baystate Medical Center, 100 Wason Ave,
Suite 210, Springfield, MA 01107, USA
e-mail: betsybjohnson@comcast.net

The social worker calls the ILDA to let her know of Nancy's call and to express concerns about a mounting family conflict.

The ILDA has a number of obligations, not the least of which is to rule out pressure or coercion. Is it possible that Susan is feeling coerced into giving a kidney to her brother? Is it possible that Susan is feeling coerced by her husband *not* to give a kidney? The ILDA reaches out to Susan. Susan indicates that her husband is still opposed to her kidney donation but she wants to continue with the workup toward donation. She states donation will be her decision and to make her own decision, she wants to follow the typical donor medical workup.

Is it solely Susan's decision to donate her kidney? Are their possible competing interests? It is the ILDA's and transplant team's obligation to do as little harm as possible to a donor. It is also their obligation to rule in or out coercion that is negatively affecting a donor's ability to make a free choice concerning his or her donation.

It is acknowledged that taking a healthy person and removing a healthy kidney is doing harm, however, this harm is balanced with the autonomous decision of the donor to donate a kidney for the benefit of another. What are the ILDA's obligations if he or she feels donation might cause emotional harm? Certainly, if an individual is noted to have an emotional or a psychiatric condition that is not currently stable, one would not want to continue with the donation process until the specific psychological issue is satisfactorily addressed. However, what are the obligations of an ILDA, who is concerned there could be future emotional harm to a donor because of entrenched family conflict? What if Susan's husband will never agree that his wife should donate a kidney to her brother? If a transplant might cause permanent harm to a marriage, should the donation process be stopped?

What are the roles of the ILDA in a case such as this? What does it mean to be an advocate for a potential living donor or to protect a donor's "best interest?" When might the imperative to protect a potential donor from harm morph into paternalism? How might the ILDA's perceived advocacy for a potential donor be in direct conflict with respect for the individual's autonomous decision making? How might the values of an ILDA effect whether a potential donor is ruled out [1]?

One of the outcomes of a National Survey of Independent Living Donor Advocates indicated 50.7% of ILDAs would rule out a potential donor, given a case scenario that involved some risk to the individual. The potential donor understood the risks and had been cleared for surgery. In addition, the person wanted to continue with donation, despite the risks. Although they had concerns and would note those concerns, only 29% of ILDAs would advocate for the potential donor's desire to move forward with kidney donation. Interestingly, of the 20.3% remaining, some of these respondents did not know they were part of the decision-making process regarding whether a potential donor moved forward with donation [2].

How might an ILDA anchor him or herself in established ethical principles, to make a recommendation about a donor moving forward or not moving forward, when there are competing issues? How might the personal and professional ethics and values of the ILDA potentially affect his or her decision regarding a donor?

One of the first ethical issues to consider is the autonomy of the potential donor. To have true autonomy, a person must have capacity to make an independent decision and must be provided with enough information to be able to give informed consent or informed refusal for a procedure. One must be able to weigh this information and seek clarification, if needed. Autonomy also considers the individual's value system and how her or his values play a key role in decision making. For example, it is well established that a competent adult who holds certain religious beliefs may accept or refuse a needed blood transfusion, even if an individual patient's refusal of a needed blood transfusion will likely cause death. Will the individual's autonomous decision not to accept a blood transfusion be overruled if a spouse does not hold the same religious belief and wants the individual to be given blood? No, the autonomous decision of the individual patient will be respected. Having said this, obviously, one wants to be sensitive to the spouse who is upset about his or her spouse's life-threatening decision not to accept a needed transfusion. In addition, acceptable medical options can and should be offered to help save the life of the individual, as long as the patient agrees. The decision not to overrule a competent person's stated wishes regarding refusal of blood transfusions is established in legal precedent as well as rooted in the ethical principle of autonomy. Then, should the ILDA be able to overrule a donor if they are competent to make a decision?

In this example, it is of importance that many medical professionals do not hold this religious belief and disagree wholeheartedly with a person who refuses a needed blood transfusion. From a medical perspective, it is *not* in the "best interest" of the individual to refuse a needed transfusion. There is a direct conflict between a patient's desired wish to forego a needed procedure and what is in the best interest of the patient, from a medical perspective.

This example illustrates the need for medical professionals to acknowledge their own value systems. One may approve or disapprove of another's treatment decision, depending on how much this decision does or does not resonate with a person's own value system. However, treatment decisions made by an individual "patient," who has capacity and understands the potential benefits and burdens of his or her decision, will typically be honored. The importance of honoring a competent person's treatment decisions was first established in the landmark case of Schloendorff v Society of New York Hospital. Justice Benjamin Cardozo wrote "Every human being of adult years and sound mind has a right to determine what shall be done with his own body…" [3]. This case challenged the prevailing medical practice of paternalism and helped create the concept of a competent person's right to give informed consent or informed refusal to any medical procedure. A "patient's" autonomous decision regarding treatment should be respected rather than overruled by the physician.

In Susan's case, among other things, we need to explore the principle of autonomy. Autonomy can, at times, be negatively affected or compromised by coercion.

What is pressure and/or coercion? There are many types of coercion, including physical, psychological, and even financial. At its base, coercion is the manipulation or pressuring of another to try to get the person to do something he or she might not truly want to do. One can use guilt, social pressure, financial incentives or disincentives, and other methods in attempts to get a person to conform to another's wishes or desires [4]. Many ILDAs have talked with a person who did not really want to donate an organ, but felt pressured or was "volunteered" by others. This type of potential donor can feel trapped and continues to move forward without really knowing how to get out of donating.

In these types of cases, it is an obligation of the ILDA to try to ferret out these concerns. Others, like transplant social workers, can also help uncover coercion. In true coercion, a person is not making a free choice to donate. Rather, the choice is based on pressure from others. An individual is unable to make an actual autonomous decision, because the person is not acting from a place of true choice.

What about a possible "reverse coercion" of a potential donor? It is really a different side to the same coin of coercion, but in this situation, the potential donor may truly *want* to donate but is feeling pressured by a loved one *not* to donate. There may be an implied or real threat to a marriage or other important relationship, if the individual moves forward with donation.

In Susan's case, we have the potential for both types of coercion. Her husband does not want her to donate, and her brother's wife wants her to donate. Can Susan make a truly free choice? She may lose her marriage if she goes against her husband's wishes that she not donate. In addition, her support system could be negatively affected. If she does not donate a kidney to her brother, Susan could cause permanent harm to the relationship she has with her brother and his wife. Is this all too much for Susan?

In Susan's case, is the ILDA to protect or advocate? Is advocating for Susan different from protecting her in this conflict? When might protecting a person morph into paternalism?

Paternalism "is a behavior, by a person, organization or state which limits some person or groups liberty or autonomy for their own good" [5]. Examples include parents knowing a certain decision will be harmful to a minor child and, therefore, not allowing the child to make a specific decision the parent(s) deem harmful. In adults, a history of paternalism includes doctors or other health professionals believing it was better not to tell a patient his or her terminal diagnosis because it would be too upsetting. The doctor believed the patient could not handle the information and would often collude with the patient's loved ones to protect the patient from worry.

While this type of paternalism can still exist, it is much less acceptable. Today, there is an expectation that a person needs enough information to fully make an informed treatment decision, even if the information is regarding a terminal diagnosis. One might even argue information is even more important if it is about a potentially fatal condition. Disclosure of benefits and burdens regarding a specific treatment option allows individuals to choose the best treatment choice for themselves. Having said this, it is true that a physician and other medical professionals will hold greater medical knowledge than a "patient" may ever possess. Noting this information gap, what are the main obligations to be met regarding informed consent or informed refusal?

It is acknowledged that the issue of informed consent and informed refusal is a broad topic, rooted in historical atrocities, such as the Holocaust and experiments on uninformed research subjects. One can find volumes written on this important issue. For the purpose of this chapter, an outline and an exploration of key elements of informed consent or informed refusal will be addressed.

First, does the person have *capacity* to understand the medical information being offered? It is not enough to say a person is competent. Competency is a legal term and simply means the person is over the age of 18 and has *not* been declared in a court of law as mentally incompetent.

Does the individual possess the ability to assimilate and weigh new information? Does he or she need an independent/professional/nonrelated translator or sign language interpreter to ensure understanding? Is the information given to the individual in a way that maximizes his or her ability to understand a procedure? It is typically not enough to just give a person a "consent" form to read and sign. A person with no medical background may need medical terms or procedures to be explained. It is important to ascertain whether the individual can explain back to the medical professional, his or her understanding of the proposed procedure. Are there gaps in knowledge that need clarification? If so, after further explanation, does the individual have a clear understanding of the proposed procedures with its potential risks and benefits? If so, one has met part of the process of informed consent.

Is the decision or desire to donate or not to donate, voluntary? As mentioned previously, pressure and coercion must be ruled out. Is the individual making a decision to donate because he or she wants to donate or because someone else wants him or her to donate? Conversely, is the individual being pressured not to go forward with donation, even though the person wants to truly donate? The issue of coercion can also include financial inducement. Is someone being offered financial incentives or disincentive in exchange for donating an organ? The key point regarding coercion is that an individual is experiencing and succumbing to some type of pressure to donate or not to donate an organ. When coercion has trumped autonomy, an individual's ultimate "decision" is based on another's wish, not on one's own independent desire to freely donate an organ.

Important in ruling out *potential* pressure or coercion is whether the individual is able to make an informed decision based on his or her own values and desires. Most humans, at some time in their lives, have felt the pressure from another to do something either against their better judgment or against their own values. However, just because a person feels this pressure, it does not mean that she or he succumbs to the pressure. A person can try to influence another, using guilt and other tactics, but this pressure does not automatically work. Is there potential that pressure will influence a decision? Certainly, but not necessarily.

It is important for the ILDA to discuss this pressure/potential coercion with a donor. Can the donor articulate what the pressure is doing to him or her? Is the potential donor able to separate his or her desires to donate or not donate from the desires of family members? What is motivating the potential donor? Does the donor have insight into his or her situation? If the donor is "motivated" to donate because of pressure or coercion from others, then his or her decision is not a free decision. The potential donor should be ruled out.

It is acknowledged that coercion can be subtle or overt. Sometimes, it is not the family that is using coercion; it can be medical professionals. Some nephrologists have been known to state to a kidney patient that they must have all their family come in for testing because the time has come to consider transplant. The kidney patient dutifully calls all family members and states that the doctor says they must get tested to see if they are a match. Imagine, if you will, a family member's potential guilt if he or she refuses to be tested? The family member, not to appear unloving, dutifully calls the transplant program to see about testing. He or she may be praying not to be a match in hopes of getting off the hook. This person, by moving forward with testing, can be seen as the family "volunteer" for the best kidney match. This coercion, and in this example it is coercion, began, not with family, but from a kidney specialist treating the person in need of a kidney transplant.

It is the role of an ILDA to explore how the decision to come forward as a potential donor transpired. Does it seem the individual wanted to come forward on his or her own, or was it strongly "suggested" to the individual? Again, one can potentially overcome coercionary tactics, but this issue must be thoroughly addressed. For example, it could be that the individual was initially asked or "volunteered" by others to be tested for compatibility. However, it turns out the potential donor truly is fine with donating. As previously stated, even though the potential exists for coercion, is the individual able to separate his or her desires from the desires of others?

It is an obligation of the ILDA to ensure that a potential donor is able to separate her or his desires from the desires of others, such as the recipient or other involved parties. As previously noted, if the "decision" to donate is not ultimately based on the potential donor's independent desire to donate, it is the obligation of the ILDA to rule out this person.

Thus far, we have explored issues of autonomy, informed consent, including voluntary decisions versus coercion. Other than concerns with the aforementioned issues, might there be other concerns that could rule out a potential donor who would like to move forward with donation?

There are times in health care when we do prevent an adult who is competent and has capacity from going forward with a desired treatment path. For example, a person may want a doctor to perform a procedure the doctor does not believe is compatible with the doctor's own values. It would be against the doctor's professional integrity to provide the treatment. Whose values prevail? A patient does have a right to accept or refuse any medical treatment, but a patient does not have a right to demand specific treatment, if it is against the professional integrity of the treating doctor or health care provider. A patient has every right to consider another doctor or hospital. Indeed, it is the treating doctor's obligation not to abandon a patient. He or she needs to try to transfer the patient to another doctor, who may be willing to provide the desired treatment.

In the field of transplant, there are times when a potential donor may want to move forward with donation but the transplant team blocks that option because of concerns. When considering ruling out a potential donor who would like to move forward, an obvious, but critical issue is the reasoning behind the rule out. Is the reasoning used in ruling out a particular donor consistent across all donors? What/ whose values trump the other?

In transplant, as noted, an ILDA and a transplant team, at times, walk a fine line between protection and paternalism when ruling out a competent adult who desires to go forward with transplant, despite concerns. It is established practice in transplant to rule out a potential donor, if he or she has unstable or inadequately treated psychiatric issues. If a person is adequately treated, a psychiatric condition is not an automatic rule out. If a person has some health concerns but the harms are not deemed too medically risky, a potential donor is not automatically ruled out. Further discussion of concerns needs to be satisfactorily addressed. For example, a potential donor's need for medication to treat high blood pressure used to be a rule out. Now, high blood pressure is not an automatic deal breaker. However, before moving forward, a potential donor's hypertension needs to be satisfactorily addressed.

As indicated, transplant practices have evolved over the years. The field of transplant continues to face new and often complex medical and ethical concerns. As noted, some of the accepted ethical "norms" in transplant are ensuring autonomy of the donor; ruling out coercion and ensuring standards of informed consent or informed refusal are met. Another linked concern is protecting the best interest of a potential donor. How might ensuring or protecting a donor's "best interest" be defined regarding the ILDA's role?

Acting in another's best interest is somewhat the other side of doing no harm or mitigating harm. As previously noted, taking a healthy kidney from a healthy person and giving it to another, is indeed doing harm to an individual. If doing physical harm to another was the only ethical consideration, all transplants would come to a screeching halt! However, we balance these harms with other values.

A main intent of the ILDA position is to ensure that the best interests and rights of the potential donor are protected. The ILDA is to be solely focused on the potential donor. Interestingly, ILDAs come from a variety of backgrounds, and depending on an ILDA's professional experience, there may be different interpretations of how an ILDA protects or ensures a donor's best interest. An ILDA who is a social worker and an ILDA who comes from a nursing background may view a donor differently. There are certain standards that are already in place to help ensure the best interest(s) of a donor. For example, there is a complete medical workup required for donors to ensure they are healthy enough to donate an organ. While it is also true that these tests will show, for example, the health of a kidney being considered for donation, the intent of the testing is to make sure the donor is not put at further medical risk if he or she donates an organ.

When exploring what is in the best interest of a particular donor, specifically when there are concerns, whose values might trump the other? Is determining what is ultimately in the best interest of a donor based on the donor's values *or* the values of an IDLA or transplant team? Is it, perhaps, at times, a mixture of both? For example, if a transplant center or ILDA strongly believes that when a potential donor comes in for an appointment to discuss donation, then he or she must come with a support person or persons. This particular ILDA or transplant center truly believes it is in the best interest of the donor to have a support person or person present, at least during the initial informational meetings. Is it good to have support from others when considering donating an organ? Yes. However, a desire by others to protect the "best interest" of the donor may, in reality, come in direct conflict with the donor's autonomy. It could be that an individual knows that others are trying to pressure him or her one way or the other regarding donation. A potential donor may want to come to transplant appointments alone to personally clarify if this is a process he or she wants to continue. There may be a variety of reasons a person wants to attend appointments alone. Is it fair to ask if the individual has enough support and to explore specific needs that may arise during various aspects of the donation process? Yes, of course. However, the caution is not to create artificial barriers for a potential donor just because an ILDA or transplant center believes a particular protocol is in *every* donor's best interest. If a donor wants to come in alone, initially or during the entire process, and the ILDA does not believe this is in the best interest of a donor, then whose values prevail?

When an individual is considering a medical procedure, such as surgery, is it typically *required* that a competent adult, with capacity, who is able to make his or her own informed decisions, bring someone with him or her to the doctor's office? In reality, it is often the opposite. One has to give expressed permission for another to be present with a doctor and his or her patient. Is it good if a trusted person comes along? It can be very good…but…it depends. It is certainly not typically required. In Western society, for better or for worse, we lean heavily toward the value of an individual's autonomy and respecting his or her *individual* treatment decision(s). Other societies may tend toward a family or group decision, and these cultural norms also ought to be respected. Conversely, if a potential donor is more comfortable coming in alone, and can clearly state why that is his or her preference, that preference ought to be respected, as well.

All this to say, an ILDA or other members of a transplant team, in a desire to protect a donor, may inadvertently be treating the donor paternalistically rather than respecting the donor's autonomy. Is it sometimes true that ILDAs may have specific experience(s) that lead them to want to set up protocols they believe are protective of the donor? Yes, however, the key point is for an ILDA to be willing to acknowledge when there is a conflict of values with the potential donor and explore possible options for resolution.

Returning to Susan's case, her husband does not want Susan to donate a kidney to her brother. It can be assumed that this discord will add significant stress to Susan's marriage. On the other hand, Thomas' spouse believes it is imperative that Susan donates. After all, she is a perfect match. Susan, herself, has expressed the desire to move forward with testing to see if she is healthy enough to donate. As mentioned, an ILDA can already foresee potentially irreparable problems that kidney donation may cause to Susan's marriage. Is this marriage conflict going to cause enough emotional harm to Susan so that the ILDA ought to rule her out? Is it in Susan's "best interest" *not* to move forward?

Considering the presenting conflict between Susan and her husband, Bill, regarding organ donation, should Susan and her husband be obligated to go to counseling before Susan can move forward? The ILDA may strongly believe this couple should go to counseling regarding their disagreement. However, the ILDA needs to remember that Susan is not required to get the consent or approval of her husband before she decides to move forward or not with donation. She is independent from her husband regarding informed consent or informed refusal for any medical procedure.

Currently, there are still ongoing, unresolved issues the ILDA needs to consider regarding Susan. For example, protecting Susan from harm(s), advocating for Susan's best interest(s), and ensuring Susan's decision, to donate or not, is free from coercion. Continued discussion with Susan is necessary to determine what her true motivation is to move forward or not move forward with donation. Might she really want to donate her kidney but ultimately decline to move forward because of her husband's pressure *not* to donate? Does she really not want to donate her kidney to her brother, but states she wants to move forward due to pressure from her sister-in-law? Could her husband know something that the team did not uncover about Susan? Would it be appropriate to interview the husband alone with Susan's permission? It might seem appropriate to try to ascertain from the husband if there are any underlying issues that the team needs to know about. He is obviously strongly opposed to her donation of a kidney. However, if the ILDA asks Susan's permission to meet with the husband alone, the ILDA risks adding his or her own pressure/coercion of Susan. Can Susan freely say "no" to the ILDA's request? Susan could believe she might be ruled out if she refuses the ILDA's request. What if Susan's husband is extremely controlling and she truly does not want him to be a part of her donation process? Does Susan really want to move forward with the donation process but now feels the ILDA does not trust her? Susan may wonder why the ILDA is asking for a private meeting. Trust between the ILDA and Susan could possibly be breached, adding additional complications to an already complex case. It is true that the ILDA and transplant team have concerns about this particular donor situation. However, asking for a private meeting with a spouse, even with "permission" from the potential donor, is fraught with potential, unintended coercive consequences. It is a very different case, if Susan, herself, requests the ILDA to meet with her husband to see if the ILDA can help her husband feel better about her donating. Does he have questions that he has not been able to ask? Susan is the driving force of this request. In order to keep the focus on Susan and her independent, competent status, the ILDA could speak with Susan and ask if it would be OK with her if Susan and the ILDA or a transplant social worker meet together with Susan's husband, so that Bill can have another chance to express his concerns about her donation and perhaps give him an opportunity to "vent." The ILDA would need to ask what, if any, concerns Susan might have with this request. The intent of the meeting would be to offer Bill an opportunity to express himself, as Susan's spouse and to have the transplant ILDA or social worker ask any questions of Bill, at that time. Susan may feel better about authorizing a meeting since she will be included. Including her in the meeting better assures she remains in control of her own process. In addition, there is no unintended, inadvertent "message" to Bill that he has any true say in Susan's decision. Susan does not need her husband's permission to move forward with donation.

Ultimately, the ILDA will need to seek Susan's true desire, based on what she really, in her heart, wants to do concerning donation. If it is clear that Susan cannot overcome the pressure from others, then she is indeed being successfully coerced and should be ruled out.

However, if Susan can clearly state her desire to either move forward or not with donation, based on *her* autonomous desire to donate, then she ought not to be ruled out just because of a concern about possible coercion and harm to her marriage. In other words, just because there can be pressure from others and concern for coercion exits, it is the obligation of the ILDA not to make any assumptions at this point. While none of us want to see a potential donor with Susan's conflicts, an ILDA needs to use extreme caution in not overlaying his or her own values onto Susan. Perhaps an ILDA would not donate an organ if it put his or her marriage in jeopardy. For the ILDA, there may be a temptation to rule Susan out at this point, because it is not in Susan's best interest to harm to her marriage.

Whether Susan moves forward with organ donation or not, she faces a dilemma. Fortunately, and possibly unfortunately, this is Susan's family. She comes to transplant with this set of circumstances.

Susan's dilemma, at this point, raises more questions rather than offering clearcut answers. What is in Susan's best interest? Is coercion having an impact on Susan's ability to make a truly autonomous decision? Ultimately, should Susan move forward with donation?

It depends greatly on Susan's responses, when the ILDA or others in transplant pose concerns about the conflicts Susan faces. First, is there good, open communication with the ILDA and others within transplant? Is the ILDA or other transplant team members comfortable with conflict? Ultimately, can the ILDA distinguish between advocacy and protection and paternalism?

Susan's Interview and Outcome

Susan initially attended an introductory transplant meeting with her husband, Bill. After that, Susan insisted on coming alone to future meetings. When the ILDA asked Susan about her support system, Susan stated it would depend on several factors, to be determined. She might or might not have the support of her husband, if she ultimately goes forward with donation. Susan indicates that she is aware she will need support after surgery, should she be able to donate. If she donates her kidney, and does not have the support of her husband, Susan says she has a cousin who understands the situation and, if needed, will help her postoperatively. Her cousin lives in the same town as Susan does.

When the ILDA explores the potential harm to Susan's marriage if she moves forward with donation, Susan states, "I know my husband is opposed to me donating a kidney to my brother. Bill is very protective of me, even when I do not want protection. He does not want me to risk my health. Also, the truth is, Bill feels I am prioritizing my brother over him. This is not a new issue in my marriage. It is just one of many conflicts we have. I love Bill and I would like our marriage to survive."

Acknowledging that Susan would like her marriage to survive, the ILDA poses concerns about the potential irreparable harm her kidney donation could have on her marriage. Can Susan reconcile this issue? As indicated, perhaps it is not in Susan's best interest to donate a kidney to her brother?

While it is acknowledged that Susan may be the best match for Thomas, he still has other options for transplant. The ILDA points out that Susan is in no way obligated to donate to Thomas. Would Susan and Bill consider marriage counseling to sort out the conflict that donation is currently causing in their marriage?

Susan states, "I have suggested marriage counseling to Bill so we can work on some issues in our marriage. Bill refuses to go. I have gone to counseling myself in an attempt to save our marriage. If I ultimately decide to donate and my marriage does not survive, I will feel awful. There is no question about that."

"However, my brother and I are very close. I would do anything I could for him. It is true that I did not have a choice about donating my bone marrow. I was 10 years old. However, even then, I knew I had done something special for my brother. Do I still feel somewhat responsible for him? Yes, I am his 'big sister' and if I can help him, I want to. However, I also want to ensure I am healthy enough to donate. I cannot unduly risk my current or future health because if my marriage does not survive, I will need to be totally prepared to support myself."

When faced with the concern about Bill and Nancy pressuring her, Susan responds, "This pressure is one reason I waited several weeks to contact your transplant center before exploring donation. I had to sort out my feelings. I know whether I donate or not, someone is going to be greatly disappointed. I do feel pressure to make the right decision. To decide what the right decision is, I am the type of person who needs to think about things, look at all the angles and then decide on the decision that feels right to me. Against my better judgment, I did come to the first meeting with Bill. I knew of his concerns and he got to express them to your transplant center. However, after he and Nancy got into even more conflict, I knew I had to explore the transplant option by myself, for myself. I know, of course, that Nancy wants me to give a kidney to my brother. She loves Tom and is desperate for him to have a transplant. On the other hand, my husband does not want me to donate. This situation has already caused huge conflict that may have a lasting negative effect on my family. I wish my circumstances were different."

The ILDA asks Susan if she can separate her true desire to donate or not from the desires of her husband and sister-in-law. In addition, the ILDA raises the issue of what her brother, Thomas, wants her to do. Is he asking Susan to donate? Is he presuming she will donate? Is Thomas using his wife, Nancy, to pressure Susan?

Susan previously stated that she and her brother share a close relationship. Of interest, but not necessarily a surprise, Susan indicates that Thomas wants her to make the best decision for herself. He knows a decision to donate may cause permanent harm to her marriage. Thomas also knows his wife wants Susan to donate. Thomas and Susan have had several heart-to-heart discussions, and Susan truly knows, no matter the decision, she and Thomas will still remain close. Susan has concern for her brother but is not feeling additional pressure from her brother.

Susan shares with the ILDA that she cannot make a totally informed decision, unless she knows she is healthy enough to undergo kidney donation. She currently feels fine and knows of no health problems. However, she understands the importance of the medical testing required of donors to ensure they are healthy enough to donate.

Considering the obligations of the ILDA to advocate for Susan's best interest(s), protecting her from harm(s) and ensuring her decision is not ultimately coerced, ought the ILDA continue to move Susan forward in the transplant process? Should the ILDA rule her out based on the circumstances of her case?

Susan does face coercive pressure from her husband and her sister-in-law. Critical to determine is whether her autonomy has been trumped by others' attempts to coerce her. Has Susan been able to separate her true desire from the wishes of others?

Susan appears to have good insight into her situation. She is aware and acknowledges pressure from her husband and sister-in-law. Susan sought counseling on her own, when her husband refused to work on the conflict in their marriage. While Susan would prefer that her marriage remain intact, she is not willing to allow pressure from her husband to automatically rule the day. Susan also is able to acknowledge the pressure from her sister-in-law. Susan has taken protective action for herself by choosing to separate herself from the conflict. She has also had private conversations with her brother and she indicates there is not pressure from her brother. He wants what is best for her.

For Susan, specifically, it has been imperative that she meet with the ILDA and others from transplant, by herself. In addition, she has explored other potential support people, should her husband choose not to help her postoperatively.

Susan demonstrates good insight about her autonomous decision-making process, because she needs to know if she is healthy enough to donate before she makes her final decision. What if medical testing were to show she is not a good candidate? Maybe, instead of going through all the medical testing, Susan would like the ILDA's help in stating there are some concerns that prevent Susan from going forward? The ILDA knows offering Susan this option might mitigate her marital harm and reduce pressure from her sister-in-law. Might this option be protective of Susan's best interest(s)?

A recipient and potential donor both know many factors go into making an ultimate decision to move forward with a specific donor. Susan could be ruled out by transplant to make it easier for Susan. The decision would be out of Susan's hands. Would this not be in Susan's best interest? Transplant could offer a vague response about the reasons Susan is being ruled out. Then, all parties could be reminded about protecting patient confidentiality by not sharing donor or recipient information. The ILDA might feel better if he or she takes responsibility for ruling Susan out. How could it be in Susan's best interest to have to choose between her husband and brother and sister-in-law? The ILDA might be tempted to protect Susan's perceived best interests in this manner. He or she could advocate for Susan not to move forward, because the ILDA needs to protect Susan from the real and potential emotional harm her situation presents. The ILDA could discuss with Susan the potential that the ILDA may not recommend for her to proceed with donation and ask how she feels about this outcome.

Surprisingly, Susan does not embrace this idea. She wants to move forward with medical testing so she can make her own decision. Susan states taking the decision out of her hands does not offer her comfort. For her, it feels less than honest and she wants to protect the integrity of her own process. Susan states that she has worked hard in counseling to be her own person. Susan states ruling her out, without her agreement, would make her feel terrible. Susan indicates that even though her personal decision to donate or not is difficult, she wants the decision to be her own. Susan emphasizes that she already faces decision-making pressure from her husband and sister-in-law, she does not want the ILDA to make a decision for her. From Susan's perspective, this would feel like one more person telling her what she ought to do.

The ILDA does not really want Susan to go forward due to the conflict of the situation. It is just not a good idea. This ILDA has the power to rule out a donor, even if the donor wants to move forward. Susan also knows this. Should the ILDA overrule Susan's desire to move forward, since the ILDA believes it is in the best interest of Susan not to go forward due to her situation?

Additional Facts

From Susan's perspective, a rule out by the ILDA will feel like just one more person telling her what to do. Is it in Susan's best interest, from her perspective, to rule her out? The answer is no. Susan will feel, in her words "terrible," if she is ruled out without her agreement. Susan agrees she could be ruled out for medical reasons, if there are true medical concerns. However, she does not yet know if there are medical concerns because she has not been through required testing.

It is true the ILDA is not comfortable with Susan's predicament. Not being comfortable with this situation is a very reasonable response. Susan's situation presents many conflicts. One has to carefully sort through the facts of this specific situation to make a final recommendation with and for Susan.

We have established that Susan has consciously distanced herself from the pressure of her husband and sister-in-law. She has insight into her how her decision, either way, may affect her relationship with her husband and/or her sister-in-law. While there are people attempting to coerce Susan, have they been successful in forcing her to make a decision against her own values? Have they been successful in influencing her decision to move forward or not move forward with donating a kidney to her brother? No. At this time, successful coercion is not present. Susan's autonomous decision-making ability is intact.

From Susan's perspective, it is in her best interest to continue to move forward with required medical testing. This is the final piece of information that Susan needs to make her ultimate decision regarding donation. As noted, Susan indicates it would make her feel terrible to be ruled out by the ILDA before going forward with medical testing, because from Susan's perspective, this would have a negative impact on the integrity of her decision-making process.

Even though the ILDA foresees emotional harm for Susan if she is not ruled out by the ILDA, in Susan's specific situation, a rule out by the ILDA creates additional harm to Susan. While many potential donors facing Susan's situation might express relief when an ILDA helps with a rule out, this is not so for Susan. Could it be that allowing Susan to continue to move forward, despite the inherent conflicts, promotes her best interest?

Unfortunately, this is not a "feel good" transplant case. No matter the decision, the ILDA or other members from transplant may never feel comfortable with conflicts like this. It is indeed tempting to rule out Susan before she is potentially put in the position of harming a marriage she would like to save. If Susan had accepted the offer of a rule out by the ILDA, it would, perhaps, be easier for the ILDA and others involved with this potential donor. Factually, though, from Susan's perspective, this option adds harm rather than reducing it. It is protective of Susan to not rule her out in this manner. Her autonomy is negatively affected by having the ILDA rule her out without her agreement. The decision to rule Susan out, based on the ILDA's concerns begins to change from perceived protection of Susan into paternalistic decision making for her.

Given all the facts of this case, what is the best way the ILDA can both protect and advocate with and for Susan? What recommendation should he or she make?

Susan is a competent adult who is able to demonstrate the ability to make an autonomous decision. She needs more information from medical testing to make a truly informed decision to opt in or out of donating a kidney. Without this medical testing, Susan is denied the ability to fully make an informed decision, even though she has the ability and capacity to make an informed decision. This is not protective of Susan and, as she has stated, this would be "terrible" for her.

On what factual basis would an ILDA depend on, to deny Susan the ability to move forward with medical testing? She is competent, her autonomy is intact, and she is willing to donate and is not being influenced by the pressures to, or not to, donate. From her perspective, it would cause her harm to be ruled out prematurely. It is in her best interest to get as much information as possible, in order for her to make the best decision for herself.

It is now time for the ILDA to present Susan's situation to the transplant team. After careful consideration, the ILDA's recommendation is to move her forward to continue the required medical workup for donation. Other members of the team express concern to the ILDA that it is not in the best interest of Susan to move forward. However, the ILDA is able to factually outline the ethical underpinnings that support the ILDA's recommendation that Susan be allowed to move forward.

Susan's autonomy is intact; she is competent, and willing to donate. Coercive attempts to change her mind have not worked. She is able to make an independent decision.

It is in Susan's best interest to move forward because she will suffer additional harm if she is declined from donation prematurely. Susan understands and agrees that if there are medical concerns discovered during testing, and these medical concerns would rule anyone else out, then she should be ruled out, as well. As indicated, Susan is simply trying to get all the facts she needs to make an informed decision.

The ILDA strongly advocates for Susan to move forward. Concerns have been explored, and Susan has addressed each concern with insight and self-awareness.

The ILDA is successful in allowing Susan to move forward. It is true the ILDA does not feel good about Susan's situation. The ILDA would have preferred to protect Susan by ruling her out. However, the ILDA recognized that transplant would be blocking a competent adult, who has good capacity for decision making. In addition, there is ultimately no effective coercion in Susan's situation.

The ILDA's initial perspective was to paternalistically protect Susan from harm that the ILDA considered was not in Susan's best interest. However, after objectively reviewing the facts of this situation, the ILDA was able to move from a paternalistic "protection" to actual protection and promotion of Susan's best interests.

Medical testing for Susan may or may not indicate a problem that will rule her out. However, what this entire process demonstrates is that Susan's integrity and the integrity of the donation process is protected. The ILDA has fulfilled the intent of this role, by ensuring attempts at coercion are not influencing the potential donor's decision. The ILDA protected and promoted the best interest of the donor. Ultimately, the ILDA advocated for Susan to move forward not because it was the easiest thing to do, rather it was the right thing to do, specifically for Susan.

The position of the ILDA is a critical, pivotal role. As this case demonstrates, it is also critical that an ILDA be aware of his or her own value system. The ILDA must be able to separate his or her own values from the values of the potential donor. Consistent ethical principles need to be applied to any donor situation, especially situations that present with complex issues.

Susan's case allowed exploration of key ethical underpinnings that informed and assisted the ILDA to traverse the complexities and pitfalls of this challenging situation. A working knowledge of pertinent ethical principles helps to ensure consistency in this critical role.

References

1. Criteria for selection of living donor needs to be consistent with general principles of medical ethics. Federal Register, Vol. 72, No. 61, March 30, 2007, Dept. of Health and Human Resources, Centers for Medicare and Medicaid Services 42 CFR parts 405,482,488,498/Rules and Regulations.
2. Steel J, Dunlavy A, Friday M, Kingsley K, Brower D, Unruh M, et al. A national survey of independent living donor advocates: the need for practice guidelines. Am J Transplant. 2012;12:2141–9.
3. Schloendorff v Society of New York Hospital, 211. N.Y. 125, 105 N.E. 92 (1914). http://en.wikipedia.org/wiki/Schloendorff_v_Society_of_New_York_Hospital. (Accessed June 24, 2013).
4. Wikipedia, The Free Encyclopedia. Coercion. http://en.wikipedia.org/wiki:coercion_persuasion. (Accessed June 24, 2013).
5. Wikipedia, The Free Encyclopedia. Paternalism. http:// en.wikipedia.org/wiki/Paternalism. (Accessed June 24, 2013).

Chapter 23
Racial Disparities in Kidney Transplant and Living Donation

Tanjala S. Purnell and L. Ebony Boulware

Disparities in the Need for Kidney Transplantation

The rapidly increasing prevalence of end-stage renal disease (ESRD), characterized by the failure of kidney function, has generated national efforts to alleviate the public health burden of this life-threatening condition. Currently, approximately 560,000 US adults are treated for ESRD, a condition that results in poor survival, poor health-related quality of life, and high health care costs [1]. Although patients with ESRD comprise less than 1 % of Medicare beneficiaries, they account for over 6 % of Medicare spending, resulting in estimated costs to Medicare of over $ 20 billion annually [1, 2].

An estimated 26 million adults in the U.S. currently have some degree of kidney damage [3], a major risk factor for the development of ESRD. Racial–ethnic minorities are substantially more likely to develop ESRD than Whites [1, 4, 5]. Adjusted rates of ESRD among African-Americans, Native Americans, and Asians are significantly higher than rates of ESRD among Whites [1] (Fig. 23.1), and ESRD rates among Hispanics are also significantly higher than rates among non-Hispanics [1] (Fig. 23.2). Compared to Whites, African-Americans experience up to fourfold greater risk of developing ESRD [1]. African-Americans and Hispanics account for approximately 47 % of the ESRD population, while comprising only 28 % of the overall US population [1, 6].

Disparities in rates of ESRD have been attributed to a multi-factorial combination of genetic, environmental, cultural, and socioeconomic influences [7]. Diabetes and hypertension are the leading causes of ESRD (accounting for over 70 % of the reported ESRD cases in the U.S.) [1], and these diseases disproportionately impact racial–ethnic minorities. Other causes include HIV infection, sickle cell disease,

---

T. S. Purnell (✉) · L. E. Boulware
Department of Medicine/General Internal Medicine, Johns Hopkins School of Medicine, 2024 E. Monument Street, Suite 2-600, 21205, Baltimore, MD, USA
e-mail: tpurnel1@jhmi.edu

L. E. Boulware
e-mail: lboulwa@jhmi.edu

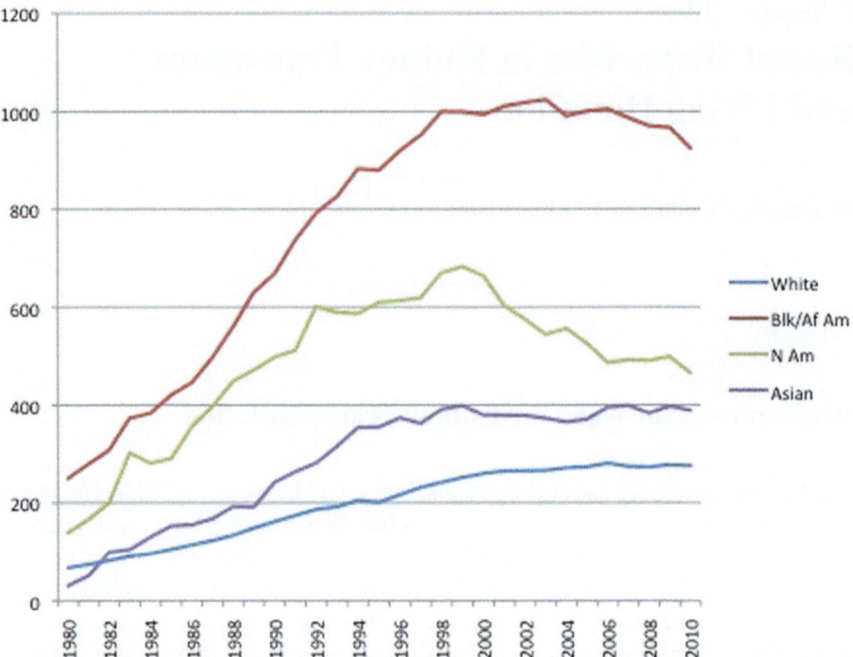

Fig. 23.1 Adjusted rates of end-stage renal disease (ESRD) by race (1980–2010). Incident ESRD patients. Adjusted for age/gender. (Reference: 2005 ESRD patients. Data Source: US Renal Data System, USRDS 2012 Annual Data Report: Atlas of Chronic Kidney Disease and End-Stage Renal Disease in the United States, National Institutes of Health, National Institute of Diabetes and Digestive and Kidney Diseases, Bethesda, MD, 2012)

systemic lupus erythematosus, heroin abuse and/or dependence, kidney stones, chronic kidney infections, and certain cancers [1].

Disparities in Access to Kidney Transplantation

Patients with ESRD require replacement of their kidney function (in the form of dialysis treatment or kidney transplantation) to sustain life. While dialysis is currently the most common therapy used to treat ESRD, kidney transplantation offers patients improved life expectancy at less cost than that for dialysis care [1, 8]. Kidney transplantation is also associated with improved mental health, physical functioning, social functioning, and other quality of life measures, such as the ability to travel and work when compared to patients receiving dialysis treatment [9–12]. Yet, the number of persons on the waiting list for a transplant greatly exceeds the number of available kidneys. Racial–ethnic minorities with ESRD have persistently lagged behind Whites with respect to both placement on the waiting list for deceased donor

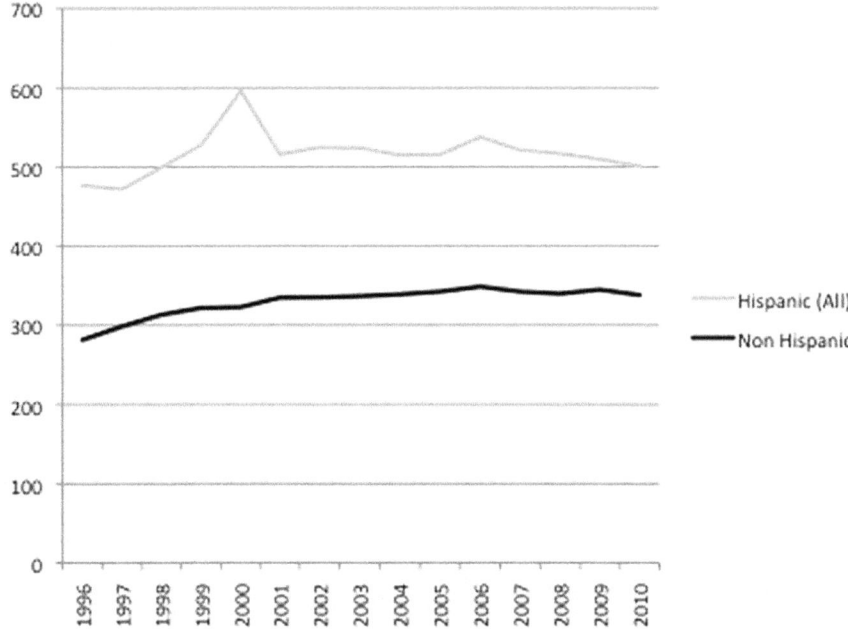

Fig. 23.2 Adjusted rates of end-stage renal disease by Hispanic ethnicity (1996–2010). Incident ESRD patients. Adjusted for age/gender. (Reference: 2005 ESRD patients. Data Source: US Renal Data System, USRDS 2012 Annual Data Report: Atlas of Chronic Kidney Disease and End-Stage Renal Disease in the United States, National Institutes of Health, National Institute of Diabetes and Digestive and Kidney Diseases, Bethesda, MD, 2012)

kidneys and receipt of deceased donor transplants [1, 4, 13–16] (Fig. 23.3). In 2010, although the rate of deceased donation was 28.1 among African-Americans compared to 21.4 among Whites, the rate of patients receiving transplants from deceased donors was only 2.0 among African-Americans compared to 2.6 among Whites [1].

Racial–ethnic disparities in rates of deceased donor kidney transplants have been attributed to several factors, including immunological incompatibility of deceased donor kidneys, lower rates of referral of racial–ethnic minorities for transplantation, inadequate transplant workup for minorities referred for transplants, human leukocyte antigen (HLA)-mismatching, sociodemographic barriers to the completion of pretransplant steps, disproportionate access to health care, and patient concerns about potential risks associated with transplantation [15–29]. Recent estimates show that American Indians/Alaska Natives, African-Americans, and Hispanics are less likely than Whites to be listed for kidney transplants [4]. Once listed for transplantation, racial–ethnic minorities have been shown to wait longer for kidneys than Whites [1]. For instance, among first-time wait-listed patients registered in 2007, 48.6% of African-Americans and 43.8% of Asians were still waiting for a transplant after 3 years, compared with only 34.5% of White patients [1]. Uninsured patients and those of lower income levels, who also tend to be disproportionately

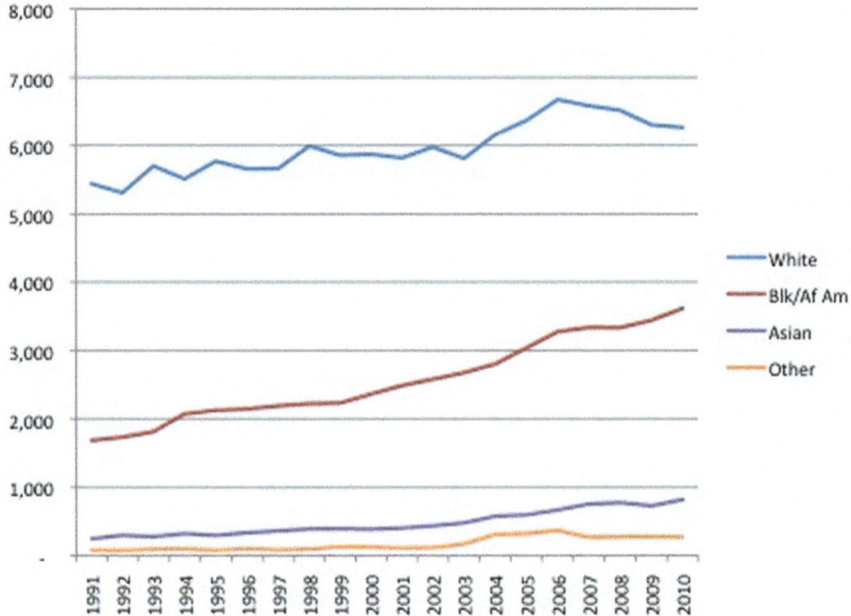

Fig. 23.3 Deceased donor transplants by race (1991–2010). Patients age 18 and older. Includes kidney-alone and kidney-pancreas transplants. (Data Source: US Renal Data System, USRDS 2012 Annual Data Report: Atlas of Chronic Kidney Disease and End-Stage Renal Disease in the United States, National Institutes of Health, National Institute of Diabetes and Digestive and Kidney Diseases, Bethesda, MD, 2012)

made up of racial–ethnic minorities [30], are also less likely to be listed for kidney transplantation.

Potential Role of Living Donation in Narrowing Disparities

Patients with progressing chronic kidney disease, those with newly diagnosed ESRD, and those already on waiting lists for deceased donor kidney transplants may increase their chances of receiving a transplant by also pursuing living donor kidney transplantation (LDKT), in which an ESRD patient receives a kidney from a living friend, family member, or other altruistic person. LDKT is the optimal therapy for many patients with ESRD providing numerous clinical benefits compared to prolonged dialysis or deceased donor kidney transplantation, including better patient and graft survival and improved quality of life [12, 31, 32]. LDKT also provides a mechanism through which patients may bypass lengthy waiting times on deceased donor kidney transplant waiting lists and therefore significantly decrease waiting times for transplants.

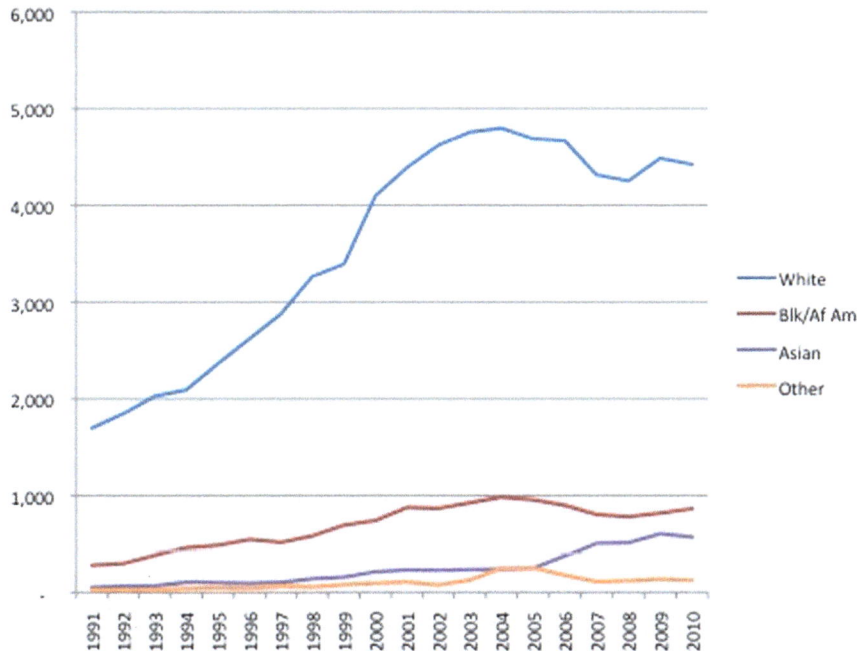

Fig. 23.4 Living donor transplants by race (1991–2010). Patients age 18 and older. Includes kidney-alone and kidney–pancreas transplants. (Data Source: U.S. Renal Data System, USRDS 2012 Annual Data Report: Atlas of Chronic Kidney Disease and End-Stage Renal Disease in the United States, National Institutes of Health, National Institute of Diabetes and Digestive and Kidney Diseases, Bethesda, MD, 2012)

Barriers to Living Kidney Donation for Racial Minorities

Despite the potential benefits of LDKT, minority ESRD patients have been consistently less likely than Whites to receive LDKT over the past two decades (Fig. 23.4), thus limiting the promise of this therapy in addressing inequities in access to kidney transplants [1, 4, 33–35]. For example, recent data show that African-Americans and Hispanics accounted for only 27.5% of the total LDKT recipients in 2012, although they account for over 47% of the ESRD patients [1, 35]. Evidence suggests that racial–ethnic minorities experience unique barriers that contribute to disparities in LDKT at the patient or potential-donor level (e.g., beliefs, concerns, and clinical characteristics) [36–44], health care provider/system level (e.g., decision support, information quality, and perceptions) [27, 45–49], and population-community level (e.g., social awareness, resource allocation, and disease burden) [50–52]. In addition, racial–ethnic minorities may experience these barriers during one or more of the four primary steps along the path to successful completion of LDKT: donor identification, transplant evaluation, kidney transplant, and posttransplant recovery [53]. The development of strategies to address disparities in receipt of LDKT requires a comprehensive understanding of these barriers that impede access to LDKT among racial–ethnic minorities in the U.S. We provide a detailed summary of barriers reported within the published literature later, and we also reference an evidence-based framework (Fig. 23.5) that contextualizes key barriers identified along the path to LDKT [53].

Patient-Related Barriers

Racial–ethnic minorities with ESRD may be more likely than their White counterparts to experience a number of patient-related barriers to receipt of LDKT, including unmet concerns about the physical, psychological, and financial risks associated with LDKT; patients' concerns about their ability to initiate LDKT discussions within their families; and less willingness to approach potential donors due to concerns about potential risks for living donors [41, 42, 46]. Studies of African-American and Hispanic patients have also identified poor LDKT knowledge, medical mistrust, and concerns about surgical risks of LDKT as potential barriers that may impede efforts to identify and approach potential live donors [37–40]. Alvaro et al. conducted focus groups of Hispanic patients and reported that lack of knowledge about living donation, concerns about potential harm to the donor, and expectations that a relative would initiate an offer to donate were identified as barriers to identifying and approaching potential donors [37]. A study by Pradel et al. also found that surgical concerns were associated with lower likelihood of considering LDKT, discussing LDKT with their family, or asking for a kidney in those receiving hemodialysis [40]. Evidence suggests that African-American potential recipients may also experience higher rates of psychological denial about the need for a kidney transplant [41, 43]. Results from a survey by Lunsford et al. suggest that African-Americans might cope with the need for a kidney transplant differently than non-African-Americans, and that African-American potential recipients may be less acceptable of and more likely to deny the need for a transplant [43]. This denial might affect persuasiveness or willingness to ask for live donation.

Concerns about the potential risks for living donors might also contribute to racial–ethnic minorities' reported difficulties identifying and approaching potential donors within their families, social networks, and communities. Boulware et al. reported that African-American patients were concerned about potential burdening of family members, potential donors' future health, and their future inability to donate a kidney to another family member who might need it, and feelings of guilt or coercing family members [41]. Within focus groups that included African-American and Asian potential transplant recipients, Waterman et al. also noted concerns about living donation, including feelings of guilt or indebtedness to the donor, harm or inconvenience to the donors, concerns that the potential donor might need the kidney later, and concerns over disappointing the donor if the transplant failed [42].

In addition to barriers encountered during donor identification, evidence suggests that higher rates of chronic illnesses, such as obesity, diabetes, and hypertension among racial–ethnic minorities may contribute to lower likelihood of completing

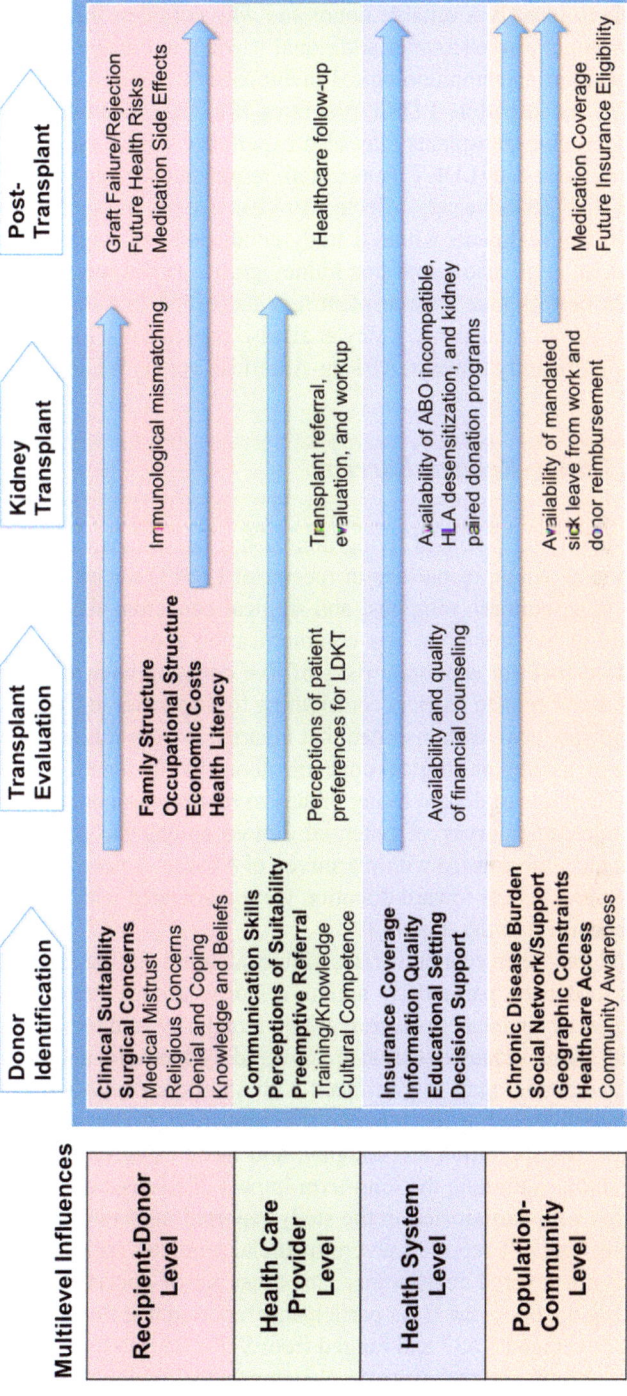

Fig. 23.5 Multilevel influences contributing to barriers to LDKT for racial–ethnic minorities. [54]

the transplant evaluation and workup process. In addition, racial–ethnic minorities who are able to identify a suitable donor and who complete the transplant evaluation process might also encounter additional barriers to transplant surgery, such as HLA sensitization and immunological incompatibility due to limited availability of blood-type incompatible LDKT programs [81]. Racial–ethnic minorities who successfully receive transplants may also experience unique barriers that threaten the long-term success of LDKT. Burke et al. found that African-American race and presence of diabetes adversely affected 10-year patient and graft survival among kidney transplant recipients within a study conducted at a single transplant center [54]. Douzdijan et al. also found that kidney graft survival was adversely affected by African-American race for transplant recipients [55]. In a study of patients who previously received transplants, Foley et al. also reported that kidney graft survival rates were significantly lower in African-American versus White recipients [56].

Potential Donor-Related Barriers

Difficulty identifying potential living donors has been shown to be a major contributor to racial–ethnic disparities in receipt of LDKT. Racial–ethnic differences in attitudes (e.g., cultural, religious, and surgical concerns) about and willingness to participate in live donation, less communication about LDKT within families, and lower tolerance for economic risks of live donation have all been implicated as potential donor-related barriers contributing to disparities in living donation [38, 39, 57]. Boulware et al. demonstrated that mistrust in hospitals and concerns about discrimination, as well as surgical concerns about living donation were associated with less willingness to donate living organs to relatives as noted within a national household telephone survey of potential donors among the general public [38]. Robinson et al. demonstrated within a survey of African-American potential donors that attitudes and beliefs toward donation were associated with self-reported willingness to become a living donor [39].

Short- and long-term economic risks of live donation may be associated with less willingness to donate, particularly among minority groups already disproportionately burdened by financial pressures. While a majority of direct medical costs associated with living kidney donation are covered by Medicare and/or private health insurance, live donors may still be faced with additional costs associated with the donation process, including lost wages due to time away from work, incidental medical expenses, transportation and lodging, and hired caregiver or child-care costs [58–61]. A study examining the long-term impact of live donation found that 19 % of live donors who participated in the study reported moderate financial problems after donating, and 4 % reported severe financial problems (such as lost work time, medical bills not covered by insurance, and other out-of-pocket expenses) [58]. In a study of living donors in the U.S., participants reported that financial costs incurred by the donor averaged $ 837 and ranged from $ 0 to 28,906 [62]. Potential donors' concerns about future insurability may also impact their willingness to donate. Findings from recent studies suggest that becoming a living donor may impact one's ability to obtain life, health, and disability insurance [60, 63]. A study of living donors in the U.S. found that while many insurance companies reported being willing to insure these individuals, a number of living donors have reported difficulties obtaining insurance coverage after donation [60]. Existing educational resources about LDKT may also lack important information that could alleviate minorities' concerns about the potential short- and long-term economic burden of LDKT.

In addition to barriers that contribute to disparities in the identification of potentially willing donors, some minorities who are actually willing to donate may not be healthy enough (i.e., clinically suitable) to complete the donor evaluation and surgical processes. Reeves-Daniel et al. performed a study of unsuccessful live kidney donations and found that African-American potential donors were more likely to be excluded due to obesity or failure to complete the transplant evaluation [49]. Tankersely et al. performed a study of inpatient donor and recipient evaluations and found that African-American patients were less likely than Whites to identify clinically suitable potential live donors at the time of evaluations due to higher rates of previously undetected comorbid medical conditions, such as hypertension among them [50]. A study of patients referred for potential live kidney donation by Lunsford et al. found that African-Americans were more likely to be lost to follow-up than non-African-Americans due to higher rates of incompatible blood types, high body mass index, or ineligible recipients [51].

Racial–ethnic minorities who complete the evaluation and surgical processes may also experience long-term risks after the transplant surgery. African-American living donors may face increased risk of developing ESRD and may be more likely than White donors to need a kidney in the future. Gibney et al. found that future risk of developing ESRD might be more exaggerated in African-American versus White donors within a study using organ procurement and transplantation network (OPTN) data [64, 65]. In a study to assess potential racial differences in posttransplant kidney function for living donors, Doshi et al. found that postdonation serum creatinine levels were slightly higher for African-American donors compared to Whites [66]. In a study of OPTN and administrative data, Lentine et al. found that after kidney donation, African-American and Hispanic donors had an increased risk of hypertension, diabetes requiring drug therapy, and chronic kidney disease, compared with White donors [67]. Nogueira et al. also found that African-American living kidney donors experienced a high incidence of hypertension and a modest drop in kidney functioning post donation in a study of long-term donor outcomes [68]. Within a study of national trends and outcomes following live kidney donation, Segev et al. reported that surgical mortality from live donation was higher in African-American donors compared with White and Hispanic donors [69].

Health Care Provider and System-Related Barriers

Racial–ethnic minorities' poorer access to routine health care, lack of provider–patient and provider–family discussions regarding LDKT, and health care providers' perceptions about minority patients' preferences and suitability for LDKT may be associated with lower rates of LDKT education and transplant referral for minority patients [27, 45–46]. Providers' views about the benefits of transplantation and beliefs about reasons for racial–ethnic differences in access to transplantation may affect how (or whether) they present LDKT as a treatment option to racial–ethnic minority patients. Ayanian et al. conducted a survey of nephrologists in the U.S. and reported that physicians were less likely to believe that transplantation improves survival for African-Americans than Whites [27]. African-American patients participating in the study were also less likely than White patients to report receiving some or a lot of information about transplantation. Within focus groups conducted to assess health care professionals' beliefs about barriers contributing to lower rates of donor identification for African-American patients, Shilling et al. revealed that providers noted lack of clinical suitability, financial concerns, reluctance to approach potential donors, surgical fears, medical mistrust, and less awareness of LDKT as potential barriers [45]. Suboptimal rates of patient–physician discussion and family–physician discussions about LDKT prior to ESRD may serve as additional barriers to donor identification among racial–ethnic minorities. Within a survey of African-Americans patients, spouses, and children, Boulware et al. found that despite most patients expressing desire for a transplant, only 68% of patients and less than 50% of their spouses had discussed transplantation with physicians [46]. These differences in provider–patient interactions may, in part, reflect variations in provider communication skills and cultural competence, knowledge about LDKT, and perceptions of patient suitability and preferences for LDKT.

Lower rates of transplant referrals and delayed receipt of nephrology subspecialty care prior to renal replacement therapy initiation have also been associated with higher rates of incomplete evaluations. Notably, Ayanian et al. found that African-American patients were less likely to be referred for evaluation at a transplant center, even after adjustment for patients' preferences and expectations about transplantation, coexisting illnesses, or socioeconomic factors [21]. Health care providers' perceptions of patients' suitability for LDKT (and their inherent biases about patients' preferences for and adherence to medical therapies) may also lead to lower rates of transplant evaluation and higher rates of incomplete workups among minority potential recipients compared to Whites [21]. Ayanian et al. conducted a survey of nephrologists in the U.S. and reported that physicians were less likely to believe that transplantation improves survival for African-Americans than Whites, and more likely to believe that disparities in rates of transplant were due to differences in patients' preferences, availability of living donors, failure to complete evaluations, and comorbid illnesses [27]. Epstein et al. examined data from five US states and reported that among patients considered clinically appropriate for transplants, African-Americans were less likely than Whites to be referred for transplant evaluations [15]. Lower rates of preemptive LDKT referrals for racial–ethnic minority patients, which result in higher rates of dialysis initiation, might also contribute to higher rates of HLA sensitization and higher burden of medical complications for minorities that impede successful LDKT [70]. Kinchen et al. conducted a national study and found that late evaluations by a nephrologist were associated with greater burden and severity of chronic illnesses and were more common among African-American men than White men [71]. Reduced health care access, including poor availability or utilization of routine follow-up medical care and less health insurance coverage may also contribute to suboptimal long-term clinical outcomes for minority patients and living donors who receive LDKT.

Population and Community-Related Barriers

Population and community-level barriers, such as suboptimal education and poor awareness about the need for living donors, neighborhood resource deprivation, and high rates of chronic illnesses within minority families and social networks also contribute to disparities in LDKT. Suboptimal quality of educational information about LDKT and lack of decision support regarding LDKT as a treatment option may lead to less awareness about the benefits of and need for LDKT within minority communities. Alvaro et al. noted that Hispanic patients reported lack of knowledge about living donation as a barrier to identifying potential donors within their networks and communities [37]. In addition, because a majority of LDKT recipients receive kidneys donated by relatives or nonrelatives emerging from recipients' close social networks, the disproportionately high burden of chronic diseases, particularly diabetes and hypertension, within racial–ethnic minorities' families and social networks may reduce the potential donor pool for many minority potential recipients. Lei et al. reported familial clustering of kidney disease within a population-based study of patients with kidney disease [47]. A study by Gaylin et al. showed that co-morbid medical conditions, such as cardiovascular disease and obesity (which are highly prevalent among US racial–ethnic minorities) were associated with lower transplant rates [72].

As evidenced by disproportionately lower kidney transplant rates in areas with higher degrees of poverty, patients and potential donors within minority populations may encounter more geographic and socioeconomic barriers to completing transplant workup. Volkova et al. found that neighborhood poverty was strongly associated with ESRD incidence, and increasing neighborhood poverty was associated with a greater disparity in renal disease rates between African-Americans and Whites [48]. Racial–ethnic disparities in community resource allocation and chronic disease burden may also contribute to racial–ethnic differences in kidney transplant rates. Stolzmann et al. found that lower community income and education levels were associated with lower likelihood of receiving transplants [73]. Within a study of United States Renal Data System (USRDS) and US census data, Hall et al. demonstrated that high levels of neighborhood poverty were associated with lower transplant rates among Asians and Pacific Islanders compared with Whites, and the degree of disparity worsened as rates of neighborhood poverty worsened [74].

Emerging research suggests lower health literacy rates within racial–ethnic minority populations may also serve as an important barrier in referral for and completion of transplant evaluations. Grubbs et al. found that inadequate health literacy among hemodialysis patients was associated with lower rates of referral for transplant evaluations [75]. It is postulated that health care providers may be less willing to refer patients with inadequate health literacy due to concerns about patients' inability to complete required steps necessary for transplanted graft survival [75]. Minimal availability and use of language and health literacy-appropriate educational resources about LDKT may contribute to minorities' higher rates of incomplete LDKT workups.

Emerging Strategies to Reduce Barriers to Living Donation

A number of promising initiatives have been recently implemented that could address some of the barriers to LDKT highlighted within this chapter [53] (Table 23.1). Current initiatives include home-based patient and family interventions, culturally sensitive educational and behavioral interventions for patients and families, standardized transplant training for non-transplant health care professionals, increased community awareness about the need for LDKT, and population-based screening programs to detect ESRD and associated risk factors [53]. A number of additional behavioral and clinical interventions have also been implemented to address barriers to completion of the LDKT process. Recent initiatives, targeted at patients and potential donors, health care providers and the health system, and population and community factors include:

Targeting Patients and Potential Donors

- Home, community, and clinic-based LDKT educational programs [76, 77].
- Involvement of patients' extended social networks in educational efforts [78, 79].
- Culturally sensitive preemptive transplant education and behavioral programs [80].

Targeting Health Care Providers and Systems

- Standardized LDKT training for non-transplant health care professionals.
- Paired kidney donation, HLA desensitization, and ABO-incompatible programs to overcome immunological barriers [81].

Table 23.1 Promising initiatives to address barriers to living kidney donation for racial–ethnic minorities [53]

	Donor identification initiatives	Transplant evaluation initiatives	Kidney transplant initiatives	Posttransplant initiatives
Recipient–donor initiatives	Culturally sensitive home and community-based education Programs to educate and engage patients' families and social networks	Financial counseling to address insurance and economic concerns	Educational/behavioral interventions to improve preemptive transplant education	Cultural, literacy, and language appropriate efforts to support patient self-care
Health care provider initiatives	Enhanced provider-patient/family LDKT education Cultural competency and racial diversity of health care providers	Educational support from heterogeneous team of health professionals	Improved health care access and continuity of care	Long-term medical follow-up for living donors Pharmacist-led counseling about medication therapy and adherence
Health system initiatives	Standardized transplant education and training for non-transplant medical professionals	Partnerships with non-health care professionals to enhance social support	Paired kidney exchange programs HLA desensitization and ABO incompatible programs	Comprehensive tracking and health-related monitoring of living donors
Population-community initiatives	Community-based partnerships to promote awareness and trust in minority communities Increased availability of healthy foods, safe physical activity space, and community health screenings	Satellite outreach transplant centers to address potential geographic barriers and enhance rates of transplant referral in rural areas	Federal and state policies to support living donors	Expanded medication coverage and access to primary health care Policies to ensure future insurance eligibility for living donors

LDKT living donor kidney transplantation, *HLA* human leukocyte antigen

Targeting Populations and Communities

- Increased availability of fresh, nutritious foods and access to safe public spaces for exercise and recreation [82].
- Increased community awareness and population-based screening programs for kidney disease and related risk factors (e.g., hypertension and diabetes) [83].
- Initiatives to bring satellite transplant clinics to rural areas to address geographic barriers.

However, many of these initiatives are relatively new. Thus, evidence of long-term effectiveness and optimal methods for implementing and disseminating the interventions are not yet clear. Continued work is needed to enhance existing initiatives and to inform the development of future interventions to overcome racial–ethnic disparities in LDKT.

Policy Initiatives to Reduce Barriers to Living Donation

Over the past decade, a number of federal and state policies have been enacted to provide support for living donors, ranging from paid or unpaid leave and from work to tax benefits for living donors [84]. The National Organ Donor Leave Act of 1999 provides additional leave time from work for living donors who are federal employees [85]. The passage of the 2004 Organ Donation and Recovery Improvement Act authorizes $ 25 million in new resources for efforts to increase donation, including establishment of the National Living Donor Assistance Program, which provides grants for reimbursement of travel and subsistence expenses and incidental nonmedical expenses incurred by low-income individuals undergoing clinical evaluation for living kidney donation [86]. The Medicare Improvements for Patients and Providers Act of 2008 aims to enhance timely provider–patient LDKT education and decision support for pre-ESRD patients. The Medicare National Transplant Education Quality Improvement Initiative, which links dialysis facility quality measures to reimbursement, is a system-level policy intervention designed to improve rates of transplant education within in-center hemodialysis facilities.

There are also a number of proposed policies, such as the Comprehensive Immunosuppressive Drug Coverage for Kidney Transplant Patients Act of 2013 (H.R. 1428, 113th) [87], which aims to amend Title 18 of the Social Security Act to terminate the 36-month limit of immunosuppressive drug coverage for transplant recipients. Additionally, the Kidney Care Quality and Improvement Act of 2005 (H.R. 1298, 109th) [88] and the Kidney Care Quality and Education Act of 2007 (S. 691, 110th) [89] both include provisions for improving the benefits of the Medicare Program for beneficiaries with kidney disease, such as increased kidney disease patient education and public awareness.

Implications and Future Directions for Living Donor Advocacy

In conclusion, racial–ethnic disparities in the prevalence of ESRD are stark, and unequal rates of transplants among minorities compared to Whites exacerbate health inequities. Barriers to kidney transplants exist at multiple levels, and interventions are slowly emerging to address these barriers. Policy initiatives to overcome some barriers exist, but have not yet demonstrated effectiveness in narrowing racial–ethnic disparities in access to LDKT. To further support LDKT and eliminate disparities in LDKT, broad dissemination of successful interventions targeting patient, physician, and health system barriers is needed. Examination of existing policies and ways in which policies might be tailored or expanded to further encourage LDKT may also be warranted. Finally, sustained partnerships among health care professionals, policy makers, patient/donor advocacy groups, and leaders within minority communities may support efforts to mitigate disparities in LDKT for racial–ethnic minorities.

Acknowledgments This work was supported in part by the National Heart, Lung, and Blood Institute (5T32HL007180) and the National Institute of Diabetes and Digestive and Kidney Diseases (1R01DK079682 and 1R01DK098759).

References

1. U.S. Renal Data System, USRDS 2011 Annual Data Report: Atlas of Chronic Kidney Disease and End-Stage Renal Disease in the United States, National Institutes of Health, National Institute of Diabetes and Digestive and Kidney Diseases, Bethesda, MD, 2011.
2. American Association of Kidney Patients. AAKP Reviews 30 Years of the Medicare ESRD Program. http://www.aakp.org/aakp-library/30-years-medicare-esrd-program. Accessed Apr 2012.
3. Coresh J, Selvin E, Stevens LA, Manzi J, Kusek JW, Eggers P, et al. Prevalence of chronic kidney disease in the United States. JAMA. 2007;298:2038–47.
4. Agency for Health care Research and Quality. 2011 National Health care Disparities Report. Rockville, MD: U.S. Department of Health and Human Services, Agency for Health care Research and Quality; March 2012. AHRQ Pub. No. 12–0006.
5. Young CJ, Gaston RS. African Americans and renal transplantation: Disproportionate need, limited access, and impaired outcomes. Am J Med Sci. 2002;323:94–9.
6. United States Census Bureau. Population Estimates. http://www.census.gov/popest/estimates.php. Accessed Apr 2012.
7. Martins D, Tareen N, Norris KC. The epidemiology of end-stage renal disease among African Americans. Am J Med Sci. 2002;323:65–71.
8. Wolfe RA, Ashby VB, Milford EL, Ojo AO, Ettenger RE, Agodoa LYC, et al. Comparison of mortality in all patients on dialysis, patients on dialysis awaiting transplantation, and recipients of a first cadaveric transplant. N Engl J Med. 1999;341(23):1725–30.
9. Purnell TS, Auguste P, Crews DC, Lamprea-Montealegre J, Olufade T, Greer RC, et al. Comparison of life participation activities among adults treated by hemodialysis, peritoneal dialysis, and kidney transplantation: A systematic review. Am J Kidney Dis. 2013 May [Epub ahead of print].

10. Ichikawa Y, Fujisawa M, Hirose E, Kageyama T, Miyamoto Y, Sakai Y, et al. Quality of life in kidney transplant patients. Transplant Proc. 2000;32(7):1815–6.
11. Manninen DL, Evans RW, Dugan MK. Work disability, functional limitations, and the health status of kidney transplantation recipients post-transplant (Los Angeles: UCLA Tissue Typing Laboratory). Clinical Transplants. 1991;2:193–203.
12. Jofre R, Lopez-Gomez JM, Moreno F, Sanz-Guajardo D, Valderrabano F. Changes in quality of life after renal transplantation. Am J Kidney Dis. 1998;32(1):93–100.
13. Eggers PW. Racial differences in access to kidney transplantation. Health Care Financing Rev. 1995;17(2):89–103.
14. Delano BG, Macey L, Friedman EA. Gender and racial disparity in peritoneal dialysis patients undergoing kidney transplantation. Am Soc Art Int Org. 1997;43:M861–4.
15. Epstein AM, Ayanian JZ, Keogh JH, Noonan SJ, Armistead N, Cleary PD, et al. Racial disparities in access to renal transplantation—clinically appropriate or due to underuse or overuse? N Engl J Med. 2000;343:1537–44.
16. Sequist TD, Narva AS, Stiles SK, Karp SK, Cass A, Ayanian JZ. Access to renal transplantation among American Indians and Hispanics. Am J Kidney Dis. 2004;44:344–52.
17. Alexander GC, Sehgal AR. Barriers to cadaveric renal transplantation among blacks, women, and the poor. JAMA. 1998;280(13):1148–52.
18. Isaacs RB, Lobo PI, Nock SL, Hanson JA, Ojo AO, Pruett TL. Racial disparities in access to simultaneous pancreas-kidney transplantation in the United States. Am J Kidney Dis. 2000;36:526–33.
19. Ojo A, Port FK. Influence of race and gender on related donor renal transplantation rates. Am J Kidney Dis. 1993;22:835–41.
20. Alexander GC, Sehgal AR. Why hemodialysis patients fail to complete the transplantation process. Am J Kidney Dis. 2001;37(2):321–8.
21. Ayanian JZ, Cleary PD, Weissman JS, Epstein AM. The effect of patients' preferences on racial differences in access to renal transplantation. N Engl J Med. 1999;341(22):1661–9.
22. Gaston RS, Ayres I, Dooley LG, Diethelm AG. Racial equity 2 renal transplantation. The disparate impact of HLA-based allocation. JAMA. 1993;270(11):1352–6.
23. Young CJ, Gaston RS. Renal transplantation in black Americans. N Engl J Med. 2000;343(21):1545–52.
24. Kasiske BL, London W, Ellison MD. Race and socioeconomic factors influencing early placement on the kidney transplant waiting list. J Am Soc Nephrol. 1998;9:2142–7.
25. Soucie JM, Neylan JF, McClellan W. Race and sex differences in the identification of candidates for renal transplantation. Am J Kidney Dis. 1992;19:414–9.
26. Navaneethan SD, Singh S. A systematic review of barriers in access to renal transplantation among African Americans in the United States. Clin Transplant. 2006;20:769–77.
27. Ayanian JZ, Cleary PD, Keogh JH, Noonan SJ, David-Kasdan JA, Epstein AM. Physicians' beliefs about racial differences in referral for renal transplantation. Am J Kidney Dis. 2004;43:350–7.
28. Gordon EJ. Patients' decisions for treatment of end-stage renal disease and their implications for access to transplantation. Soc Sci Med. 2001;53:971–87.
29. Hicks LS, Cleary PD, Epstein AM, Ayanian JZ. Differences in health-related quality of life and treatment preferences among black and White patients with end-stage renal disease. Qual Life Res. 2004;13:1129–37.
30. Hall YN, Rodriguez RA, Boyko EJ, Chertow GM, O'Hare AM. Characteristics of uninsured Americans with chronic kidney disease. J Gen Intern Med. 2009;24(3):917–22.
31. Cecka M. Clinical outcome 2 renal transplantation. Factors influencing patient and graft survival. Surg Clin North Am. 1998;78:133–48.
32. Nanovic L, Kaplan B. The advantage of live-donor kidney transplantation in older recipients. Renal Web and Nature Clinical Practice Nephrology. 2008;5:18–19.
33. Purnell TS, Xu P, Leca N, Hall YN. Racial differences in determinants of live donor kidney transplantation in the United States. Am J Transplant. 2013 June;13(6):1557–65.

34. Gore JL, Danovitch GM, Litwin MS, Pham PT, Singer JS. Disparities in the utilization of live donor kidney transplantation. Am J Transplant. 2009;9:1124–33.
35. United Network for Organ Sharing. Organ Procurement and Transplantation Network Data: Kidney Transplants in the US: 1988–2013. http://optn.transplant.hrsa.gov/latestData/rptData.asp. Accessed May 2013.
36. Weng FL, Reese PP, Mulgaonkar S, Patel AM. Barriers to living donor kidney transplantation among black or older transplant candidates. Clin J Am Soc Nephrol. 2010;5(12):2338–47.
37. Alvaro EM, Siegel JT, Turcotte D, Lisha N, Crano WD, Dominick A. Living kidney donation among Hispanics: a qualitative examination of barriers and opportunities. Prog Transplant. 2008;18(4):243–50.
38. Boulware LE, Ratner LE, Sosa JA, Cooper LA, LaVeist TA, Powe NR. Determinants of willingness to donate living related and cadaveric organs: identifying opportunities for intervention. Transplant. 2002;73:1683–91.
39. Robinson DHZ, Borba CPC, Thompson NJ, Perryman JP, Arriola KRJ. Correlates of support for living donation among African American adults. Prog Transplant. 2009;19:244–51.
40. Pradel FG, Suwannaprom P, Mullins CD, Sadler J, Bartlett ST. Haemodialysis patients' readiness to pursue live donor kidney transplantations. Nephrol Dial Transplant. 2009;24:1298–305.
41. Boulware LE, Hill-Briggs F, Kraus ES, Melancon JK, Senga M, Evans KE, et al. Identifying and addressing barriers to African American and non-African American families' discussions about preemptive living related kidney transplantation. Prog Transplant. 2011;21;97–105.
42. Waterman AD, Stanley SL, Covelli T, Hazel E, Hong BA, Brennan DC. Living donation decision making: recipients' concerns and educational needs. Prog Transplant. 2006;16:17–23.
43. Lunsford SL, Simpson KS, Chavin KD, Hildebrand LG, Miles LG, Shilling LM, et al. Racial differences in coping with the need for kidney transplantation and willingness to ask for live organ donation. Am J Kidney Dis. 2006;47:324–31.
44. Lunsford SL, Shilling LM, Chavin KD, Martin MS, Miles LG, Norman ML, et al. Racial differences in the living kidney donation experience and implications for education. Prog Transplant. 2007;17:234–40.
45. Shilling LM, Norman ML, Chavin KD, Hildebrand LG, Hildebrand LG, Lunsford SL, Martin MS, et al. Health care professionals' perceptions of the barriers to living donor kidney transplantation among African Americans. J Natl Med Assoc. 2006;98(6):834–9.
46. Boulware LE, Meoni LA, Fink NE, Parekh RS, Kao WH, Klag MJ, et al. Preferences, knowledge, communication, and patient-physician discussion of living kidney transplantation in African American families. Am J Transplant. 2005;5(6):1503–12.
47. Lei HH, Perneger TV, Klag MJ, Whelton PK, Coresh J. Familial aggregation of renal disease in a population-based case-control study. J Am Soc Nephrol. 1998;9:1270–6.
48. Volkova N, McClellan W, Klein M, Flanders D, Kleinbaum D, Soucie JM, et al. Neighborhood poverty and racial differences in ESRD incidence. J Am Soc Nephrol. 2008;19:356–64.
49. Reeves-Daniel A, Adams PL, Assimos D, Westcott C, Alcorn SG, Rogers J, et al. Impact of race and gender on live kidney donation. Clin Transplant. 2009;23:39–46.
50. Tankersely MR, Gaston RS, Curtis JJ, Julian BA, Deierhoi MH, Rhynes VK, et al. The living donor process in kidney transplantation: influence of race and comorbidity. Transplant Proc. 1997;29:3722–3.
51. Lunsford SL, Simpson KS, Chavin KD, Menching KJ, Miles LG, Shilling LM, et al. Racial disparities in living kidney donation: is there a lack of willing donors or an excess of medically unsuitable candidates? Transplantation. 2006;82:876–81.
52. Clark CR, Hicks LS, Keogh JH, Epstein AM, Ayanian JZ. Promoting access to renal transplantation: the role of social support networks in completing pre-transplant evaluations. J Gen Intern Med. 2008;23:1187–93.
53. Purnell TS, Hall YN, Boulware LE. Understanding and overcoming barriers to living kidney donation among racial and ethnic minorities in the United States. Adv Chronic Kid Dis. 2012;19(4):244–51.

54. Burke G, Esquenazi V, Gharagozloo H, Roth D, Strauss J, Kyriakides G, et al. Long-term results of kidney transplantation at the University of Miami. Clin Transpl. 1989;215–228.
55. Douzdijan V, Thacker LR, Blanton JW. Effect of race on outcome following kidney and kidney-pancreas transplantation in type I diabetes: the South-Eastern Organ Procurement Foundation experience. Clin Transplant. 1997;11:470–5.
56. Foley DP, Patton PR, Meier-Kriesche HU, Li Q, Shenkman B, Fujita S, et al. Long-term outcomes of kidney transplantation in recipients 60 years of age and older at the University of Florida. Clin Transplant. 2005; 101–9.
57. Purnell TS, Powe NR, Troll M, Wang NY, Haywood C, LaVeist TA, et al. Measuring and explaining racial and ethnic differences in willingness to donate live kidneys in the United States. Clin Transplant. [Epub ahead of print]
58. Clarke KS, Klarenbach S, Vlaicu S, Yang RC, Garg AX. The direct and indirect economic costs incurred by living kidney donors-a systematic review. Nephrol Dial Transplant. 2006;21:1952–60.
59. Jacobs C, Thomas C. Financial considerations in living organ donation. Prog Transplant. 2003;13:130–6.
60. Wolters HH, Heidenreich S, Senniger N. Living donor kidney transplantation: chance for the recipient—financial risk for the donor? Transplant Proc. 2003;35:2091–2.
61. United Network for Organ Sharing. Costs related to living donation. http://www.optn.org/about/donation/livingDonation.asp#costs. Accessed Apr 2012.
62. Johnson EM, Anderson JK, Jacobs C, Suh G, Humar A, Suhr BD, et al. Long-term follow-up of living kidney donors: quality of life after donation. Transplantation. 1999;67:717–2.
63. Spital A, Jacobs C. Life insurance for kidney donors: another update. Transplantation. 2002;74(7):972–3.
64. Gibney EM, King AL, Maluf DG, Garg AX, Parikh CR. Living kidney donors requiring transplantation: focus on African Americans. Transplantation. 2007;84:647–9.
65. Gibney EM, Parikh CR, Garg AX. Age, gender, race, and associations with kidney following living kidney donation. Transplant Proc. 2008;40:1337–40.
66. Doshi M, Garg AX, Gibney E, Parikh C. Race and renal function early after live kidney donation: an analysis of the United States Organ Procurement and Transplantation Network Database. Clin Transplant. 2010;24:E153–57.
67. Lentine KL, Schnitzler MA, Xiao H, Saab G, Salvalaggio PR, Axelrod D, et al. Racial variation in medical outcomes among living kidney donors. N Engl J Med. 2010;363(8):724–32.
68. Nogueira JM, Weir MR, Jacobs S, Haririan A, Breault D, Klassen D, et al. A study of renal outcomes in African American living kidney donors. Transplantation. 2009;88:1371–6.
69. Segev DL, Muzaale AD, Caffo BS, Mehta SH, Singer AL, Taranto SE, et al. Perioperative mortality and long-term survival following live kidney donation. JAMA. 2010;303(10):959–66.
70. Kasiske BL, Snyder JJ, Matas AJ, Ellison MD, Gill JS, Kausz AT. Preemptive kidney transplantation: The advantage and the advantaged. J Am Soc Nephrol. 2002;13:1358–64.
71. Kinchen KS, Sadler J, Fink N, Brookmeyer R, Klag MJ, Levey AS, Powe NR. The timing of specialist evaluation in chronic kidney disease and mortality. Ann Intern Med. 2002;137:479–86.
72. Gaylin DS, Held PJ, Port FK, Hunsicker LG, Wolfe RA, Kahan BD, et al. The impact of comorbid sociodemographic factors on access to renal transplantation. JAMA. 1993;269:603–8.
73. Stolzmann KL, Bautista LE, Gangnon RE, McElroy JA, Becker BN, Remington PL. Trends in kidney transplantation rates and disparities. J Natl Med Assoc. 2007;99(8):923–32.
74. Hall YN, O'Hare AM, Young BA, Boyko EJ, Chertow GM. Neighborhood poverty and kidney transplantation among US Asians and Pacific Islanders with end-stage renal disease. Am J Transplant. 2008;8:2402–9.
75. Grubbs V, Gregorich SE, Perez-Stable EJ, Hsu CY. Health literacy and access to kidney transplantation. Clin J Am Soc Nephrol. 2009;4:195–200.

76. Rodrigue JR, Cornell DL, Kaplan B, Howard RJ. A randomized trial of a home-based educational approach to increase live donor kidney transplantation: effects in blacks and whites. Am J Kidney Dis. 2008;51:663–70.
77. Waterman AD, Hyland SS, Goalby C, Robbins M, Dinkel K. Improving transplant education in the dialysis setting: the "explore transplant" initiative. Dialysis Transplantation. 2010;39(6):236–41.
78. Clark CR, Hicks LS, Keogh JH, Epstein AM, Ayanian JZ. Promoting access to renal transplantation: the role of social support networks in completing pre-transplant evaluations. J Gen Intern Med. 2008;23:1187–93.
79. Garonzik-Wang JM, Berger JC, Ros RL, Kucirka LM, Deshpande NA, Boyarsky BJ, et al. Live donor champion: finding live kidney donors by separating the advocate from the patient. Transplantation. 2012;93(11):1147–50.
80. Boulware LE, Hill-Briggs F, Kraus ES, Melancon JK, Falcone B, Ephraim PL, et al. Effectiveness of educational and social worker interventions to improve pursuit of preemptive living donor kidney transplantation: a randomized controlled trial. Am J Kidney Dis. 2013;61(3):476–86.
81. Warren DS, Montgomery RA. Incompatible kidney transplantation: lessons from a decade of desensitization and paired kidney exchange. Immunol Res. 2010;47(1–3):257–64.
82. Sallis JF, Bauman A, Pratt M. Environmental and policy interventions to promote physical activity. Am J Prev Med. 1998;15(4):379–97.
83. National Kidney Foundation. The Kidney Early Evaluation Program (KEEP). http://www.kidney.org/news/keep/KEEPabout.cfm. Accessed May 2013.
84. National Conference of State Legislatures. State Leave Laws Related to Medical Donors. http://www.ncsl.org/programs/employ/Leave-medicaldonors.htm. Accessed Apr 2012.
85. United States Public Laws. Organ Donor Leave Act. 5 USC 9601: H.R. 457. http://thomas.loc.gov/cgi-bin/query/z?c106:H.R.457.
86. United States Public Laws. Organ Donation and Recovery Improvement Act. 42 USC 201: 108 H.R. 3926. http://www.govtrack.us/congress/bills/108/hr3926c.
87. Comprehensive Immunosuppressive Drug Coverage for Kidney Transplant Patients Act of 2013. H.R. 1428, 113th. http://www.govtrack.us/congress/bills/113/hr1428/text.
88. Kidney Care Quality and Improvement Act of 2005. H.R. 1298, 109th. http://www.govtrack.us/congress/bills/109/hr1298.
89. Kidney Care Quality and Education Act of 2007. S. 691, 110th. http://www.govtrack.us/congress/bills/110/s691.

Chapter 24
The Evolution of the Role of the Independent Living Donor Advocates: Recommendations for Practice Guideline

Jennifer L. Steel, Andrea C. Dunlavy, Maranda Friday, Kendal Kingsley, Deborah Brower, Mark Unruh, Henkie P. Tan, Ron Shapiro, Mel Peltz, Melissa Hardoby, Christina McCloskey, Mark L. Sturdevant and Abhinav Humar

J. L. Steel (✉)
Department of Surgery, Psychiatry, and Psychology,
University of Pittsburgh Medical Center, 3459 Fifth Avenue,
MUH 7S, Pittsburgh, PA 15213, USA
e-mail: steeljl@upmc.edu

A. C. Dunlavy
Department of Surgery,
University of Pittsburgh School of Medicine,
3459 Fifth Avenue, Montefiore 7S, Pittsburgh, PA 15213, USA
e-mail: adunlavy@gmail.com

M. Friday
Department of Surgery,
University of Pittsburgh Medical Center, Montefiore Hospital,
7S, 3459 Fifth Ave., Pittsburgh, PA 15213, USA
e-mail: fridaymn@upmc.edu

K. Kingsley
Department of Surgery, UPMC Montefiore Hospital,
3459 Fifth Ave, Pittsburgh, PA 15213, USA
e-mail: Kingsleyka@upmc.edu

D. Brower
Department of Surgery, University of Pittsburgh,
Kaufman Building, Suite 601, 3471 Fifth Ave.,
Pittsburgh, PA 15213, USA
e-mail: browerds2@upmc.edu

M. Unruh
Department of Nephrology, Internal Medicine, University of New Mexico,
MSC 10-5550, Albuquerque, NM 87131-0001, USA
e-mail: mlunruh@salud.unm.edu

H. P. Tan
Department of Surgery, Division of Transplant Surgery,
University of Pittsburgh Medical Center, Veterans Hospital of Pittsburgh, 3459 5th Ave,
Pittsburgh, PA 15213, USA
e-mail: tanhp@upmc.edu

J. Steel (ed.), *Living Donor Advocacy*, DOI 10.1007/978-1-4614-9143-9_24,
© Springer Science+Business Media New York 2014

Living donors contribute to nearly half of all kidney transplants and increasing numbers of liver, lung, and intestine transplants [1]. In 2000, a consensus statement recommended that all transplant centers that perform living donor surgeries retain an independent living donor advocate (ILDA) "whose only focus is on the best interest of the donor." In 2007, the Department of Health and Human Services (DHHS) and the United Network for Organ Sharing (UNOS) required all transplant centers to retain an ILDA [2]. According to the UNOS and the DHHS, the primary elements of the ILDA's role include: (1) ensuring the protection of current and prospective living donors (DHHS); (2) being knowledgeable about living organ donation, transplantation, medical ethics, and the informed consent process (DHHS and UNOS); (3) not being involved in the transplant recipient activities on a routine basis (DHHS and UNOS) and being independent in the decision to transplant the potential recipient (UNOS); (4) representing and advising the donor, protecting and promoting the interests of the donor, respecting the donor's decision, and ensuring that the donor's decision is informed and free of coercion (DHHS); and (5) assisting the potential living donor in understanding the consent and evaluation process, surgical

---

R. Shapiro
Division of Transplantation, Department of Surgery, Starzl Transplant Institute,
University of Pittsburgh Medical Center, 3459 Fifth Avenue,
UPMC Montefiore 7S, Pittsburgh, PA 15213, USA
e-mail: shapiror@upmc.edu

M. Peltz
Department of Surgery, University of Pittsburgh,
2014 Wightman Street,
Pittsburgh, PA 15217, USA
e-mail: melecheitan@gmail.com

M. Hardoby
UPMC, 4401 Penn Avenue, Pittsburgh, PA 15224, USA
e-mail: mlh804@yahoo.com

M. Hardoby · C. McCloskey
Department of Surgery, University of Pittsburgh,
4605 Amsterdam Street, Pittsburgh, PA 15201, USA

C. McCloskey
e-mail: cmccloskey@chahtam.edu

M. L. Sturdevant
Department of Surgery, Starzl Transplant Institute,
University of Pittsburgh, 3459 Fifth Avenue,
15213, Pittsburgh, PA, USA
e-mail: Sturdevantml2@upmc.edu

A. Humar
Department of Surgery, University of Pittsburgh, Room 725,
3459 Fifth Ave., Pittsburgh, PA 15213, USA
e-mail: humara2@upmc.edu

procedures, and the benefit of and need for postsurgical follow-up (UNOS) [3, 4]. Although the evaluation of living donors is a multidisciplinary process, the ILDA can have a significant impact on the donor, and indirectly the transplant candidate, particularly if the ILDA has "veto" power with regard to the surgery as recommended in the consensus statement.

A recent national survey of ILDAs in the U.S. found that a wide range of educational backgrounds, disciplines (e.g., social workers, physicians, and clergy), and practices exist across ILDAs [5]. The recommendations for the development of practice guidelines are outlined in Table 24.1 and were, in part, based on the results of a national survey of ILDAs [5]. The details of the survey results can be found elsewhere; however a summary of the findings, followed by recommendations for practice guidelines, can be found earlier in book (see Chap. 8) [5].

Recommendations for Practice Guidelines

Practice guidelines, including uniform training of ILDAs, would greatly improve the consistency of practice across transplant centers, which is of particular importance if the ILDAs are involved in the selection process and/or have the ability to "veto" the surgery [2, 5]. The impact of a donor being "vetoed" from surgery would likely affect the life of the donor and recipient significantly, possibly resulting in the candidate's death.

Practice guidelines may be defined as generally accepted, informal or formal, standardized or evidence-based techniques, methods, or processes [6]. The goals of developing practice guidelines for ILDAs are to set standards, delineate the division of labor, create boundaries, and educate patients and health care professionals regarding the practices of ILDA. Regardless of these benefits, practice guidelines also have disadvantages. For example, those spearheading the guidelines may bring biases from their own disciplines, and recommendations may not reflect the local or regional needs or circumstances of the center. Practice guidelines may also limit innovation and advances in the field and standardize practice based on the "average," rather than "best" practice. Furthermore, practice guidelines can result in a more cumbersome and/or restrictive process and if not developed appropriately, may have legal implications. Table 24.1 provides a list of the areas that warrant further discussion and consensus by the transplant community to improve consistency across ILDA practices and to ensure appropriate service delivery.

Qualifications and Role of the ILDA

At this time, the only qualifications to serve as an ILDA is "being knowledgeable about living organ donation, transplantation, medical ethics, and the informed consent process" [3, 4]. The definition of "knowledgeable" in areas can range from

Table 24.1 Recommendations for practice guidelines

Area	Recommendations
1 Qualifications and definition of role	Define minimal qualifications and professional boundaries
	Define roles and responsibilities
2 Training and continuing education	Consistent and formal training of ILDAs
	Continuing education for ILDAs
	Certification process of ILDAs
	Peer supervision
	Development of measures of practice standards and outcomes
3 Practice	Timing of ILDA evaluations (e.g., screening, evaluation, and postoperation)
	Content of evaluation
	Attendance and participation in selection committee meetings
	Documentation of donor evaluation and follow-up
	Contracts and educational information provided to donors
	ILDA involvement in the selection process of donors
	Long-term follow-up of donors by ILDA
4 Ethical issues	Types of donors and exclusions (e.g., valuable consideration)
	Resolution of disagreements between transplant center and ILDA
	Informed consent regarding ILDA–donor communication
	Limits of confidentiality in disclosure of donor evaluation
	Limits of confidentiality in documentation of donor evaluation
5 Fiscal issues	Malpractice insurance for ILDAs
	Financial reimbursement for ILDA services

an individual who has no formal training in these areas (e.g., volunteer who has donated an organ) to a transplant surgeon who has years of specialized training in the area of transplantation. The ILDA training should include a basic foundation of knowledge in transplantation, organ donation, bioethics, and the guidelines of governing bodies such as UNOS and DHHS, and the informed consent process is recommended.

Both UNOS and DHHS have made recommendations with regard to professional boundaries. The recommendation is that the ILDA cannot be routinely involved in transplant candidate activities, so as to reduce potential bias while evaluating the living donor for surgery. However, only 54% of the ILDAs at the time of the survey interpreted "independent" with reference to this professional boundary.

Furthermore, more than half of the ILDAs reported a dual role (e.g., social worker, nurse, or physician and ILDA). The advantages of a dual role may include that the ILDA may have greater breadth and depth of knowledge of the donor by performing a full psychosocial or medical evaluation and/or have more frequent contact with the donor, as with a nurse coordinator. As reflected in the findings of the survey, disadvantages may be the lack of differentiation between the two roles, particularly if the ILDA is involved in the selection process. It was apparent that some ILDAs may make recommendations for the donors' suitability for surgery based on their non-ILDA role. Further clarification is recommended regarding the role of the ILDA in the selection process as well as the separation of roles when dual roles exist.

Training and Continuing Education

The lack of formal training of ILDAs was evidenced by the national survey of living donor advocates. The majority of ILDAs reported that they were trained by a member of the transplant team (48.5%), which may be considered a conflict of interest but potentially the most relevant training with regard to the region and/or center practices. The remaining ILDAs reported various other methods of being trained, which included training themselves, or receiving little or no training [5]. This lack of consistent training translates to the significant variability in practices observed across centers. Ideally, a separate organization or subcommittee within an organization (e.g., UNOS and American Society Transplant Sugeons (ASTS) that is not connected to the ILDA's own transplant center would provide training to ILDAs. The standards of training may include a certain number of hours and/or an examination and certification process to provide evidence of at least a minimum knowledge base. The content and duration of training as well as fiscal issues associated with training should be carefully considered. Web-based training may be optimal as the wide range of ILDA disciplines (e.g., nursing and clergy) makes annual meetings a potential venue for training and continuing education challenging. Continuing education for ILDAs is also recommended as the field of living donation evolves, as do the guidelines and requirements set forth by the DHHS and the UNOS. Similar to other professions, a certain number of continuing education credit hours could be required every 2 years to facilitate the ongoing education of ILDAs.

Once practice guidelines have been developed and consistent training across ILDAs has been established, performance standards and methods to measure performance can be implemented. Without practice guidelines, it is difficult for transplant centers, governing bodies, and the donors themselves to know if donors are receiving the appropriate services from the ILDA.

Practice of ILDAs

According to the results of the national survey, the timing of the evaluation varied across ILDAs greatly, with some ILDAs being involved in the screening process of donors and others being involved in the evaluation. Some ILDAs reported being involved with all phases of the processes. Only 56% of ILDAs were involved in the postoperative follow-up period. At a minimum, it is recommended that ILDAs be involved in the evaluation and the immediate postoperative phase of donation. The ILDA's involvement during the screening process could be cost-effective if the donors who did not meet the ILDA criteria were screened out prior to the completion of several medical tests and meetings with the transplant team members.

It is also recommended that the ILDA be available after the face-to-face evaluation but before the surgery in case issues arise prior to the surgery in which the donor needs the ILDA's assistance (e.g., decision not to proceed with surgery). Furthermore, the ILDA should follow-up some donors after being declined from donation as new medical (e.g., cancer) or psychiatric conditions (e.g., bipolar disorder) may have been diagnosed during the evaluation and warrant treatment. The donor may need further clarification with regard to his/her diagnosis or may experience barriers to accessing the treatment that was recommended. Furthermore, in instances where donors lose their loved one during the surgery or shortly after transplant, a longer follow-up of donors is recommended by the ILDA or other transplant team members (e.g., psychology and social work).

Consensus regarding the content of the evaluation, follow-up of donors, as well as the documentation is warranted. At the minimum, the ILDA evaluation should include the criteria that the donor: (1) is willing to donate and displays competence to make the decision to donate; (2) has been explained the potential medical, psychosocial, and financial risks of donation; (3) appears to be free from pressure or coercion to donate; (4) has not reported that he/she will profit from donating their organ; (5) has been explained the informed consent process; and (6) has been educated about the importance of long-term postsurgical follow-up. In addition, it is recommended that ILDAs also assess the donor's motives to donate. An ILDA may provide a donor with a document describing the laws related to valuable consideration and have the donor sign it if there are any concerns regarding compensation for donating their organ. Understanding if there are any family members or friends who may not be supportive of the donation is also important to prevent potential psychosocial consequences to the donor.

The documentation of the ILDA–donor evaluation in the medical record may include only a checklist of the items above (yes or no) with a separate confidential file that includes the details of the ILDA–donor discussion. If the ILDA–donor evaluation is not confidential, the donor should be informed that the information he/she shares may be placed in the medical record which the transplant team and other health care professionals may view and may be discussed with the transplant teams.

The consistency and quality of educational materials given to donors should be addressed, as printed information can have an impact on the donor's decision to proceed with surgery, and the accuracy of the document is essential. Although some of the ILDAs reported use of contracts with the donor, this seems contrary to the role as the "advocate." For example, a contract stating that the donor needs to complete the 2-year follow-up recommended by UNOS may be viewed as pressure and cannot be enforced. Nonetheless, the long-term follow-up should be encouraged by all members of the transplant team and the donor should be allowed flexibility on where the medical follow-up can be performed.

Due to the importance of the ILDA being present to hear the discussion regarding donor suitability for surgery, it is recommended that the ILDA attend the selection committee meetings during at least the donor presentations. The ILDA should be present so that he/she can serve as the donor's voice, present the donor's concerns, ask questions, and understand the reasons the donor is declined, if applicable. In rare cases, understanding the family dynamics including the donor–candidate relationship may be important and having the ILDA meet other family members and/or discuss the donor–candidate relationship with the donor and recipient teams may be warranted.

If the ILDA is to be a part of the selection process (e.g., authority to "veto" the surgery), the donors' understanding of the ILDA's role in the selection process should be made known to them so that they are aware that what is said to the "advocate" may be used in the decision for determining their suitability for donation. Optimally, the informed consent should include information about the ILDA's role and if it is decided that the ILDA be involved in the selection process, then this should also be included in the donor's informed consent process.

Ethical Issues

While there are several ethical challenges within the field of transplantation that warrant further discussion and consensus (e.g., valuable consideration and competence to make informed decisions), several ethical issues directly related to the role of the ILDA remain unresolved. First, consistent training of all ILDAs in the principles of bioethics and decision making would be optimal. Second, in cases where the ILDA may be obligated to disclose the reasons to the transplant team for recommending against surgery, verbally during the selection committee meeting and/or as part of the donor's medical record, the donor should be made aware of the ILDA's role. This could be done similarly to the other transplant team members by including a description of the ILDA's role in the informed consent process as well as the ILDA explaining this to the donor. Furthermore, if the details of the evaluation are included in an electronic medical record system where other health care professionals outside of transplantation may have access to this information, the donor should be made aware of the fact that this would occur.

The DHHS recommends that the ILDA "protects" as well as "respects" the donor's decision for surgery. Based on the results of the national survey, the majority of ILDAs favored "protection" of the donor (e.g., the ILDA believes that it is not in the donor's best interest to proceed with surgery even if the donor wants to proceed, and the ILDA recommends against the surgery; 51%), while the minority of ILDAs may "advocate" for the donor (e.g., the ILDA recommends surgery if the donor wants to proceed despite the risks; 29%) [6]. While "protection" of the donor is important under certain circumstances (e.g., pressure or coercion), a paternalistic role of the ILDA was not likely the intention of those who suggested that donors have an "advocate" that act in their best interest.

Further, if the ILDA can "veto" the surgery, and the donor wants to proceed despite understanding the potential risks, it also calls into question whether the ILDA is an "advocate" for the donor if the donor understands the risks and still wants to proceed with surgery [6]. The ILDA should let the donor know if there is the ability to "veto" the surgery. However, in the case in which an ILDA does decline a donor from surgery and the donor wanted to proceed, the donor–ILDA relationship may be negatively affected and the donor may no longer want assistance from the "advocate."

The survey queried the ILDAs regarding how they managed conflicts between the ILDA and transplant team if they did not agree with the decision for the donor to proceed with surgery. The majority of the ILDAs reported that a consensus was reached (34%), while others reported that they had not experienced a disagreement (18%) or that the ethics/compliance committee/psychiatrist was consulted (17%). A national ombudsman connected with UNOS or the DHHS could be appointed for cases in which a disagreement cannot be reached or due to pressure experienced by the ILDA (e.g., political and financial), creating a higher level of protection for the ILDAs' autonomy.

Fiscal Issues

The implementation of an ILDA has considerable costs associated with it, and on average each center pays approximately US$ 80,000 per year for this service [4]. New guidelines or changes in existing policies concerning the ILDA recommended by governing bodies may be associated with an increased number of hours per week for the ILDA as well as increased costs to the transplant or medical center supporting the ILDA. Although few ILDAs reported billing for their services, it is unclear whether the services provided by the ILDA should be billable services reimbursed by insurance companies or Medicare and Medicaid. If a donor is billed and the services are not reimbursed, the candidate and/or donor may become responsible for the costs. This was not likely intended when this role was conceptualized and it remains unclear if the candidate and/or donor or their insurance company should pay for an "advocate." In addition, although most medical professionals who are employed by the transplant center and/or hospital may be covered with the hospital's malpractice insurance, those ILDAs practicing independently may want to consider the liability associated with their position, particularly if involved in the selection process or postsurgical follow-up.

Conclusion

The practice recommendations discussed here are based on the findings of the national survey summarized previously as well as the opinions of the authors. The recommendations that are proposed here are not exhaustive and are aspirational in intent and are likely to evolve with time. Practice guidelines are recommended for legal and regulatory issues (e.g., state or federal laws), consumer or public benefit (e.g., improving service delivery, avoiding harm to the patient, and decreasing disparities in underserved or vulnerable populations), and professional guidance (e.g., new role, professional risk management issues, and advances in practice) [5]. Without such practice guidelines, donors, and indirectly the candidates, may be at increased risk for possible bias or undue harm.

Acknowledgments We would like to thank all the living donor advocates who participated in the survey. The response rate to the survey was reflective of the enthusiasm and commitment to donors.

References

1. Health Resources and Services Administration. U.S. Department of Health and Human Services, April 18, 2012. http://www.unos.org/.
2. Abecassis M, Adams M, Adams P, Arnold RM, Atkins CR, Barr ML, et al. Consensus statement on the live organ donor. JAMA. 2000;284:2919–26.
3. Department of Health and Human Services, Part II. Centers for Medicare & Medicaid Services 42 CFR Parts 405, 482, 488, and 498 Medicare Program. Hospital Conditions of Participation: Requirements for Approval and Re-Approval of Transplant Centers To Perform Organ Transplants. Final Rule Federal Register/Vol. 72, No. 61/Friday, March 30, 2007/Rules and Regulations, 15198–280.
4. United Network for Organ Sharing has also modified its bylaws the same year. Appendix B, Section XIII, 2007.
5. Steel JL, Dunlavy A, Friday M, Kingsley K, Brower D, Unruh M, et al. A national survey of living donor advocates: A need for practice guidelines. Am J Transplant. 12(8):2141–9.
6. American Psychological Association. Criteria for Practice Guideline Development and Evaluation. Am Psychol. 2002;57(12):1048–51.

Index

A
ABO blood group compatibility
  determination of, 78
Active-duty military
  as live organ donor, 144, 145
Advisory Committee on Organ
  Transplantation (ACOT), 112
Advocacy, 135
  levels of, 131
  role of, 137
Affordable care act, 297, 298
African American living kidney donors, 335
African American potential donors, 335
Altruistic donor, 247
American Society of Transplantation, 105, 111
Amsterdam Forum on the Care of the Live
  Donor, 9
Anonymous donation, 163
Army/Navy organ transplant service, 144
Autonomy, 131, 270, 271
  assessment of, 307, 310
  Berofsky's view of, 306
  concept of, 302, 303, 305, 307
  Dworkin's view of, 306
  Frankfurt's views on, 303, 306
  Kantian notion of, 304
  philosophic literature on, 305
  responsibilities of, 307
  senses of, 303, 307
  understanding of, 310

B
Barriers, 336
Bilateral living donor lung transplantation, 78,
  87, 88
Biliary complications, 38
Bioethics, 350
  in ILDA, 353

Blood-type distribution system, 20
Bone marrow transplant, 311
Bronchial anastomosis, 84
Bronchoscopy, 79, 84, 86

C
Cadaveric transplantation, 78
Center for Medicare and Medicaid Services
  (CMS), 207, 267, 269
Chest tube dance, 86
Coercion, 197, 198
  aspects of, 232
  signs of, 198
Comorbid illness, 8
Comorbidity, 4, 5
  of donors, 6
Comorbid medical conditions, 337
Compatibility, 25
Complications
  Clavien grading system of, 38
Conflict, 223, 224, 225, 227, 228
Continuous epidural infusions, 85
Crossmatch compatibility, 25

D
Deceased donor liver transplants (DDLT), 29,
  30, 39
Decisional capacity
  assessment of, 310
Decision-making capacity, 266
Department of Health and Human Services
  (DHHS), 110
Domino paired donation, 22
Donation
  benefits vs. risks of, 162
  health consequences of, 164
  psychological benefit of, 160
  risks of, 267

Donor, 231, 232, 238, 250
    coercion of, 126
    emotional support for, 85
    impact of, 128
    postoperative care of, 95
    radiologic evaluation of, 93
    standard preoperative testing of, 93
    stories of, 231
Donor advocacy, 104, 133
    origin of, 106
    standards of, 107
Donor advocate, 103, 113
Donor assistance, 295
Donor candidates, 125, 275–278, 281, 283–290
Donor coercion, 276, 277
Donor evaluation, 3, 11, 30, 126, 133, 207–209, 212, 215
Donor identification
    barriers in, 332
Donor–ILDA relationship, 354
Donor influence, 275–279
Donor left lower lobectomy, 82
Donor lobectomies
    technical aspects of, 79
Donor lobe preservation, 82
Donor morbidity
    studies on, 38
Donor mortality, 37
Donor postoperative management, 85, 86
Donor pressure, 276–279, 281, 282
Donor right lower lobectomy, 80
Donor safety, 30, 35
Donor selection, 76, 77, 212
Donor's motivation, 198, 199, 201, 203
Donor surgery, 256

E
Education, 197, 199–201, 203
End-stage renal disease (ESRD), 328
    disparities in, 327
    effect on kidney function, 328
    in racial-ethnic minorities, 332
    prevalence of, 327
    risk factors of, 327
    role of living donation in, 330
    treatment of, 328
End-stage renal disease (ESRD)
    process, 5, 98, 108
Ethical issues, 152
Ethics, 312
Evaluation, 131–135, 205, 206, 212, 217
    guidelines for, 11

of transplant candidate, 4
risks associated with, 215
role of team members in, 135
Exchange donation, 160

F
Family and Medical Leave Act (FMLA), 294, 296
Financial assistance, 293, 296
Financial concern, 299
Financial contraindication, 294
Financial gain, 298
Financial hardship, 297
Financial risks, 293, 294, 296, 299
    levels of, 294
Formal evaluation, 217
Fundraising opportunities, 297

H
Health care financing, 107
Health care provider, 253–255, 257, 282, 336, 338
Health care team, 222
Health insurance, 294, 295, 297
Health risk factors, 13
Higher power, 239, 241, 243, 249
Histocompatibility testing, 20, 23
HLA donor-recipient match, 87

I
ILDA-donor evaluation, 352
    documentation of, 352
Immunosupression, 104, 105, 109
Independent advocate
    role of, 205
Independent living donor advocacy team (IDAT), 293
    goals of, 293
Independent living donor advocate (ILDA), 115, 120, 121, 131, 197–203, 205, 206, 208–210, 212, 215, 217, 223–228, 267, 268, 270, 275–283, 285, 286, 288, 289, 311, 312, 314, 348
    advantages of, 351
    aspects of, 205
    assessment of, 211, 215, 285
    benefits of, 289
    case studies of, 278, 318–325
    challenging aspects of, 289
    collaborative approaches of, 289
    concept of, 104
    concerns of, 226
    conflicts of, 354

Index 359

controversies of, 126
disadvantages of, 351
documentation of, 198
donation process in, 226
ethical issues of, 353
ethics of, 126
evaluation of, 197–199, 201–203, 210, 352
fiscal issues of, 354
guidelines for, 217
guidelines of, 120
interviews of, 217
LaPointe Rudow's conception of, 125
objective of, 317
obligations of, 312, 314, 316, 322
participation of, 217
perspective of, 209, 215
practical guidelines for, 349
practice of, 352
practices of, 124, 125, 126
psychological aspects of, 226
quantification of, 349
responsibilities of, 122
risks of, 200, 202
role in ambivalence, 209
role in donor candidate selection, 217
role in selection process, 353
role of, 120, 121, 124, 126, 131, 132, 199, 203, 206, 209, 212, 213, 215, 217, 221–223, 228, 288, 316, 348, 353, 354
significance of, 353
surveys of, 121, 124, 125, 223, 349
training standards of, 351
understanding of, 126, 213
Informed consent, 149, 152, 159, 162, 165, 209, 210, 261, 263, 264
aspects of, 270
assessment of, 217
concept of, 205, 207, 261
criterias for, 272, 273
elements of, 205, 208, 210, 266
for live kidney donation, 207
history of, 264
in living donation, 262, 266, 269, 270
models of, 261, 270
process of, 268
prominence of, 265
provisions of, 206, 215
quality of, 208
role in health care, 261
use of Nuremberg Code in, 265
violation of, 265
voluntariness in, 267

Informed decision making, 198, 203
Inherent risks, 201, 202
International Society for Heart and Lung Transplantation (ISHLT), 87

J
Johns Hopkins Hospital Incompatible Kidney Transplant program, 20

K
Kidney disease, 253, 254
Kidney donation, 141, 151, 161, 275, 279, 280, 282, 283
financial consequences of, 298
impact of, 278
Kidney donor, 253, 255, 257, 293, 295
surgery of, 253, 258
Kidney paired donation (KPD), 17, 18, 20–25, 141
current landscape of, 18
definition of, 20
development of, 140
fiscal aspects of, 24
growth of, 140
nondirected donors in, 22
programs of, 140, 145
registries of, 19
types of, 17
Kidney transplant, 91, 98, 140, 141, 144, 255, 316, 329, 331, 332
barriers to, 341
evaluation of, 254
graft survival rates for, 142
Kidney transplantation, 10, 103–106, 108–111
advances in, 109
factors in, 109

L
Laparoscopic distal pancreatectomies, 92
Laparoscopic donor nephrectomy, 92
Laparoscopic pancreatectomy, 98
case studies of, 96
evolution of, 99
recipient outcomes of, 98
LD pancreas recipient, 97
Left lateral hepatectomy, 37
Left lateral lobectomy, 35
Life insurance policies, 297
Listening, 307–309
Live donor, 91, 137
evaluation of, 134
program of, 135
Live organ donor, 112

Liver transplantation
  factors affecting, 29
Living donation, 3, 6, 8, 11, 13, 120, 124, 126,
    197–201, 205–207, 209, 210, 215, 217
  assessment of, 201
  consensus guidelines for, 11
  controversies of, 126
  decisions related to, 203
  donor related-barriers in, 334
  economic risks of, 334
  effects of, 202
  evaluation of, 197, 202
  goals of, 201
  impact of, 213, 334
  issues in, 121
  risks of, 197, 201, 215
  role of ILDA in, 351
  safety of, 163
  studies on, 334
  types of, 199
Living donor, 4, 5, 7–9, 11, 21, 23, 25, 33, 75,
    77, 87, 103, 109–111, 114, 221–228,
    293, 296, 297, 311
  advantages of, 39
  consent form of, 255
  documentation of, 115
  experiences of, 253
  history of, 103
  informal consent for, 103
  medical selection of, 4
  morbidity studies on, 4
  outcomes of, 6
  practices of, 104
  procedure of, 37
  transplantation of, 104
Living donor advocate (LDA), 200, 201,
    232, 255, 302, 305, 307
  assessment of, 231, 310
  purpose of, 232
  tools in, 233, 307
Living donor advocate team (ILDT),
    134, 135
  aspects of, 133, 137
  benefits of, 132
  donors in, 137
  role of, 135, 136
  roles and responsibilities of, 133
Living donor kidney transplantation
    (LDKT), 330
  advantages of, 331
  barriers in, 331, 334
  ethical disparities in, 334
  fiscal issues of, 332
  surgical risks of, 332

Living donor kidney transplantion (LDKT),
    106, 141, 280
Living donor (LD) pancreas transplantation,
    91, 92, 98
Living donor liver transplant (LDLT),
    29, 39
  concept of, 29
  concerns of, 37
  evaluation of, 30
  positive outcomes of, 29
Living donor lobar lung transplantation
    (LDLLT), 75
Living donor lobectomy, 88
Living donor–recipient relationship, 139
Living donors, 120, 125, 139, 233, 261, 263,
    267, 270, 272
  medical selection of, 4, 13
  use of, 145
Living donors advocate (LDA), 126
Living donor team, 105, 113, 121, 275, 276,
    282, 286, 289
  concept of, 104
Living donor team (ILDT), 289
Living donor transplantation, 120, 207, 310
  benefits of, 210
Living kidney donors
  guidelines for, 11
Living organ donation, 275, 276, 282, 289,
    290, 301
  advantages of, 301
  ethical factors of, 301
  in education, 283
Living Organ Donor Expense Reimbursement
    (LODER) program, 299
Living organ donors, 139, 145
Long-distance kidney exchanges, 23
Long-term dialysis, 225
Lost wages, 296
Lung allocation score (LAS) system, 87, 143
Lung transplantation, 143
  cadaveric donors for, 75, 76, 82, 87, 88

M

Magical thinking, 217
Medical ethics, 3, 263, 348, 349
  commitments of, 301
Medical evaluation, 3, 11, 30
  goals of, 4
Medical outcomes, 13
Medical team, 137
Military donors, 144
Motivation, 231–233, 239, 241
  for organ donation, 243

Index

N

National Institute of Allergy and Infectious Diseases (NIAID), 88
National Living Donor Assistance Center (NLDAC), 297
National Organ Transplantation Act (NOTA), 110, 126, 211, 296, 298
National Survey of Independent Living Donor Advocates
  outcomes of, 312
Nondirected/altruistic donors, 17, 21, 22
  prevalence of, 22
  role of, 21
Non-judgmental regard, 310
Nonjudgmental regard, 307
Non-simultaneous extended altruistic donor (NEAD) chain, 22

O

OPTN/ UNOS notified transplant programs, 11
Organ donation, 164, 267, 296
  Air Force guidelines for, 145
  ot of costs related to, 297
Organ donor evaluation, 6
Organ Procurement and Transplantation Network (OPTN), 110, 131, 139, 335
  regulations of, 134
Organ transplantation, 103, 104
  advances in, 105
Overwhelming post-splenectomy sepsis (OPSS), 94

P

Paid time off, 294, 296
Paired donation
  concept of, 25
  factors of, 20
  programs of, 18, 24
  registries of, 23, 24
Paired exchange programs, 284
Pancreas donor, 92, 93, 98
Pancreas transplantation, 92, 97, 98
  case studies in, 96
  donor considerations in, 92
  purpose of, 91
Patient-related barriers, 332, 334
Patients' advocate, 221, 222
  Schwartz's conceptions on, 222
Population and community-level barriers, 337
Post-donation
  benefits of, 165
  medical evaluation of, 145
  outcomes of, 163, 165
Post-surgical
  assistance of, 201
Potential donor
  participation of, 217
Potential donors, 31, 34, 75, 78, 85, 88, 198, 200
  reproductive concerns of, 10
Practice guidelines, 349, 351, 355
  advantages of, 355
  disadvantages of, 349
Practice recommendations, 355
Preoperative pulmonary function testing (PFT), 9
Prospective donors, 7, 197–200, 202, 206, 211, 212, 215, 217
  strategies of, 209
Psychosocial evaluation, 134, 149, 152–154, 162, 165, 210
Psychosocial outcomes, 149, 150, 164
Psychosocial status risk profile, 217

Q

Quality Assurance and Performance Improvement (QAPI) process, 135

R

Racial-ethnic disparities, 337
Racial-ethnic minorities, 327, 328, 331, 334, 335
  donor identification in, 336
  risks of, 332
Recipient operation, 84
Recipient outcomes, 162
  concerns of, 164
Recipient pneumonectomies, 84
Recipient postoperative management, 86
Recipient selection, 76
Related living donors, 139, 140
  for kidney transplants, 142
Relationship, 231–233, 239, 241, 243, 245, 246, 247, 249
Research ethics, 265
Responsibility
  Aristotle and the Stoics' conception of, 302
Right lobectomy, 36
Risks
  assessment of, 289
  quantification of, 13
  understanding of, 217
Robotic-assisted laparoscopic donor nephrectomy, 99

S

Sacred story, 231, 232, 251
Simultaneous pancreas-kidney (SPK),
   91, 96, 98
   donors in, 96, 97
   transplants in, 97
Sociodemographic barriers, 329
Socioeconomic barriers, 337
Surgery, 254–258
   recovery process in, 257
System-related barriers, 335, 336

T

Team approach, 132, 135, 137
Team members, 134
Thromboembolic complications, 32
Transplant, 314, 320, 322
Transplantation, 105, 253, 254, 257
   developments in, 105
   policies of, 112
Transplant cases, 324
Transplant center, 120, 121, 126, 206,
   284, 294–296, 317, 318, 321
   case studies of, 295
   role of, 298
Transplant clinic, 86
Transplant facility, 207
Transplant organs, 227
Transplant practices, 317
Transplant programs, 207, 209, 224,
   227, 301
Transplant surgery
   barriers in, 334

Transplant teams, 131, 208, 209, 212,
   221–228, 318, 324
   concerns of, 319
Transplant tourism, 211

U

Undocumented recipients, 144
   role of medicare in, 144
United Network for Organ Sharing (UNOS),
   110, 120, 124, 126, 211, 221
   guidelines for, 120, 207, 211
   policies of, 215, 225, 227, 228
   role of ILDA in, 121
Unrelated living organ donors, 139, 140, 142,
   144, 145, 149–152, 162–165
   acceptance of, 152
   benefit to risk ratio in, 162
   concept of, 152
   concerns of, 152
   evaluation of, 155
   informed consent of, 159
   psychosocial evaluation of, 150, 154, 155
   psychosocial issues in, 152
   significance of, 162
   types of, 153

V

Voluntariness, 301, 302, 307
   Aristotle and the Stoics' conception of, 302
   assessment of, 308
   concept of, 303
   of donation decision, 307
   understanding of, 310

MIX
Papier aus verantwortungsvollen Quellen
Paper from responsible sources
FSC® C105338

If you have any concerns about our products,
you can contact us on
ProductSafety@springernature.com

In case Publisher is established outside the EU,
the EU authorized representative is:
**Springer Nature Customer Service Center GmbH
Europaplatz 3, 69115 Heidelberg, Germany**

Printed by Libri Plureos GmbH
in Hamburg, Germany